Communicating Quality and Safety in Hea

As health services are becoming more complex, communication is critical to enable healthcare clinicians to provide safe and high-quality care. In response to the growing emphasis on clinicians' capacity to practise effective communication, *Communicating Quality and Safety in Health Care* provides real-life communication scenarios and inter-professional case studies. The book engages healthcare trainees from across medicine, nursing and allied health services in a comprehensive and probing discussion of the communication demands that confront today's healthcare teams.

This book explains the role of communication in mental health, emergency medicine, intensive care and a wide range of other health service and community care contexts. It emphasises the ways in which patients and clinicians communicate, and how clinicians communicate with one another. The case studies explain why and how communication is critical to good care and healing. Each chapter analyses real-life practice situations, encourages the learner to ask probing questions about these situations, and sets out the principal components and strategies of good communication.

Written by prominent and internationally renowned scholars, *Communicating Quality and Safety in Health Care* helps both learners and instructors contextualise the practical exemplars by identifying the connections to relevant accreditation and policy requirements.

Additional resources for instructors are available online at www.cambridge.edu.au/academic/qualitysafety

Rick Iedema is Professor of Healthcare Innovation at the University of Tasmania and has a dual appointment with the New South Wales Ministry of Health's Agency for Clinical Innovation.

Donella Piper is a private consultant for Donella Piper Consulting Ltd.

Marie Manidis is a Postdoctoral Research Fellow at the University of Technology, Sydney.

Communicating Quality and Safety in Health Care

Edited by

Rick Iedema   Donella Piper   Marie Manidis

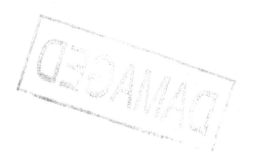

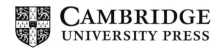

CAMBRIDGE
UNIVERSITY PRESS

CAMBRIDGE
UNIVERSITY PRESS

477 Williamstown Road, Port Melbourne, VIC 3207, Australia

Cambridge University Press is part of the University of Cambridge.

It furthers the University's mission by disseminating knowledge in the pursuit of
education, learning and research at the highest international levels of excellence.

www.cambridge.org
Information on this title: www.cambridge.org/9781107699328

First published 2015

Cover designed by Sardine Design
Typeset by Aptara Corp.
Printed in Singapore by Markono Print Media Pte Ltd

A catalogue record for this publication is available from the British Library

*A Cataloguing-in-Publication entry is available from the catalogue
of the National Library of Australia at* www.nla.gov.au

ISBN 978-1-107-69932-8 Paperback

Additional resources for this publication at
http://www.cambridge.edu.au/academic/qualitysafety

Cambridge University Press has no responsibility for the persistence or accuracy of URLs for
external or third-party internet websites referred to in this publication and does not guarantee
that any content on such websites is, or will remain, accurate or appropriate.

*Please be aware that this publication may contain several variations of Aboriginal and Torres Strait
Islander terms and spellings; no disrespect is intended. Please note that the terms 'Indigenous Australians'
and 'Aboriginal and Torres Strait Islander peoples' may be used interchangeably in this publication.*

....

Every effort has been made in preparing this book to provide accurate and up-to-date
information that is in accord with accepted standards and practice at the time of publication.
Although case histories are drawn from actual cases, every effort has been made to disguise the
identities of the individuals involved. Nevertheless, the authors, editors and publishers can make
no warranties that the information contained herein is totally free from error, not least because
clinical standards are constantly changing through research and regulation. The authors, editors
and publishers therefore disclaim all liability for direct or consequential damages resulting from
the use of material contained in this book. Readers are strongly advised to pay careful attention
to information provided by the manufacturer of any drugs or equipment that they plan to use.

Foreword

In my previous role as Director General of NSW Health and, more recently as Chief Executive Officer of the Australian Commission on Safety and Quality in Health Care, I have reviewed many serious adverse events. These events, leading to serious patient harm, were frequently precipitated by inadequate communication between clinicians, and between clinicians and their patients.

Over the years, I have listened to many patients and their families tell stories about their healthcare experiences. Whether their experiences were positive or not often depended on the quality of communication they received from clinicians. This included the type of information, how they received that information and the interactions they had with their clinicians.

We know that communication problems are a major contributing factor in serious adverse events. As a result, there has been a great deal of effort in Australia and internationally to understand the genesis of communication failures as a strategy to improve the effectiveness of communication, reduce preventable patient harm and increase patient satisfaction in their care.

Effective and respectful communication is critical to the quality and safe delivery of patient care. Achieving this is not a simple task, as the system in which health care is delivered is complex. Clinicians require highly developed communication skills to negotiate this complexity. Clinicians need to develop these skills from strong a evidence base, starting at undergraduate level.

This textbook, edited by three leaders and researchers in this field, provides an excellent evidence base for students to start developing their communication skills. Each chapter has been written by prominent and internationally renowned health educators, practitioners and scholars. The textbook presents theories, useful strategies and tools to assist clinicians to communicate effectively in various clinical scenarios and settings. Clinical scenarios are illustrated with real-life examples, contextualised to the Australian setting. These examples will have resonance with readers, providing both context and relevance to their own practice, thus enhancing their learning opportunities.

This textbook is an important foundational resource for undergraduate healthcare students to develop the knowledge and skills to communicate effectively across service sectors, clinical specialties and clinical situations. It highlights the importance of respect, ethical practice, honesty, openness and patient centredness as essential elements of effective communication. In addition, the textbook provides useful patient-centred communication strategies and tools about how to partner with patients in shared decision making, informed consent and open disclosure.

Understanding the needs of patients and providing patient-centred communication will not only increase satisfaction but minimise distress and potentially reduce patient harm.

Adjunct Professor Debora **Picone AM**
Chief Executive Officer
Australian Commission on Safety and Quality in Health Care

Foreword

Over the past decade, I have listened to the healthcare experiences of health consumers. Healthcare consumers, who come from all walks of life, who as patients, family members and carers of patients, trust that their healthcare professionals will act in their best interests at all times.

As a facilitator at forums, and as a healthcare consumer advocate, I have listened to people recount their healthcare experiences. I have listened to unsolicited personal accounts of healthcare experiences from people while waiting at bus stops, while sitting on airplanes, and in the supermarket checkout line. I have listened as healthcare experiences are relived. And, regrettably, people's experiences had been less than optimal.

The experiences I hear about are those of people as patients being traumatised by the healthcare system. They, or the person they cared for, had experienced harm in the course of receiving their health care.

It is evident that, despite the differing healthcare settings and the specific healthcare needs of each person, there are commonalities across these experiences.

Many patients had alerted members of their healthcare team to their changing health status. Family members had informed healthcare staff of their family member deteriorating, before their very eyes. There were reports of 'raising the alarm' that 'things were amiss' or 'just weren't 'right''. All the expressed concerns were subsequently dismissed by the health professionals caring for them.

The most significant recurring theme was of not being listened to, not just once, but repeatedly. Not only did I recognise these themes, I myself had experienced them all too well when my son died in hospital twelve and a half years ago.

Regardless of their healthcare need or the setting health care is provided in, people come to health care as patients with a reciprocal expectation of trust. Trust is really the only lifebuoy that a patient has to hold on to in the tumultuous ocean of health care. Each interaction a healthcare provider has with a patient, no matter how brief, builds on that trust or erodes it. When patients are not listened to, or are objectified as just a body part, physical and/or psychological harm are the inevitable outcome.

I often hear it said that patients expect too much these days. Each one of us as a human being innately expects to be valued and treated with respect by another, whether that is in our daily lives, our workplace or within the interaction we have with our healthcare providers. A personal responsibility to valuing and respecting the patient as a person and authentically listening and hearing their voice enables the atmosphere for trust to grow.

It is widely accepted now that patients play a key role in their own safety and in the mitigation of harm and also in their own care and healing. Their insights can also inform improvements to both the safety and quality of overall healthcare provision.

Not only do patients bring a unique perspective, but they also provide the missing link to the improvements required to the overall safety and quality of health care. The progress of this improvement depends on optimising the communication between all healthcare professionals and the people that they care for.

This book makes a welcome and timely contribution, as a resource to attain the environment that enables healthcare providers to maximise their interactions with patients in ways that matter to patients and increase the safety and quality of the care they receive.

Stephanie Newell
**Australia's Patients for Patient Safety Representative
to the World Health Organization**

Contents

Contributors

About the editors

Rick Iedema manages the research portfolio at the New South Wales Ministry of Health's Agency of Clinical Innovation. He is also Professor of Healthcare Innovation at the University of Tasmania's Faculty of Health. He has published across a wide range of journals about the organisational and communication dimensions of health care, including his most recent book, *Visualising healthcare improvement: Innovation from within* (Abingdon: Radcliffe Publishing, 2013, with Jessica Mesman and Katherine Carroll).

Donella Piper is a consultant to the healthcare industry and is a lawyer by background. Donella has lectured in the School of Law and the School of Health at the University of New England and the Law School at Flinders University of South Australia. Her research interests, grants, publications and consultancies focus on health and medical law, safety and quality, and patient-centred care including consumer engagement, open disclosure and experience-based co-design.

Marie Manidis has worked in the private, public, vocational and higher education sectors for the past 30 years. In these sectors Marie has held numerous management and specialist positions working on state and national level projects. Marie's current interests are in social, organisational and professional practices in the health sector. She is now a Postdoctoral Research Fellow at the University of Technology, Sydney.

About the contributors

Douglas Bellamy is District Cancer Clinical Nurse Consultant, Hunter New England Cancer Services, Hunter New England Health Local Health District. With more than 27 years of experience in clinical, management, project management and research in cancer settings, Douglas Bellamy is a strong advocate for interdisciplinary evidence-based practice.

Deidre Besuijen (nee Cornes) qualified as a radiation therapist at the Central Institute of Technology, New Zealand in 1994, receiving a postgraduate Diploma of Public Health from the University of Otago, Wellington, NZ in 1999 and a BSc Therapeutic Radiography degree (with First Class honours) from Anglia Polytechnic University, Cambridge, UK in 2002. In late 2012 she became Radiation Oncology Information Technology Project Manager for the new North West Cancer Centre in Tamworth.

Kate Bower is a research fellow at the University of Tasmania, Sydney. She is currently undertaking a study into communication in healthcare incident disclosure funded by an ARC Discovery Grant, awarded to Professor Rick Iedema. Kate has a strong commitment to interdisciplinary work, with a background in sociology, higher education, and women's and gender studies.

Phyllis Butow is Professor and NHMRC Senior Principal Research Fellow in the School of Psychology at the University of Sydney. She is Chair of the Australian Psycho-Oncology Co-operative Research Group (PoCoG) and a co-director of the Centre for Medical Psychology and Evidence-based Decision-making (CeMPED). Phyllis has worked for over 20 years in the areas of doctor–patient communication and psycho-oncology, conducting a large body of research on patient involvement in cancer consultations and decision-making.

Katherine Carroll is a medical sociologist and Assistant Professor of Health Services Research in the Division of Health Care Policy and Research at Mayo Clinic, US. She uses ethnographic, visual and qualitative methodologies to engage with health professionals, patients and their families in order to improve the delivery of health care in complex and high-technology settings. Her previous position as an Australian Research Council Postdoctoral Fellow in the Faculty of Arts and Social Sciences, University of Technology, Sydney, examined human milk donation for use in neonatal intensive care units as part of the broader tissue economy in Australia and the US.

Tina Cockburn is an Associate Professor at the Queensland University of Technology Faculty of Law and an active researcher within the Australian Centre for Health Law Research. Her health law research focuses on patient safety law and in particular medico-legal issues arising out of adverse medical outcomes and the communication of information, including patient consent and post-treatment open disclosure. She has published extensively, nationally and internationally, about current issues in medical litigation.

Aileen Collier is Lecturer in Palliative Care at Flinders University in Adelaide. She has a clinical background as a palliative care nurse in a diverse range of settings in the UK and Lao PDR as well as Australia. Aileen's scholarly interests are focused on improving access to quality palliative and end-of-life care. Her PhD thesis was the winner of the 2013 International Institute of Qualitative Methods award and examined the links between where dying people are and the extent to which spaces enable or constrain their agency and contribute to the quality of the care they receive.

Sam Davis is a social gerontologist and experienced researcher. Dr Davis is Course Coordinator for the Applied Gerontology postgraduate program in the School of Health Sciences, Flinders University, South Australia. She is a core member of the Global Action on Personhood (GAP). Her current major project, funded by Department of Social Services, Aged Care Service Improvement and Healthy Ageing Grants Fund, focuses on dementia care education for Australian residential aged care staff.

K. J. Farley graduated from the University of Melbourne in 2004 and is an intensive care specialist at Western Health. K. J. is also a general physician, with an interest in perioperative medicine, ICU outreach and improving the care of long stay ICU and hospital patients. K. J. has also completed the University of Melbourne's Postgraduate Certificate in Clinical Ultrasound.

Gerard J. Fennessy is an intensive care specialist at Western Health, Melbourne, and specialist retrieval physician with Adult Retrieval Victoria. He has 15 years experience as a doctor, having worked in many hospitals in New Zealand and Australia. He has interests in both online and face-to-face education for medical students, trainee doctors, nursing staff, advanced trainees and fellows.

Cindy Gallois is Emeritus Professor of Psychology and Communication at the University of Queensland. She is a Fellow of the Academy of the Social Sciences in Australia, International Communication Association, Society of Experimental Social Psychology, International Association of Language and Social Psychology, and International Academy of Intercultural Relations. Her research focuses on intergroup communication in health, including the impact of communication on safety and quality of patient care. She has a special interest in communication accommodation in health.

Natalya Godbold is a Sessional Lecturer in Information Behaviour at the University of Technology, Sydney, with a focus on the everyday practices of living with chronic disease. She examines how people with chronic illnesses translate medical advice into everyday self-care practices and is interested in the dynamics of healthcare provision from the perspectives of patients and their families. Her PhD examined how people make sense of kidney failure in online discussion boards.

Jane Gray is Director of Research, Innovation and Partnerships for Hunter New England Local Health District in NSW, Jane joined Hunter New England Health as the Director of Innovation Support in November 2009. Before this, she led NSW Health's Patient and Carer Experience Program for the Health Services Performance Improvement Branch from 2006 to 2009. She is passionate about understanding and improving staff, patient and carer experience of the public health system.

George Hayden is a Njaki Njaki man from the eastern Wheatbelt region of the Noongar Nation in the south-west of Western Australia. George has a vast history of working with his Mob throughout his career, be it in the public or private arena. For the past four years he has been a Cultural Consultant to the Building Mental Wealth team at Curtin University (School of Psychology and Speech Pathology). His current role, as an Associate Lecturer at the Centre for Aboriginal Studies at Curtin University of New Technology, requires him to provide members of the research team with appropriate cultural guidance.

Nick Hopwood is a Senior Research Fellow at the University of Technology, Sydney. He has been conducting research about learning and education for over a decade. Most recently he has explored learning and pedagogy in relation to child and family health professional practices, and in medical and nursing clinical education. Nick is interested in investigating connections between learning and health.

Caris Jalla is a researcher who has worked at the University of Western Australia, Edith Cowan University and the Telethon Kids Institute and is currently working at the Centre for Cerebral Palsy. In her early career she was awarded the Faith Stewart Book Prize in Health Sciences at UWA. Her current research project focuses on the improvement of service delivery of disability supports and services for Aboriginal families in regional Western Australia.

Daryl Jones graduated from the University of Melbourne in 1996 and is an Intensive Care Specialist at Austin Health. Daryl is also an Adjunct Research Fellow at Monash University, an Adjunct Associate Professor at the University of Melbourne and an advisor to the Australian Commission on Safety and Quality in Health Care. He has completed a doctor of medicine in aspects of the rapid response team (RRT) and has recently completed a PhD on the RRT that assesses the characteristics and outcomes of patients who are reviewed by the RRT, and details of resource utilisation of the medical emergency team (MET) in ICU-equipped hospitals throughout Australia.

Christine Jorm is based at Sydney University. She has doctorates in neuropharmacology and sociology and worked as an anaesthetist for more than 15 years before moving to full time work in patient safety and quality. Her book, *Reconstructing medical practice: Engagement, professionalism and critical relationships in health care* (Aldershot: Gower Publishers, 2012) suggests that doctors' delicate self-esteem, collegiate relationships and cherished connections with patients reduce their ability to admit to error or engage with the system. Christine's range of publications reflects both the complexity inherent in safety and her enthusiasm for interdisciplinary collaboration. After four years assisting medical students to develop professionalism, her current work is focused on interprofessional and interdisciplinary education.

Benn Lancman is a specialist anaesthetist and human factors specialist. Benn served as a junior doctor representative with the Clinical Excellence Commission in NSW, and currently has an appointment at the University of Sydney in the Workforce Education and Development Group working on projects that impact trainee performance and the acquisition of expertise. Benn is also a passionate educator who instructs on EMST courses and runs workshops at clinical conferences, on issues of communication, incident investigation and clinical error. His current work is exploring how process redesign and the intelligent application of technology can develop safer, more efficient healthcare systems.

Bill Madden is an accredited specialist in personal injury law in practice at Slater and Gordon Sydney. He is Adjunct Professor at the Queensland University of Technology (Australian Centre for Health Law Research) and Adjunct Fellow at the University of Western Sydney (School of Law). He is also co-author of *Australian medical liability* (Sydney: LexisNexis Australia, 2014) and of *Health care and the law* (Pyrmont: Thomson Reuters Lawbook Co, 2010). He is further an editorial board member of the journals *Australian Health Law Bulletin* and *Australian Civil Liability*.

Elizabeth Manias is Research Professor at the School of Nursing and Midwifery at Deakin University. She is also an Honorary Professor at the Melbourne School of Health Sciences, the University of Melbourne, and Adjunct Professor of the Department of Medicine at the Royal Melbourne Hospital. Elizabeth is a registered nurse and registered pharmacist. In 2014, Elizabeth was inducted in the International Nurse Researcher Hall of Fame by Sigma Theta Tau International for making an outstanding research contribution to health care. Her area of interests include medication safety, medication adherence, communication processes between health professionals, patients and family members, organisational and environmental aspects associated with patient safety, and consumer participation in care.

Kirsten McCaffery is a Professor at Sydney University's School of Public Health and Co-Director of the Centre for Medical Psychology & Evidence-based Decision-making. Her research interests include psychosocial aspects of screening, decision-making and health literacy. Her recent work examines the issues around communicating overdiagnosis and overtreatment in cancer screening, and the development and evaluation of interventions to increase health literacy.

Janine McIlwraith is a highly accomplished health lawyer who has co-authored two prominent medical law texts, *Health care and the law* (4th edition 2006; 5th edition 2010; Pyrmont: Thomson Reuters Lawbook Co) and *Australian medical liability* (2008, 2102; Sydney: LexisNexis Australia), in addition to having edited several chapters of *Halsburys laws of Australia* focusing on professional negligence in the health arena. In addition to her academic accomplishments, Janine is currently undertaking a PhD in the area of patient safety through the Centre for Health Innovation at the University of NSW. Janine practises as a specialist medical lawyer and is currently working with Slater and Gordon, Melbourne.

Catherine O'Grady, Honorary Associate of the Department of Linguistics at Macquarie University, is a teacher and researcher with an abiding interest in the application of discourse analytical findings in clinical education. Catherine was awarded the Vice Chancellor's Commendation for outstanding achievement for her PhD thesis, *The nature of expert communication as required for the general practice of medicine – a discourse analytical study*. Her recent publications, that focus on themes of empathy and trust in primary care and surgical contexts, appear in high-ranking peer-reviewed journals including *Discourse & Society* and *Health Communication*.

Vicki Parker is Professor of Rural Nursing at the University of New England and Hunter New England Local Health District. Vicki has experience in practice-based research with particular focus on experiences of illness and health care, models of care, interprofessional practice, nursing and rural workforce. Vicki has designed and implemented numerous education units within undergraduate, postgraduate nursing programs and industry, developed and taught interprofessional units and played a key role in the professional development of health professionals across disciplines, including design and delivery of clinical supervision resources and workshops, and mentoring of staff.

Jennifer Plumb is a medical anthropologist and mental health policy specialist currently working at the Australian Commission for Safety and Quality in Health Care. Her research background is in the ethnography of mental healthcare settings as a method for deepening our understanding of how staff in those environments conceptualise and attempt to enact patient safety. Recent professional projects outside of academia have included work for the Australian government on stakeholder perspectives on mental health reform, and an initiative to develop nationwide indicators of patient experience.

George Ridgway is a lecturer in the Learning Centre at the University of Sydney. He received his PhD in biochemistry from the University of London and his Masters in Applied Linguistics at Sydney. He taught communication skills at the University of Leeds and the Yorkshire Deanery in the UK, working with medical students, junior doctors, specialists and general practitioners. He has co-authored a book, *Making it real: A practical guide to experiential learning* (Abingdon: Radcliffe Publishing, 2006), and a book chapter titled 'The content and process of simulated patient-based learning activities' in Nesterl, D. and Bearman, M., *Simulated patient methodology: Theory, evidence and practice* (Chichester: John Wiley & Sons, 2014), which focuses on working with simulated patients.

Luke Slawomirski is a health economist who has held senior policy and analyst positions with state, national and international agencies and organisations. His most recent position was Program Manager, Implementation Support, at the Australian Commission on Safety and Quality in Health Care. Luke has a clinical background in physiotherapy, having practised in Australia and the UK for close to a decade before completing his Master's degree and moving onto the policy arena. He speaks regularly at national and international conferences and events on healthcare policy issues including open disclosure, appropriateness of care, efficiency and equity, and healthcare funding. His areas of interest include the political economy of health, clinical governance and quality improvement.

Jill Thistlethwaite is a health professions education consultant and general practitioner, Adjunct Professor at the University of Technology Sydney and academic titleholder at the University of Queensland. She trained as a GP in the UK and has worked as a health professional academic in the UK and Australia. Her research interests include interprofessional education and practice, professionalism, shared decision-making and women's health. In 2014 Professor Thistlethwaite was a Fulbright senior scholar at the National Center for Interprofessional Practice and Education at the University of Minnesota, US.

Prue Vines is a Professor at the Faculty of Law, University of New South Wales and Visiting Professor, University of Strathclyde, Glasgow. Her specialisms include the attribution of responsibility in the law of torts and the impact of the legal system on end of life decision-making for Aboriginal people. She is the author of numerous publications on the law of torts, particularly on apologies in civil, including medical, liability. She has published widely in all her areas of interest.

Acknowledgements

The authors and Cambridge University Press would like to thank the following for permission to reproduce material in this book.

··

Artwork

Figures 1.1, 1.2 and 1.3: Reproduced with permission of the Bureau of Health Information. **1.4:** Reprinted from Street, R. L., Makoul, G., Arora, N.K. & Epstein, R.M. (2009). How does communication heal? Pathways linking clinician-patient communication to health outcomes, *Patient Education and Counseling*, 74, 295–301, with permission from Elsevier. **2.1:** Reproduced with permission of Groeningemuseum Brugge © Lukas-Art in Flanders. **2.2:** Reproduced with permission of Rijksmuseum, Amsterdam. **4.1:** Reproduced with permission of the Australian Bureau of Statistics. **4.2:** Reproduced by permission, NSW Ministry of Health © 2015. **5.2:** Reproduced with permission of *The Medical Journal of Australia*. **8.1:** Reproduced with permission of the World Health Organization. **8.2:** Reproduced with permission of Royal Australasian College of Surgeons. **18.1:** Reproduced with permission of Taylor & Francis Ltd. **21.1:** Reprinted from Healy J. & Braithwaite, J. (2006). Designing safer health care through responsive regulation. *Med J Aust*, 184, S56–S59. © Copyright 2006 *The Medical Journal of Australia* – reproduced with permission. *The Medical Journal of Australia* does not accept responsibility for any errors in translation. **22.1:** Reproduced with permission of the Australian Commission on Safety and Quality in Health Care.

··

Text

Chapters 2 and 5: ACSQHC material reproduced with permission. **Chapters 2, 5 and 22:** ACSQHC material reproduced with permission. **Chapter 14:** (Table 14.1) Shared decision making: What do clinicians need to know and why should they bother? *Med J Aust 2014; 201*(1): 35–39. © Copyright 2014 *The Medical Journal of Australia* – reproduced with permission. The Medical Journal of Australia does not accept responsibility for any errors in translation. **Chapter 15:** SPIKES protocol republished with permission of AlphaMed Press, from Baile, W. F., Buckman, R., Lenzi, R., Glober, G., Beale, E. A. & Kudelka, A. P. (2000). SPIKES – A six-step protocol for delivering bad news: Application to the patient with cancer, *The Oncologist*, 5(4), 302–311, permission conveyed through Copyright Clearance Center, Inc. Practice example 15.1 reproduced with permission of Cancer Australia. **Chapter 18:** Excerpt in practice example 18.1 reprinted from Butow et al. (2013), Inferior health-related quality of life and psychological well-being in immigrant cancer survivors: A population based study, *European Journal of Cancer*, 49(8), 1948–1956, with permission from Elsevier. Excerpt from Butow et al. (2010) in practice example 18.1 reproduced with kind permission from Springer Science+Business Media. Excerpt from Butow & Baile (2012), copyright © 2012 John Wiley & Sons, Ltd. **Chapter 19:** Practice example 19.1 and accompanying analysis is reproduced with some changes and with the permission of Emerald Group Publishing. It was previously published in O'Grady, (2011b) and first appeared in O'Grady (2011a). **Chapter 21:** Text in practice example 21.1 reproduced from Ramsay et al. (2014), Governing patient safety: Lessons learned from a mixed methods evaluation of implementing a ward-level medication safety scorecard in two English NHS hospitals, *BMJ Quality & Safety*, 23, 136–146, with permission from BMJ Publishing Group Ltd.

Online instructor resources

Available at www.cambridge.edu.au/academic/qualitysafety.

The 🌐 icon indicates that there are related instructor resources.

Instructor resources include:
- links to videos, with accompanying questions
- podcasts, with accompanying questions
- multiple-choice questions
- short-answer questions

These resources are available to adopters of the book, and require a username and password. Please contact Cambridge University Press (academicmarketing@cambridge.edu.au with the subject 'Communicating Quality and Safety in Health Care password') if you require a access to these resources, and provide details of course, semester and enrolment as well as your name, university and position. If you do not wish to be added to our contacts database and receive email marketing, please state this in your email.

Part 1

Communication in health care, and its role in quality and safety

1

Introduction: communicating for quality and safety

Rick Iedema, Donella Piper and Marie Manidis

Learning objectives

This chapter will enable you to:
- identify the reasons for communication becoming more and more important in health care;
- describe the role of (inadequate or non-) communication in clinical errors and patient complaints;
- list the strategies that have been proposed for improving healthcare communication;
- set out the direct and indirect benefits of good communication.

Key terms

Clinical incident
Complaints
Continuity of care
Patient-centred
Quality of care
Safety of care
Shared decision-making

Overview

In this introductory chapter, we talk about why communication is so important in health care. Indeed, we believe that communication is central to safe and good quality health care. We know that for many people communication is something we do naturally. It is taken as given, and not considered worthy of very much attention. People may also think there are more urgent things to worry about, such as technical precision, clinical knowledge and professional skills.

Communication has been defined in different ways. A recent NHS document defines communication in these terms:

> Communication is a process that involves a meaningful exchange between at least two people to convey facts, needs, opinions, thoughts, feelings or other information through both verbal and non-verbal means, including face-to-face exchanges and the written word. (National Health Service, 2010)

The above definition of communication suggests that communication takes place face-to-face, non-verbally and in writing. We know, however, that communication also increasingly relies on information and communication technologies (ICTs). ICTs harness all kinds of visual and numerical information, as well as language. Further, communication can occur according to well-established formats (procedures or checklists), but it can also move through channels that can be quite hidden and hardly perceptible, like machines talking to one another and initiating actions on the basis of pre-set instructions. In this digital environment, communication is bolstered by a seemingly infinite number of channels (reaching right across the globe), resources (real-time communication as well as historic records) and genres (training clips, speeches, documentaries, publications).

And yet it is becoming increasingly clear, too, that ineffective *in situ* communication can defeat high levels of technical precision, knowledge and skills. For example, a missed medication may undo the success of a surgical intervention. Equally, and by contrast, effective *in situ* communication can alleviate the adverse effects of inadequate knowledge and skills. For example, clinicians and patients are able to help and support one another through communicating about the details of care. For this reason, *how* health professionals communicate with their patients and with each other is becoming an increasingly prominent issue for policy-makers, managers, patients, and for health professionals themselves.

Why is this so? Think back to your own encounters with your health service when you or a loved one were a patient. Think about how people communicated with you, and how you felt about it. You may fondly remember clinicians communicating with you in a way that showed interest and made their care memorable. They took you seriously and looked after you by communicating about matters in ways that involved you and made you feel they took time to understand you as patient. Decisions made sense, conversations were considerate and respectful, and the care felt safe.

You may also have witnessed quite hurried conversations by what appeared to be doctors at the end of your or your relative's bed, or nurses huddling and talking in quiet voices and in a language that was difficult to understand. Different clinicians may have come past in quick succession, all addressing issues whose purpose or relevance was not immediately clear to you. Decisions may have been made in ways that were surprising, contradicting prior decisions and plans, ignoring previous information, or plainly not intended for you, or your relative, but for another patient altogether.

These examples make clear the following principle that anchors the chapters in the present book: *in situ communication is where care happens in the first and last instance.*

Of course, care happens in many other things that clinicians do with and for patients. Normally, however, communication precedes, accompanies and follows on from clinical actions and interventions. But communication establishes bonds and renders those care activities understandable. Research has shown that effective *in situ* communication is critical to patients' healing. Achieving such effective and healing communication across a variety of settings is what this book is about.

While perhaps not always an immediate cause of an incident or an injury, inadequate communication can render care unsafe or counterproductive. Such care can limit your comprehension of how a health service works, of what you're supposed to do as a patient or a clinician, or how you're to respond to clinicians' advice. For all these reasons, communication plays a central role in how we enact healthcare practices and relationships.

So these are the three principles that are at the heart of this book:

1. communication is where care happens in the first and last instance;
2. communication goes beyond ensuring that the clinician–patient interaction is empathetic and informed, as it encompasses processes that enable and encourage the patient and clinician to discuss both the personal-treatment and the service-organisational dimensions of care; and
3. communication is therefore at the heart of healthcare service quality and safety.

Because communication is where care happens in the first and last instance, and because communication structures care practices and relationships, the quality of communication determines the quality and safety of care. Quality is concerned with whether patients are satisfied with the care they receive. Patients' safety is concerned with the absence of unintended harm, and with making patients feel safe. While health care is more able to conduct invasive procedures nowadays than in the past, the more frequent use of dangerous technologies, treatments and medications, and the increased reliance on institutional and cross-specialty collaboration, have made health care more complex and more dangerous than ever before, rendering patients' safety a critical concern. First and foremost, clinical decisions and actions are safe and of high quality thanks to not only technical skill, but also principally to effective, respectful and attentive communication.

Communicating for quality and safety

It appears that, in most domains of life, we communicate with more people and more frequently than we used to in the past. We may be listening to someone speak and typing a text message on our phone at the same time. Or we may be partaking in a teleconference while reading an email and leafing through a report. One important reason for this intensification of communication is that there are now more channels of communication. Many of these channels can operate simultaneously: talk, text, vision. These various channels of communication inform us about different things, at different speeds, and in different formats. Aside from communicating what others do elsewhere, these channels also increasingly provide feedback about where we are and what we do ourselves: they may tell us where we are located geographically, or how we are performing against a particular benchmark.

While it might appear that all this communication and feedback help make life easier, it actually makes life more complex. We are invited to rethink what we are doing more frequently. We are encouraged to ask more questions about more aspects of who we are and what we do than occurred in the past.

Health care has not remained immune to this intensification of communication. We are now in email contact with our general practitioners (GPs) and specialists. We may have their mobile numbers. When we visit them they will be using computers that display test results and diagnostic reports. When we are admitted to a ward as a hospital patient, we can liaise verbally with ward staff, we can Skype with family, and we can post messages on PatientVoice, a website that enables patients to post comments about the care they receive. Professionals will liaise using mobile phones, email, and a host of other ways of communicating: electronic records, video- and teleconferencing, Facebook, and so forth. The care that patients receive, seek and request is increasingly influenced by and structured around these new channels of communication.

The speed of connection and communication has changed what it means to be a patient and a professional. Patients are increasingly communicatively engaged, even if at the moment a large proportion of patients still expect their healthcare professional to make decisions for them.

Professionals are having to make a greater effort to communicate with patients who come from a greater range of socio-cultural backgrounds: people have less in common and less can now be taken for granted. To counteract this reduction in shared socio-cultural values and practices, **patient-centred** care has now become the new standard. This means acknowledging we need to communicate with individual patients to establish what they want and need. Professionals are also increasingly having to reflect on how they communicate with their colleagues. Hierarchy and status are becoming less viable resources for deciding how to speak with people.

> **patient-centred**
> putting the needs of the patient at the centre of processes and priorities.

Problems in healthcare communication

Only about 50% of patients recently surveyed by the Commonwealth Fund in the US feel that their doctor spends enough time with them. Consider Figure 1.1, which is taken from a recent Bureau of Health Information (New South Wales) report. The figure shows the approval rating of how long Australian medical staff spend with their patients (60%) to be level with UK and US ratings:

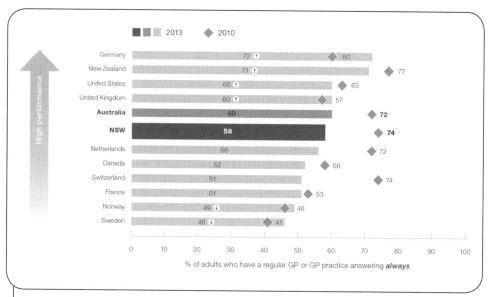

Figure 1.1 *Commonwealth Fund survey 2010 and 2013* When you need care or treatment, how often does the regular doctor/GP or medical staff you see spend enough time with you? (BHI, 2014)

Of interest here is that the 2013 approval rating of Australian and New South Wales medical clinicians is considerably lower than its 2010 equivalent. Does this mean patients are becoming more demanding? Or are doctors becoming busier?

Now consider Figure 1.2. This figure shows that a slightly greater percentage of patients (67% in 2013) find their doctor easy to understand. But this percentage too is down from 77% in 2010.

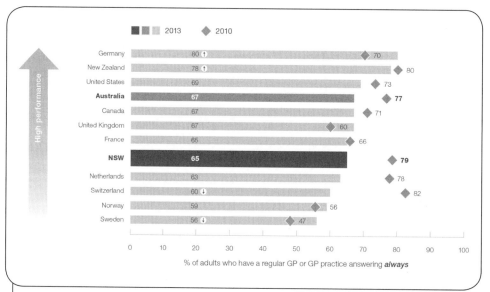

Figure 1.2 *Commonwealth Fund survey 2010 and 2013* When you need care or treatment, how often does the regular doctor/GP or medical staff explain things in a way that is easy to understand? (% answering *always*) (BHI, 2014)

Why is this so? Does the lower 2013 percentage result from rising patient expectations? Or is it because more patients and practitioners have arrived from overseas, needing to work harder on clear explanations? And what might explain patients' view that only in about 53% of cases their provider 'always knows' their medical history (Figure 1.3)? Could this be an effect of greater 'patient mobility' – do patients move house, state and country more often? Could it also result from the growing amounts of information that practitioners need to gather and process? And what might be the effect of the rising complexity of patients' diseases, now that more people are chronically ill, and also more often now have multiple diseases, or 'co-morbidities'?

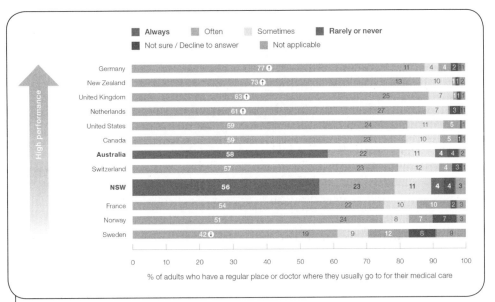

Figure 1.3 *Commonwealth Fund survey 2013* When you need care or treatment, how often does the regular doctor/GP or medical staff you see know information about your medical history? (BHI, 2014)

When we look at health care from the perspective of what patients complain about, we also note that shortcomings in communication are high on the list (Robins, Fasih & Schweitzer, 2014). A review of 59 studies reporting on a total of 88 069 patient **complaints** found that one of the two primary factors underlying complaints was communication (the other being treatment problems (Reader, Gillespie & Roberts, 2014)). For patients generally, good, open and honest communication has been found to be a critical component of effective care (Iedema et al., 2011).

> **complaints**
> a person's expressions of dissatisfaction with care services received.

We can also look at healthcare communication from the perspective of healthcare incidents, or care gone wrong (see Chapter 22). Here it becomes even more apparent that inadequate communication creates high levels of dissatisfaction and tension (Sutcliffe, Lewton & Rosenthal, 2004).

Furthermore, a number of studies have now shown that inadequate communication itself may cause communication failures, and that these failures have real consequences for patients' health: they *harm* patients (Iedema et al., 2008). Much of this communication harm has been shown to be avoidable. For example, more effective ward round and clinical handover communication contributes to avoiding communication failures. A study of Danish incident reports revealed that 52% of the incidents identified in a review of 84 error investigation reports were caused by 'avoidable communication problems' (Rabøl et al., 2011). This finding that inadequate communication or non-communication is a prominent cause of patient harm in health services, particularly for patients from linguistically and culturally diverse backgrounds, is now a common one (Gu, Itoh & Suzuki, 2014; Siu, Maran & Paterson-Brown, 2014).

For patients who come into care with communication challenges due to mental health issues, speech disability, dementia or delirium, the situation is markedly worse still. They have a 46% higher chance of experiencing a clinical error (Bartlett et al., 2008). We address each of these challenges in the chapters that follow.

Improving healthcare communication

The Commonwealth Fund and New South Wales Bureau of Health Information data presented above were derived from surveys asking patients for feedback. In the not-so-distant past, these kinds of feedback were rarely sought from patients. Patient feedback surveys have become prominent only in the last decade or so (Jenkinson, Coulter & Bruster, 2002). Patients' views on their care and on how practitioners communicate with them are considered increasingly important (Weissman et al., 2008). Regular patient satisfaction surveys are now done across Western industrialised countries, a trend that was started by the Picker Institute in the UK (Jenkinson, Coulter & Bruster, 2002). Many government agencies now use 'patient trackers' or on-the-spot feedback surveys using electronic tablets which communicate with a central database that can process thousands of surveys at a time.

But understanding how patients are experiencing care is only one side of the coin. The other side of the coin is how we address the communication shortcomings that patients help us identify. In recent years, a range of strategies has emerged for ensuring that clinician–patient communication improves. One is 'informed consent' (Chapter 14). Informed consent ensures that clinicians ask patients for permission before they initiate treatments. Likewise, **shared decision-making** is a strategy that calls attention to the importance of clinicians sharing decisions with patients, rather than imposing decisions on them (Chapter 12). A much more recent initiative is 'open disclosure', a policy that requires clinicians to be open and honest about mishaps in care (Chapter 22).

> **shared decision-making**
> decision-making in which patients and clinicians make treatment plans and decisions together. Shared decision-making discussions take account of best scientific evidence available, as well as patient's values and preferences.

The reason communication is now considered so important is not just that patients are becoming more assertive about their rights, less tolerant of problematic service standards, and more vocal in their criticism of inadequate health care. Better communication is needed not just to satisfy patients' 'service expectations' but is also critical to delivering good care, to minimising avoidable readmissions, and to maximising patients' ability to manage their own care.

The centrality of communication to care is due to the rising complexity of care: more aspects of care need to be negotiated 'on the spot'. Complexity means this: events have many different dimensions, events are less easily categorised and acted on than they were before, and more communication is now necessary to determine what to do next, even if sometimes events can pose 'wicked problems'. Wicked problems are problems where there is no easy solution. In these circumstances, stakeholders need to be given the opportunity to come to terms with the 'size' of the problem, with the potential lack of a solution altogether, and with the kind of compromise solution that may need to be adopted. The 'wicked problem' described in practice example 1.1 exemplifies what we mean.

Practice example 1.1

A 'wicked problem' – a palliative care patient in an Australian teaching hospital[1]

While still living at home, a 78-year-old female patient is under palliative care treatment at an Australian teaching hospital. Last week, she needed to go into hospital as her lungs have been filling with fluid and she was finding it difficult to breathe. This was her second visit to the hospital in two weeks. This is how she talks about what happened: 'My palliative care doctor happened to be away last week, [since he was] having a minor operation, so no one really "owned" me when I arrived on the Tuesday.' I identified that she felt like a medical orphan.

For an unknown reason, possibly as a consequence of her own doctor being away, the hospital staff took three days to determine that a drain should be inserted in one of her lungs instead of just draining it. The drain would help solve her breathing problem, and would mean that she didn't need to keep coming back for treatment. Before the procedure on the Friday morning, she was 'nil by mouth' (fasting). At about 10:30 a.m., they took her down to surgery, prepped her, covered her with green sheets and placed her lying on her side. This meant she was lying on the leg which had the tumour that was in fact the cause of her impending death, and the pain it caused had been treated with morphine for quite some time. She was left lying on the tumour for an hour. She was in agony, she said. No one was aware of her agony, and no one explained to her what was happening.

Then, suddenly, there was a mad flurry and someone came to tell her that 'they couldn't find a drain'. It seemed that the person whose job it was to check 'the equipment' in question had not done so.

continued ›

> **Practice example 1.1** continued ›
>
> Next, a number of senior doctors came and spoke to her and 'explained' how they were getting in touch with the drain supplier. They expressed regret, but did not apologise to her. They explained the mishap again, and they also said that 'they themselves were very shaken by the whole experience'. After that, a nurse dressed her and returned her to her room.
>
> Then at 4 p.m., she was once again wheeled down to surgery. Once there, she was left waiting for another hour, during which time no one communicated with her about what was going on. Eventually, at 5 p.m., she was given another anaesthetic and the operation commenced. The surgeons and anaesthetists had decided to give her not a local but a general anaesthetic, due to the patient's now highly stressful state. The drain insertion operation went well.
>
> The patient had been nil by mouth since that Friday morning, and, following the surgery, she was not given dinner. The following morning, the Saturday, she was not given breakfast. She had now gone without food for more than 24 hours. Only after she created a fuss requesting some food was she brought something to eat.

The vignette in practice example 1.1 highlights communication to be critical to at least three important dimensions of care:

continuity of care
care such that the patient does not face avoidable delays, cancellations and other access barriers; continuity results from practitioners ensuring that their care integrates with the care provided by colleague practitioners.

quality of care
refers to whether healthcare services provide the right care at the right time to the right person, achieving the best possible outcomes for those people every time they come into contact with the healthcare system.

safety of care
the prevention of errors and adverse effects resulting from care provided to patients.

1. **continuity of care:** There was inadequate handover between the treating physician (who went on leave for an operation) and the clinical team receiving the patient on the Tuesday. This omission resulted in care discontinuity: the patient's treatment and management took two full days to be worked out.

2. **quality of care:** The patient was not given explanations, she was kept lying on her tumour, causing excessive pain, and she was not fed from Thursday night until Saturday morning, when she was finally obliged to ask the clinicians for food. Each of these three problems detracted from the quality of her care.

3. **safety of care:** The palliative care doctor had not left adequate instructions to the clinicians taking over from him, raising the risk of an inappropriate decision being taken. In addition, the surgical equipment had not been inspected before the patient's operation, and the anaesthetic procedure was changed from local to general due to the patient's raised anxiety. Each of these latter three problems are safety problems.

In all, had the clinicians communicated more effectively and attentively, with each other as well as with the patient, every single one of these problems could have been avoided. The palliative care doctor knew the patient was going in for elective surgery and should have briefed his colleagues about the patient's problem and needs. The admitting clinicians should have taken charge on the Tuesday and worked out how to manage the patient's surgical needs, rather than waste two (expensive) bed days. The surgical staff should have checked the equipment or put processes in place to make sure the surgical equipment was up to date. The postoperative handover from theatre should have clarified the patient's nutrition needs. Someone should have communicated with the patient to clarify what was going on reassure her and lessen her anxiety, and ensure she did not need a general anaesthetic.

> **clinical incidents**
> situations where the patient experiences an unintended outcome from the care received; they may involve short-term or lasting harm, or even ('healthcare-caused') death. Also known as 'adverse events'.

Here, as in most **clinical incidents** and patient complaints in health care, inadequate communication is evident right across the care trajectory.

What is good healthcare communication?

The chapters in this book address good healthcare communication in a large range of care domains. By way of definition, we can say that good healthcare communication presumes that you:

- are respectful towards colleagues and patients;
- are ethical in your use and sharing of healthcare information;
- have awareness of others such that you are able to respond to their communication, knowledge and information needs;
- involve others in decision-making about what is done for and with patients;
- are open and honest about the intended and unintended outcomes of your practices.

The healthcare and organisational benefits of good communication

There are many benefits of good communication for the care of the patient and for the organisation of that care. Too often, clinicians regard themselves as autonomous experts. Positioning yourself as an autonomous expert often implies that you regard communication as a non-essential luxury. The detrimental effect of this view is that it limits your involvement with and responsibility for how patients travel through a whole episode of care that relise on various kinds of expertise.

For example, a patient is referred to hospital by a GP, and that GP hears nothing about that patient's progress until after the patient has been discharged from hospital. Another frequent example is of the patient's discharge being inadequate, and those in the community have insufficient information about how to continue the patient's medication regimen. While the care provided in each specific setting may have been exemplary, the lack of care continuity threatens its overall aim of ensuring the patient's healing.

Problems in communication also frequently affect service and internal processes. At times, patients are unable to move from the emergency department into a specialty ward due to staff refusing to communicate ethically about patients' problems (Nugus, 2009). Or clinical handover and ward round communication falls short, in that the outgoing team does not systematically update the incoming team about the various issues affecting their patients (Jorm, White & Kaneen, 2009). Good healthcare communication is critical to ensuring seamless transitions in patients' care, both within a service, and across services.

In health care, communication protocols and checklists are often used to 'force' clinicians to address clinically or interpersonally important matters. But good communication goes much further than healthcare professionals adhering to checklists and ticking off technical issues. Good communication is as much about attentiveness, respect and flexibility as it is about precision, accuracy and comprehensiveness. Attentiveness, respect and flexibility are critical to ensuring the patients' care is integrated and continuous, keeping them safe, and making them feel safe.

Good communication is critical to managing complex situations, particularly when such situations present as 'wicked problems'. Wicked problems are problems that are very difficult to resolve, and that sometimes can't be resolved. Wicked problems offer only compromises or tragic choices.

Tragic situations are when you aren't able to decide what is wrong with a patient. You have to acknowledge the patient presents with a 'medically unexplainable symptom' (a 'MUS'), and you can't offer help. Tragic choices occur when you have to determine and negotiate with a family (and maybe the patient) whether to extubate the patient (extract an endotracheal tube, a catheter, a drain or a feeding tube from the patient's body) because it is apparent the patient is dying.

These situations may mean that you have to reconcile yourself as a clinician to compromised decisions. When these compromised decisions are likely to have only tragic outcomes, they require intense communication with those involved. Failing to communicate about challenging or tragic issues may be detrimental both to clinicians' well-being and to patients' and families' ability to accept their fate.

As the chapters in the present volume point out, attentiveness, respect and flexibility are a pre-condition for good communication. Without attentiveness, respect and flexibility, your judgments about what is precise, evidence-based, accurate and comprehensive – however well-informed and technically and scientifically defensible – may remain misguided. In short, good communication is as much about being sensitive to the needs and problems of others as it is about following rules, displaying expertise, and applying evidence.

The healing effects of communication

In a landmark article published in 2009, Street and colleagues point out that good healthcare communication *heals* (Street et al., 2009). The healing power of good healthcare communication has both direct and indirect outcomes (see Figure 1.4). Direct outcomes include survival, less suffering, emotional well-being and faster recovery. Indirect outcomes are satisfaction, understanding, agreement, trust and feeling known. These indirect outcomes are likely to convert into better access to care, patients' commitment to treatment, and better self-care skills.

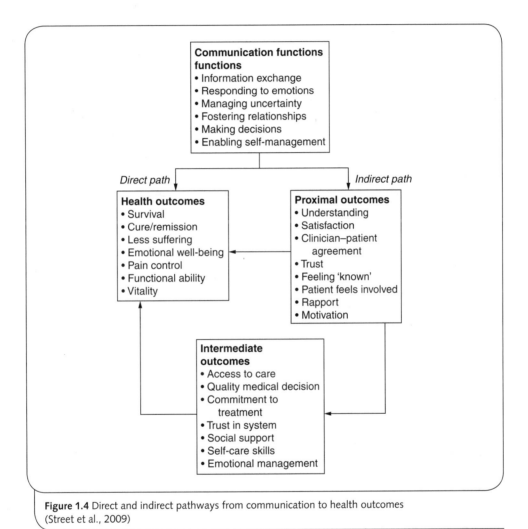

Figure 1.4 Direct and indirect pathways from communication to health outcomes (Street et al., 2009)

These claims are equally relevant for clinicians' well-being. Good communication is healing for them, too. Junior clinicians will feel respected, in spite of their not yet fully developed skills. They will feel safe, knowing that there are others to whom they can turn with questions and concerns. They will feel protected because there are others who are attentive to their problems and dilemmas, and who will help out or jump in when necessary. All these benefits of good communication for clinicians' well-being translate readily into greater patient safety, and higher quality of care.

The importance of Street et al.'s 2009 article is that it emphasises the role of communication in (1) raising patients' satisfaction ('indirect path'), and (2) ensuring the accuracy of the clinical–technical dimensions of care ('direct path'). The conclusion Street and colleagues enable us to draw is that no longer can we regard communication as a side issue, or as a merely subjective transaction, tangential to good care and healing. We now know communication is itself a clinical intervention, and it ties medical and surgical interventions to what needs to happen in the future for the patient to benefit from them. In short, communication *heals*.

Conclusion

We are reading more and more about the importance of good communication for effective and high-quality healthcare provision. Prominent agencies around the world have begun to report on the shortcomings of how clinicians communicate with their patients and with each other. Inadequate communication has also been found to play an important role in clinical incidents and patients' complaints.

Good communication has been found to enhance patients' safety, their well-being, their chance and pace of healing, and their knowledge and adoption of medical and drug therapy regimens. On the other hand, good communication enhances relationships among staff, strengthens teamwork, and spreads information that is critical to the care of patients. Good communication associates with better continuity of care within and across institutions, higher levels of safety, better junior staff training, and less clinical uncertainty and staff isolation.

Communication is now among the most critical things in health care. Complex patients and complex care trajectories cannot be navigated on the strength of linear roadmaps and simple checklists. Increasingly, we need to talk about how to go on together, to make sure we all understand what is now necessary and possible. It is for that reason that the chapters that follow all make use of vignettes of real-life care events and situations. By reading these vignettes, you should become attentive to the dilemmas that may affect patients and clinicians alike, and how communication is your most important resource for determining how to go on together.

Practice example 1.2

You work on a cardiac unit in a major hospital. The patients on the unit are mostly older patients, and many of them have secondary illnesses in addition to their heart problems (their 'primary diagnosis'). A colleague of yours speaks up during a meeting, saying, 'I wish we could provide proper cardiac care in this hospital. Most of our patients need all sorts of additional kinds of care, and they should really be in geriatrics or in respiratory care. Why doesn't anyone recognise they should not send those patients to us?'

continued ›

Practice example 1.2 continued ›

The manager of the unit responds to this as follows: 'Do you really think that we will ever again be getting patients whose care will be simple and straightforward? You may have trained in cardiac care, but to say you dislike looking after patients with complex needs is like saying you would prefer to work in a service where the processes are simple and linear. But health care will never again be simple and linear. Our patients will always be complex, and they will become only more so as time goes on. We won't ever have a ward full of nice 40-year-old patients with only easy-to-fix heart problems, even though that is what your training may have prepared you for.'

Reflective questions

1. Why do you think your colleague was complaining – what bothered him?
2. What do you think are the consequences of looking after older patients with multiple diseases – how will the clinical work differ from that provided to 'a ward full of nice 40-year-olds'?
3. How does the cardiac unit define itself, in the eyes of your colleague – as a specialty unit concerned with maintaining its specialty orientation, or as a patient care facility?

References

Bartlett, G., Blais, R., Tamblyn, R., Clermont, R. J., & MacGibbon, B. (2008). Impact of patient communication problems on the risk of preventable adverse events in acute care settings. *Canadian Medical Association Journal*, 178(12), 1555–1562.

Bureau of Health Information. (2014). *Healthcare in focus 2013: How well does NSW measure up? April 2014*. Sydney: Author.

Gu, X., Itoh, K., & Suzuki, S. (2014). An error taxonomy system for analysis of haemodialysis incidents. *Journal of Renal Care*. doi:10.1111/jorc/12081

Iedema, R., Allen, S., Britton, K., & Gallagher, T. H. (2011). What patients know about problems and failures in care. *BMJ Quality and Safety*, 21(3): 198–205. doi:10.1136/bmjqs-2011-000100

Iedema, R., Sorensen, R., Manias, E., Tuckett, A., Piper, D., Mallock, N., Williams, A., & Jorm, C. (2008). Patients' and family members' experiences of open disclosure following adverse events. *International Journal for Quality in Health Care*, 20(6), 421–432.

Jenkinson, C., Coulter, A., & Bruster, S. (2002). The Picker Patient Experience Questionnaire: Development and validation using data from in-patient surveys in five countries. *International Journal for Quality in Health Care*, 14(5), 353–358.

Jorm, C., White, S., & Kaneen, T. (2009). Clinical handover: Critical communications. *Medical Journal of Australia*, 190(11), S108–S109.

National Health Service. (2010). *Essence of care 2010: Benchmarks for communication*. London: The Stationary Office.

Nugus, P. (2009). Selling patients. *British Medical Journal, 339*, 1444–1446.

Rabøl, L. I., Andersen, M. L., Østergaard, D., Bjørn, B., Lilja, B., & Mogensen, T. (2011). Descriptions of verbal communication errors between staff. An analysis of 84 root cause analysis-reports from Danish hospitals. *BMJ Qual Saf, 20*(3), 268–274.

Reader, T. W., Gillespie, A., & Roberts, J. (2014). Patient complaints in healthcare systems: A systematic review and coding taxonomy. *BMJ Quality & Safety, 23*(8), 678–689.

Robins, J. A., Fasih, N., & Schweitzer, M. E. (2014). Looking back, moving forward: An analysis of complaints submitted to a Canadian tertiary care radiology department and lessons learned. *Canadian Asociation of Radiology Journal.* doi:10.1016/j.carj.2014.02.003

Siu, J., Maran, N., & Paterson-Brown, S. (2014). Observation of behavioural markers of non-technical skills in the operating room and their relationship to intra-operative incidents. *The Surgeon.* doi:10.1016/j.surge.2014.06.005

Street, R. L., Makoul, G., Arora, N.K., & Epstein, R. M. (2009). How does communication heal? Pathways linking clinician-patient communication to health outcomes. *Patient Education and Counseling, 74*, 295–301.

Sutcliffe, K. M., Lewton, E., & Rosenthal, M. M. (2004). Communication failures: An insidious contributor to medical mishaps. *Academic Medicine, 79*(2), 186–194.

Weissman, J. S., Schneider, E. C., Weingart, S. N., Epstein, A. M., David-Kasdan, J., Feibelmann, S. *et al.* (2008). Comparing patient-reported hospital adverse events with medical record review: Do patients know something that hospitals do not? *Annals of Internal Medicine, 149*(2), 100–108.

Note

1 Permission to relate this story was given by the patient soon after the event, and after her death consent was obtained from her closest family members.

2

A brief history of communication in health care

Rick Iedema, Donella Piper and Marie Manidis

Learning objectives

This chapter[1] will enable you to:
- understand the historical evolution of how healthcare professionals have communicated with patients;
- contextualise and compare the modern approach to communicating with patients with historical approaches;
- understand what is now required to communicate effectively with patients in today's more complex configurations of healthcare work.

Key terms

Birth of the clinic
Complexity
Healthcare communication
Medicalisation
Public expectations

Overview

This chapter provides a brief history of how communication developed within the context of healthcare provision. The chapter describes this history by referring to how the problem of human disease has been approached over time, and how this reshaped the ways we have communicated about care. We start our account at the time when care began to be institutionalised by people with increasing specialist training and with rising levels of financial and governmental support.

First, then, we discuss the lead up to the emergence of Western healthcare institutions. Caring for the sick was common throughout the ages, of course, with different cultures developing their own unique ways of caring for the unwell (Porter, 1999). For centuries, religious orders had specialised wards attached to monasteries where male nurses specialised in looking after the diseased. The Middle Ages saw the rise of charitable guesthouses and alms houses where people suffering from a wide variety of afflictions were admitted and nursed (Risse, 1999).

These early nursing practices were gradually complemented with medical approaches to disease treatment. Medicine emerged during the Renaissance from a fusion of two different fields. One was the practice of dissecting corpses, already evident in Greek times, and then only intermittently allowed under later Christian regimes. The other was the practice of drug administration, combining sophisticated folk knowledge of herbal treatments with pharmacological experimentation and clinical observation.

These twin endeavours made possible medical and surgical interventions that rapidly increased in effectiveness, not least thanks to their increasing reliance on modern science (Bliss, 2011). In essence, however, this Western approach to health care progressively constructed the diseased human body as an object to be repaired. This meant that disease and thereby also the patient were 'medicalised'. By promoting scientific experimentation and medical–surgical techniques to the exclusion of others, this kind of medicine risks losing sight of the diseased patient's individual and unique responses to their suffering, and downplays the patient's right and frequent desire to be involved in the negotiation of their own care.

Second, we discuss the emergence of a different, more communicative approach to providing health care. Healthcare practitioners have communicated with their patients through the centuries, but in Western nations **medicalisation** has had depersonalising effects, which this second development counterbalances. Emerging only relatively recently, this second development aims to acknowledge patients as central players and decision-makers, and not just position them as informants about their own bodies and diseases. This 'rise of the speaking patient' marks the beginning of what later became known as the 'biopsychosocial' or 'patient as person' philosophy characteristic of late twentieth century health care.

Finally we describe the twenty-first century reality of high levels of healthcare **complexity**, and of the kinds of communication that it entrains. Central here is the increasingly complex character of healthcare institutions; fraught care trajectories; constantly changing medical, clinical, diagnostic and information technologies; rising levels of bureaucratic monitoring, intervention and regulation; and migrating professionals and patients on top of a rise in care consumers' assertiveness and public participation in healthcare decision-making.

Healthcare communication in the present century cannot be understood without taking account of all these developments and factors, and the complexities they create for providers, policy-makers and consumers.

---

medicalisation
how human problems are increasingly framed within a medical framework. That is, problems are given a medical (rather than a social, cultural or educational) diagnosis and response.

complexity
a term used to describe situations that unfold in (seemingly) random or inexplicable ways. Complex situations do not resemble anything we are familiar with, and they do not allow us to act as we commonly do. They require new kinds of behaviours, new thinking and new solutions.

healthcare communication
the exchange of knowledge, information, feelings and meanings that takes place in and around healthcare settings and services.

Introduction

To understand communication in health care, we need to look back to the time when medicine began to organise itself into formal institutions. Care had been institutionalised to a degree in religious settings throughout the ages. But the Renaissance saw a number of significant new developments, together creating a radical change in the care given to ill people. Among these developments, noteworthy are the rise of secular (non-religious, charitable) shelters for the unwell, and the beginning of scientific medicine thanks to a fusion of anatomical knowledge with pharmacological expertise.

Towards the end of the Middle Ages, European societies began to isolate people into separate spaces because they were considered to be 'different': they were orphans, paupers, invalids, the old, the blind, the deaf, beggars, the mad, prostitutes or criminals. These people were progressively sequestered in sick houses, prisons, and mad houses and the like. These 'modern' institutions all emerged around the beginning of the Enlightenment in the seventeenth and eighteenth centuries – the time when the practice of categorising and classifying phenomena came into full swing. Collectively, these new institutions marked the beginning of a Europe-wide response to managing the risk and spread of disease (notably leprosy, the plague and, later, syphilis), deviancy (particularly crime), and madness (individuals' inability to conform to new and more intense **public expectations**).

As time went on, the sick house began to evolve from a place of social isolation into a place of rehabilitation, and then into a place where the diseased began to be subjected to innovative cures. These new cures were administered in places that Michel Foucault associates with the **birth of the clinic** (Foucault, 1973). The word 'clinic' derives from the Greek word *kline* meaning 'bed', and from the Latin *clinicus*, 'a person who attends to a patient'. Foucault's point was that the West was unique because there a new healthcare practice developed as the core of an entirely new institution: the hospital. This new institution had two defining features: it brought together people who were not well, and it was staffed with people who had developed and were actively developing new skills in deploying novel technologies on living bodies in ways never before attempted.

The clinic was further unique in that the new cures practised there involved a novel collaboration among practitioners with different specialisations. First, from as early as the fourth century, there were those whose religious orientation inclined them to nurse the diseased and disadvantaged in dedicated wards attached to their monasteries (Miller, 1985). Second, there were the anatomists who descended from a long line of people who, for centuries, had done quite simple forms of surgery to gather knowledge about the human body from dissecting corpses. Then there were those who experimented with and dispensed drugs and potions, combining folklore and nascent science.

> **public expectations**
> the norms and values that we as citizens hold up as important. Whereas 50 years ago our public expectations with regard to receiving health care were quite modest, twenty-first century healthcare consumers place very high expectations on professionals and services.

> **birth of the clinic**
> Michel Foucault's phrase for the emergence of a new medicine in the nineteenth century. This new medicine became possible thanks to 'a new medical gaze': a much more systematic and invasive way of subjecting the living human body to diagnosis and treatment than had been possible and acceptable previously.

The fusion of these three specialisations proved revolutionary, producing what is now known as Western health care. It is important to remember here that this developmental trajectory has steered health care more and more towards detecting and treating pathological lesions, and away from dealing in holistic ways with the human body and its life circumstances. This trajectory defines to an important extent how modern medicine now positions its consumers: as people who are tolerant and willing to wait, or be (a) *patient*. From its inception, then, medical practice has tended to regard and treat patients as 'inert anatomical creatures', rather than as living and speaking persons (Armstrong, 2002).

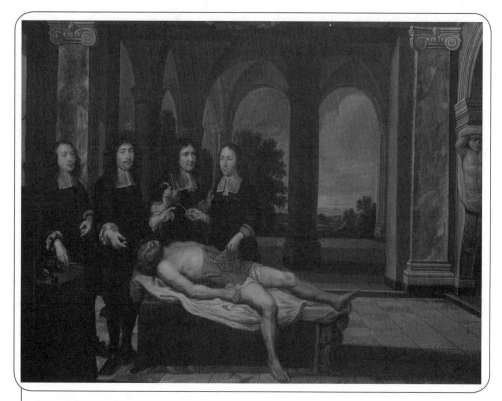

Figure 2.1 *The Anatomy Lesson*, Anonymous Master, Bruges, 1679. As published in the Europeana database: Groeningemusuem Brugge © Lukas-Art in Flanders

At a result of a period of rapid scientific progress and successes in medicine over the last two centuries, what the patient had to say became increasingly immaterial to what the doctor did and knew. The patient's voice became increasingly displaced by machine readings, test results and print-outs. What the doctor might want to communicate became increasingly defined by their technical knowledge about and clinical actions on the diseases of the body. This situation was further exacerbated with the rapid escalation in the number and power of technologies enabling clinical investigations into patients' diseases.

Initially, these techniques were quite simple: inspection (scanning the body with the eye), palpation (laying on hands to identify abnormalities), percussion (to identify different densities of the lesion) and auscultation (listening to internal processes) (Armstrong, 2002). Soon, they became more technological: think of X-rays, pathology reports, and blood tests, all emerging during the late nineteenth century and early twentieth century.

Because they were so powerful in what they revealed about the diseased human body, these investigative techniques lent the now rapidly expanding array of medical interventions special significance (Bliss, 2011). This status was consolidated by medicine becoming associated with – and legitimated by – two increasingly prestigious institutions: the

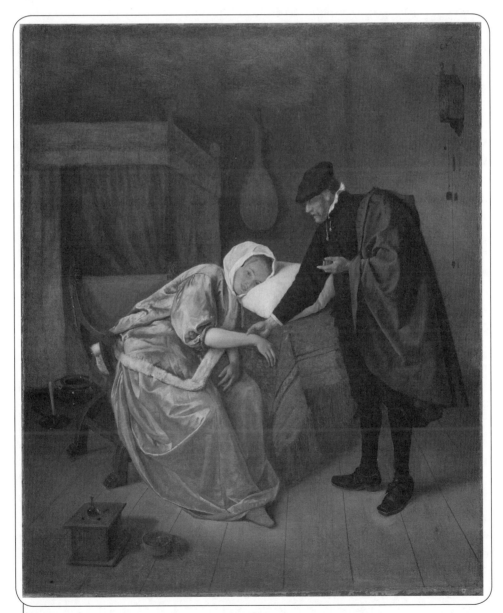

Figure 2.2 *The Sick Woman*, Jan Steen (1663–66), Rijksmuseum, Amsterdam

modern hospital and the university academy (Abel-Smith, 1964; Porter 1999; Szasz & Hollender, 1987 [1956]). The training and certification of doctors provided by the academy bolstered the status of the modern hospital. In turn, the research on actual subjects made possible by their connection with hospital consolidated the scientific prestige of medicine.

Increasingly, medicine prided itself – and continues to pride itself! – on the self-sufficiency of its methods and science. For medicine, personal, social and cultural influences became less and less relevant to its scientific truths and knowledge, and thus to its patient consultations (Good, 1994). The patient's object status was reinforced in 'clinical teaching manuals that were published in the nineteenth and early twentieth centuries … [which] … barely mention[ed] the process of obtaining reports of symptoms ("the medical history") from the patient' (Armstrong, 2002, p. 59). For medical science and medical practice, then, knowledge had become quite disconnected from the 'patient as person'. Patients were to be informed, rather than communicated with.

For its part, nursing prides itself on a long history of caring for the unwell without the intervention of elaborate cures. Nursing reaches back to the time of the early religious orders whose monasteries institutionalised separate shelters for sick people. The practice of nursing was, of course, greatly influenced by the rise of clinical medicine, its institutionalisation in the modern clinic, and its annexation of nursing as 'hand-maiden' (Thompson & Stewart, 2007). This annexation required nursing to shift from a charitable institution providing custodial care to an institution that complemented and increasingly extended the new doctors' medical and surgical expertises into curative care. Nurses were now expected to be submissive towards the 'paternal' doctor and 'maternal' towards the patient, producing frequent interprofessional tensions that could have damaging consequences for patients' care (Wicks, 1999).

Allowing the patient to speak

In the second half of the twentieth century, people became more educated and socially mobile, thanks to a host of technological, social and cultural developments. Armstrong describes the twentieth century as the time when disease became seen not as purely a body issue, but also a person issue: disease was 'released from its prison of the body' (Armstrong, 2002, p. 149). With this, doctors began to realise that patients, too, could have important insights about their own bodies and about the underlying and circumstantial factors of their disease.

This realisation was accompanied by medicine's appreciation that patients' health could be affected by socio-cultural factors – not just intrinsic anatomical and bio-physiological ones. This helped soften doctors' view of patients, and made them realise they needed a different way of communicating with patients. As medical practitioners began to acknowledge that afflictions were not fully explainable with reference to body-internal lesions alone, they understood that patients had biographies that warranted being explored for clues as to the origin and trajectory of their disease.

Around the 1950s and 1960s, this development culminated in patients being formally inaugurated as an important and credible source of information in medical training.

Indeed, patients were now expected to assist doctors in their quest to identify and explain the signs, symptoms and progress of their disease. Perhaps as much due to general societal change as to developments in medicine proper, patients were now expected to assume a role as informants about the world external to them and about how it affected them, their behaviour, their bodies and their disease.

We must not think, however, that this heralded the advent of open communication between the patient and the doctor. On the contrary, healthcare practitioners continued to be advised that they needed to maintain an 'objective view' of the patient's body. To achieve this, they were to practise 'detached concern' (Lief & Fox, 1963). Instead of letting themselves be swept along by the patient's account, doctors were to practise detachment while at the same time communicating to the patient that their focus was on their cure.

Communication here served not to nurture an intimate interpersonal relationship, but to achieve scientific–medical accuracy through careful elicitation and intelligent interpretation of patients' talk. This accuracy was best assured when the health practitioner kept their distance from the patient as person. It was left to nursing to attend to the subjective and emotional needs of the patient (Radcliffe, 2000; Stein, 1967).

As patients were increasingly expected to report on their diseases and each patient's specific 'life world' circumstances, healthcare practitioners were encouraged to realise that the patient's disease, at least in part, might be an expression of the individual's personal lifestyle and unique psychology. Encouraged by forward-looking post-war thinkers and educators like Michael Balint, clinicians were encouraged to understand the patient and their motivations, as well as their behaviour.

This necessitated an entirely new approach to how healthcare practitioners were to communicate with their patients. In this new schema, for example, the doctor–patient consult was to consider not just the patient's physical environment and habits, but also their social and practical circumstances. Critical here became the patient's employment history and their living circumstances. This meant giving the patient the opportunity to discuss their job worries, interpersonal adjustments and disappointments, and even their marital history (Armstrong, 2002, p. 62). This was the birth of the 'bio-psycho-social' approach to clinician–patient communication (Engel, 1977).

The 'biopsychosocial' approach was first evident in Michael Balint's work (Balint, 1955). During the 1950s and 1960s in the UK, Balint began to promote an approach to patient–health practitioner communication that emphasised the psychological dimension of their relationship as being at the heart of the healthcare process. There was much more at stake here than eliciting biopsychosocial issues from the patient. Balint emphasised the importance of health practitioners enabling the patient to speak, but this was on top of the health practitioners paying attention to *themselves*. They now were to communicate in a reflexive manner, assessing their own responses and their effects on the patient. Here, the healthcare professional was to ask questions not just of the patient, but also about their own behaviour, their own communication. All this was in order to avoid 'objectifying' the patient and their disease.

To a large degree, the rise to prominence of the biopsychosocial patient occurred as a counterpoint to the overwhelming and taken-as-given paternalism (a father-like attitude) that prevailed among doctors at the time, paralleled by nurses' maternalism (a mother-like attitude) (Wilson-Barnett, 1986).

As Peter Ubel explains, doctors' paternalism meant that they routinely made decisions for patients:

> In the pre-revolutionary days of physician paternalism, [a prostate cancer] patient's urologist would have told him that he had a small growth in his prostate and needed surgery. Or, if the surgeon felt that the patient was too frail to benefit from the surgery, he would have withheld information about the tumour and monitored it without the patient's knowledge. (Ubel, 2012, p. 3)

This paternalistic relationship between the doctor and the patient meant moreover that the doctor could consider the patient 'too fragile' for bad news and therefore withhold it to protect the patient.

> If the patient were deemed too fragile for bad news, the doctor would turn to euphemism or out-and-out evasion. The tumour would be described as 'an X-ray shadow' or 'an infection'. In those days, doctors made decisions and patients were expected to follow orders. (Ubel, 2012, p. 3)

The post-war years – the 1950s and 1960s – introduced new and probing questions about how medicine, nursing and hospitals generally conducted their healthcare processes, relationships and communication. A prominent example of this questioning was Glaser and Strauss's work, asking why patients (or their relatives) were not or were rarely informed about their impending deaths (Glaser & Strauss, 1965). In a study done over three years, Glaser and Strauss reassessed the degree to which health practitioners discussed dying with their patients. They concluded that only limited progress towards open information sharing had been achieved in the intervening years (Glaser & Strauss, 1968).

This change in attitude towards patients' role in their care arose from a post-war dissatisfaction with established institutions (Marcuse, 1991 [1964]). This post-war sentiment turned people away from all kinds of institutional authority, and reoriented them towards interpersonal relationships. For Balint and colleagues, this involved identifying medicine as 'illness-centred' and doctors' approach as paternalistic. What they saw as needed instead was 'person-centred' medicine, defined as paying increasing attention to patients' unique needs, circumstances and preferences. Questioning the priorities of illness-centred medicine, person-centred care necessitates very different communicative skills on the part of the healthcare practitioner (Balint et al., 1970) – skills that to date had not been a priority in medical and nursing training (Stewart, 1995).

Balint's 'illness-centred versus patient-centred' distinction became the origin of a new range of 'patient-centred' communication practices that began to make their way into healthcare communication in the second half of the twentieth century. Prominent among these are 'informed consent' and 'shared decision-making'. More recently still, we have begun to talk about the importance of 'patient choice' and 'patient involvement'. Common to these new concerns is that healthcare practitioners and health systems generally are to become more attentive to their patients, and more responsive to their needs and preferences.

Health system responsiveness

Health system responsiveness became an important concern for healthcare policy-makers and healthcare services during the 1980s and 1990s. This concern culminated in the publication in 2000 of the World Health Organization (WHO) report on this issue (see http://www.who.int/responsiveness/en).

The WHO's interest in service and system responsiveness paralleled growing interest around the Western world in enhancing healthcare professionals' and services' responsiveness towards their patients. This attitude was promoted to counterbalance the increasingly scientific, supply-driven and disease-centric orientation on the part of most health practitioners and services towards their patients. Responsiveness was promoted to attune care and care communication more to the patient's 'life world' (Mishler, 1984). This responsiveness and attentiveness aimed to ensure that patients' personal needs, preferences and desires were acknowledged and accommodated in their care. Responsiveness practised by practitioners and services renders care more congenial to the patient and better aligned with their circumstances, leading to better clinical outcomes.

The new frontier: complex care

Now, in the first part of the twenty-first century, we are witnessing the emergence of yet another kind of patient–health practitioner relationship, and another kind of patient–health practitioner communication. This is because twenty-first century care – and therefore also healthcare communication – is increasingly confounded and complicated by the following factors:

- the multiplication of diseases and attendant multi-morbidity, particularly for patients with chronic diseases;
- the rising number of chronic disease patients;
- the increasing specialisation and technologisation of care (providing health practitioners and patients with more options for testing and treating, and more channels for communicating);
- the rise of the 'informed consumer': patients and carers becoming better informed due to their access to internet resources;
- the intensification of social and linguistic difference due to migration and mobility, and therefore health practitioners and services having to accommodate a broader range of service users (including those with low levels of health literacy due to migration and those with very high levels of literacy and access to health-related information, resulting in rising levels of social–professional expectation);

- the rise in the number of stakeholders claiming a say in the dynamics of care provision (including the bureaucracy, policy-makers, the media, academic researchers, pharmaceutical companies, consumer interest groups, and others).

Together, these factors produce situations where patients and health practitioners have to communicate more frequently about a greater range of challenging circumstances, also known as 'wicked problems'. Wicked problems (as explained in Chapter 1) are understood as those that are difficult or even impossible to solve. They involve contradictory, incomplete and/or changing information and requirements. One example of this is that around 50% of patients now present in primary care with medically unexplainable symptoms (Nimnuan, Hotopf & Wessely, 2001).

Wicked problems produce tragic choices when treatments are unlikely to return a positive result, or when patients need or desire treatments that a service or clinician may not be in a position to deliver. These circumstances necessitate delicate conversations and negotiations. Instead of being able to communicate about a particular treatment, its evidence and its likely outcomes, the clinician has the task of communicating that there is no certainty about what is wrong with the patient, that no known treatment is available for the patient, or that no available treatment is likely to return the outcome requested or expected by the patient.

These dilemmas become particularly visible with patients who are chronically ill and who need ongoing and uniquely tailored care, and whose chance of a cure is nil or limited. End-of-life care is another domain where increasingly complex communication takes place. End-of-life care navigates through increasingly technology-based medicine and the unpredictable ethical implications of applying technological interventions that lack a substantial curative effect (Kearney, 2000). Especially in intensive care, dying may require curative options to be balanced against and at times harnessed to palliative care options, resulting in very complex conversations (Seymour, 2000). Leadbeater and Garber (2010) articulate this problem with some urgency in their recent report, *Dying for Change*:

> Unless we can devise ways to get people to talk about how they want to live while they are dying, our efforts to improve services will be like groping in the dark.

Likewise, complex ethical dilemmas arise from the increasingly detailed information that is now available for pregnant mothers about their foetuses, their birthing conditions, their neonatal states, genetic test results, and so forth. Not just pregnant mothers but all of us are encouraged to engage in more frequent screening, particularly when family members are found to suffer from specific diseases. This screening may generate knowledge not just about existing symptoms, but also about as-yet-unrecognised health risks. Were we not to know about those dangers, we might not see the need to have them addressed with dangerous medications or invasive surgery whereas, knowing about these dangers, we may want to see them alleviated through proactive care. All these situations require highly sophisticated and deeply complex kinds of communication about risk percentages, curative options, life chances and spiritual or philosophical stances.

In sum, the patient is now increasingly likely to present as a complex problem in need of a complex solution achieved through delicate negotiation. The patient and the clinician face considerable uncertainty, and a host of tentative choices. At the same time, and confounding this already challenging situation even more, the clinician answers to a growing number of stakeholders: health service managers, the bureaucracy, medico-legal lawyers, healthcare complaints commissions, academia, consumer groups, the media, and so forth. Patient–health practitioner communication is no longer a two-way conversation but is a multi-party conversation, even if most stakeholders are not physically present. Inevitably, this communication has to face in numerous directions at the same time.

Practice example 2.1   What happens in contemporary practice[1]

To understand the complexity that is inherent in communicating with today's patients, consider Garth's story below. Garth (P) is a patient in his mid-forties and is in need of emergency care after his finger has been severely ripped in a stable door. He presents one morning to a local emergency department (ED). On his arrival there, the triage nurse (N1) establishes quickly that Garth needs to be seen by a doctor and will most likely need to be operated on that day. She first administers first aid and tells him what she is doing, reassuring him all the time:

N1:   What I'm going to do it just put a cold wet dressing on.

P: OK.

N1:   Don't be concerned if it seems to be bleeding a lot through it …

P: OK.

N1:   … just a lot of fluid here but it's just saline.

P: OK.

N1:   Just rest your hand out. I'm not going to put it over the end.

P: No worries.

N1:   It will just help keep it clean.

P: Thank you very much.

N1:   And keep it moist.

Garth then sees a second triage nurse who goes over some of his story again. She organises for Garth to have an X-ray. After that, another nurse (N3) arrives and introduces herself to Garth, (re)checks his name and begins his admission to the hospital, asking him more detailed questions including some that have been asked before. N3 shifts effortlessly between obtaining information (communicating with Garth as the source of objective medical information and as a 'person'):

N3:   You're not allergic to anything?

P: Except needles.

continued ›

Practice example 2.1 continued ›

N3   OK. Well, can't promise you anything about that. [Cuffs him]

P: I know, that's scaring me.

N3:   Um …

P: I'm an asthmatic.

N3:   Asthma? OK.

P: Yeah.

N3:   Any other medical problems?

P: No.

N3:   No? Um, ever had any other operations?

P: Ah, no.

N3:   No? No, still got your tonsils?

P: Yep.

N3:   You've got your appendix?

P: Yep, should have had them out. Should have had them out, yeah, but
      I didn't.

N3:   Alright. Who do you live with?

P: Ah, my son. And a friend, [name], and his daughter.

N3:   Yeah. Just because – we ask that question just because if you need to stay in
      hospital or something …

P: Yeah.

N3:   … then we need to make sure …

P: Yeah, that's right.

N3:   … you know, if you're a carer of somebody, if somebody to care for that …

P: Yeah, well I've got sons, yeah. We have – I've got, oh well I'll have to make a
      phone call, but yeah, I'll be able to arrange it.

N3:   Yes, that's alright. We can get you the phone afterwards.

P: They're not babies.

N3:   OK. Um, do you drink any alcohol?

P: Sure do. Got one?

N3:   How – (much) do you drink every day?

P: Oh, no. No, don't do that.

N3:   No. How much would you drink a week?

P: Oh, well …

N3:   Half a carton?

P: No.

N3:   Less?

P: Yeah, quarter – I – I might have one or two every evening.

N3:   OK.

N3 then tells Garth that he is going to go into surgery later.

continued ›

Practice example 2.1 continued ›

Just over an hour after Garth's arrival at the ED, the junior doctor (D1) arrives. He introduces himself to Garth, identifies himself as one of the doctors in the hospital, and begins history-taking. Notice how he shifts to and fro between getting medical information from Garth and attending to him as a 'person'.

D1 arrives as N3 is assisting Garth with sling.

D1:   Hi, Mr [last name], I'm [name], one of the doctors.

P: Hello, how are you?

D1:   What did you do?

P: I, um, I was working a horse and, um, I went to bring it through …

N3:   Do you want to sit down for me, mate, so I can …

P: Yeah.

D1:   I've got some gauze on here.

P: Yeah. I had to, um, bring it through and the door just shut on my hand.

D1:   Yeah.

P: And I think I've – it jammed in there and I pulled it out and virtually pulled my finger off.

D1:   A door, what kind of door was it?

P: It's just a – it was a, like a gate, a gate with rubber but on the back sort of had steel, and then it went into an external angle of a – a timber angle.

D1:   Right. OK, got your finger caught.

P: So it was, yeah. Yeah, just, there was no room to …

                    …

D1:   Yes. Now, just have a little look. Have you had any pain relief yet?

P: No.

D1:   No.

N3:   I just need a line and stuff put in.

D1:   Yeah. OK.

N3:   If you want to just RAT [Rapid Assessment Team] him off, maybe?

D1:   Yeah.

Analysis and reflection

What is unique about this communication addressing Garth's care? We see above and in the continuation of the conversation below that Garth's injury, personal circumstances and his care are complicated. He requires surgery and the surgeons must be advised; he needs an X-ray and the radiographers must be told; he has two blood tests so the pathology laboratory is involved; he requires someone to care for his son while he is in hospital; he requires several health practitioners working with him using clinical instruments and makeshift bandaging and slings; and he needs immediate care for the bleeding and to take care of the pain due to his injury. These factors require his health practitioners to listen closely to him; to listen to and cooperate with each other; to check on whether the surgeon has received the information about Garth; to think about Garth as a patient and as a person simultaneously; to observe and respond to his behaviour and that of each other; and to give feedback rapidly to him and to each other as his care progresses.

As the care unfolds, the junior doctor and the nurses don't just provide clinical and technical information and build a relationship with the patient. Importantly, they work in a much broader, more extended and far more complex process involving not just themselves and the patient, but also multiple teams of professionals: the surgeons, pathologists and radiographers.

As is evident in the transcript, aspects of the talk focus on history-taking and information-giving, and on the accuracy and comprehensiveness of what is said. Here, what is in focus is the patient's complaint, not the person. The 'patient as object' approach concerns itself with health practitioners asking questions and negotiating answers in such a way as to obtain correct and specific information from patients so that they can make well-informed clinical and technical decisions. Here, the person in need of information is the health practitioner, not the patient.

By informing Garth of what is going to happen to him, the doctor acknowledges that Garth may want to know (and have a say in, if appropriate) what happens next. Although Garth is not a patient presenting with multiple diseases like many of today's emergency department patients do (Australian Institute of Health and Welfare, 2012), even his relatively straightforward care necessitates the involvement of several practitioners and constant feedback between them.

Reflective questions

1. What aspects of patient–health practitioner communication in Garth's consultation are timeless? In other words, what do doctors and nurses do and say that helps you to recognise their clinical roles?
2. Similarly, what aspects of Garth's responses make him a typical patient?
3. How has Garth been allowed to participate in his own care?
4. Has Garth's participation made it easier for the nurses and doctors caring for him? If so, how; if not, why?
5. How do the junior doctor's and staff nurses' conversations differ? Are the nurses still submissive to the doctor's medical authority?

Implications for practice

What are the implications for practice from how clinical conversations have developed and changed over time? While there are several dimensions of patient–healthcare practitioner interaction that are enduring over time, such as the one-on-one consultation (Roter, 2000), there are also many technological, social and medical changes that influence their interaction (Buetow, Jutel & Hoare, 2009).

The difficulty that arises here is that even simple kinds of care become complex. In complex situations, and particularly in 'wicked' situations that lack solutions, you will no longer be able to rely on pre-scripted approaches to conversing with your patients and your colleagues. Instead, you will need to develop ways of responding to families, carers, patients, and other professionals *in the moment*. This requires a new responsiveness: a way of responding to others that recognises and addresses their unique circumstances (Iedema & Manidis, 2013).

Each chapter in this book deals with what this 'communicating in the moment' means for the various healthcare domains where we provide patient care. Most important for 'communicating in the moment' will be your ability to reflexively adapt communication strategies to accommodate and negotiate with the person at the centre of the encounter, rather than take them for granted and reduce your interaction to a well-rehearsed routine. You will have to respond in ways that recognise the unique wishes of the family members who are present, people's cultural predispositions, colleagues' professional prerogatives, and know how to create common ground among stakeholders about the as-yet uncertain or contested goals of treatment.

Theoretical links

Over the centuries, the hospital grew from a simple refuge for the diseased and the dying to a place of rehabilitation and haphazard cures following the Middle Ages, and an increased focus on teaching and research since the eighteenth century, culminating in places of medical scientific and technological progress during the nineteenth and twentieth centuries (Risse, 1999). Each of these phases had its unique ways of positioning clinicians and patients, and each was characterised by its own unique ways of communicating among those providing care, and with those receiving the care.

Now, after centuries of scientific and technological development, we are in a time where health care has become very complex due to the availability of multiple curative technologies. But this has also produced more complex care circumstances: patients with chronic diseases and multiple co-morbidities. Here, we encounter high levels of uncertainty about what to do for patients, and about the effects of our clinical interventions (Lillrank & Liukko, 2004). Because of this, we must involve patients more closely in deciding how to structure their care, and in managing their care.

This last development points to a new way of providing care: namely, *co-producing* care. The notion of *care co-production* was coined to draw our attention to the changing role that is now played by patients in their own care, and to care requiring an *ongoing* relationship between health practitioners and patients (Wanless, 2004). Here, communication shifts from 'making and informing the patient of a curative decision', via 'ensuring patients are recognised as people with needs and preferences', towards 'care as ongoing multi-party negotiation process' (Mol, 2008).

Conclusion

In summary, to really understand healthcare communication, we need to consider more than merely the clinical and interpersonal dimensions of the patient–health practitioner encounter (de Haes & Bensing, 2008). An entirely new way of communicating is now becoming evident, one that encompasses much more than single care and consult episodes where information is shared or where relationships are shaped. Future patients are more likely to want to orient their communication with healthcare practitioners towards their own trajectories through services, their own roles, and their personal expectations and aspirations.

Practice example 2.2

The health department has developed a new policy that applies to care for the confused hospitalised older person. Older patients may experience confusion for a number of reasons: a lack of food, medications, an unfamiliar environment, and so forth. The policy advises that it is important to differentiate confusion (a temporary state) from dementia (a permanent condition). It is important to differentiate confusion from dementia because confusion can be reversed provided patients are not treated as if they have dementia. Where dementia treatment tends to rely on medication (and may even resort to restraints), the treatment of confusion relies (or should rely) in a significant way on communication with the patient.

You are employed on an orthopaedic ward, and you are juggling several patients each waiting for a hip fracture operation. The operation needs to occur within 48 hours to be maximally effective, so there is pressure to move patients through. One of the patients is called Emma. Emma shows signs of confusion and you realise you need to spend time with her to reassure her everything is OK. After a while, you have to calm Emma because she is becoming increasingly disoriented and fearful. You also still have to provide care to the other patients on the ward. You know that medicating Emma may not help.

Reflective questions

1. How might you prepare yourself as a health practitioner for communicating with patients like Emma and Garth?
2. How might you prepare for not always being able to do everything that is needed for your patients, and what actions could you undertake to mitigate this?
3. How might you prepare yourself as a patient for health care, given what you now know about the complexity of care?

Further reading

Mol, A. (2008). *The logic of care. Health and the problem of patient choice.* London: Routledge. Annemarie Mol takes issue with patient choice as a major cornerstone of good care. She concludes: '[G]ood care is not a matter of making well-argued individual choices but is something that grows out of collaborative and continuing attempts to attune knowledge and technologies to diseased bodies and [people's] complex lives.'

References

Abel-Smith, B. (1964). *The hospitals 1800–1848.* London: Heinemann.

Armstrong, D. (2002). *A new history of identity: A sociology of medical knowledge.* Basingstoke: Palgrave.

Australian Institute of Health and Welfare. (2012). *Multiple causes of death: An analysis of all natural and selected chronic disease causes of death 1997–2007.* Canberra: Author.

Balint, M. (1955). The doctor, his patient and the illness. *The Lancet, 265*(6866), 683–688.

Balint, M., Hunt, J., Joyce, D., Marinker, M., & Woodcock, J. (1970). *Treatment or diagnosis: A study of repeat prescriptions in general practice.* London: Tavistock.

Bliss, M. (2011). *The making of modern medicine: Turning points in the treatment of disease.* Chicago: Chicago University Press.

Buetow, S., Jutel, A., & Hoare, K. (2009). Shrinking social space in the doctor-modern patient relationship: A review of forces for, and implications of, homologisation. *Patient Educ Couns, 74*(1), 97–103. doi:10.1016/j.pec.2008.07.053

de Haes, H. C. J. M., & Bensing, J. M. (2008). Endpoints in medical communication research: Proposing a framework of functions and outcomes. *Patient Education & Counseling, 74*(2009), 287–294.

Engel, G. (1977). The need for a new medical model: A challenge for biomedicine. *Science, 196*, 129–136.

Foucault, M. (1973). *The birth of the clinic: An archeology of medical perception.* New York: Vintage.

Glaser, B., & Strauss, A. (1965). *Awareness of dying.* London: Weidenfeld and Nicholson.

Glaser, B., & Strauss, A. (1968). *Time for Dying.* Chicago: Aldine.

Good, B.J. (1994). *Medicine, rationality and experience.* Cambridge: Cambridge University Press.

Iedema, R., & Manidis, M. (2013). *Patient-clinician communication: An overview of relevant research and policy literatures.* Sydney: Australian Commission on Safety and Quality in Health Care and University of Technology, Centre for Health Communication.

Kearney, M. (2000). *A place of healing: Working with suffering in the living and dying.* Oxford: Oxford University Press.

Leadbeater, C., & Garber, J. (2010). *Dying for change.* London: DEMOS.

Lief, H. I., & Fox, R. C. (1963). Training for 'detached concern' in medical students. In H. I. Lief, V. F. Lief, & N. R. Lief (Eds.), *The psychological basis of medical practice* (pp. 12–35). New York: Harper Row.

Lillrank, P., & Liukko, M. (2004). Standard, routine and non-routine process in health care. *International Journal of Health Care Quality Assurance, 17*(1), 39–46.

Marcuse, H. (1991 [1964]). *One-dimensional man: Studies in ideology of advanced industrial society*. London: Routledge.

Miller, T. S. (1985). *The birth of the hospital at the Byzantine empire*. Baltimore: Johns Hopkins University Press.

Mishler, E. G. (1984). *The discourse of medicine: Dialectics of medical interviews*. Norwood, N.J.: Ablex.

Mol, A. (2008). *The logic of care. Health and the problem of patient choice*. London: Routledge.

Nimnuan, C., Hotopf, M., & Wessely, S. (2001). Medically unexplained symptoms: An epidemiological study in seven specialities. *Journal of Psychosomatic Research, 51*(1), 361–367.

Porter, R. (1999). *The greatest benefit to mankind: A medical history of humanity from antiquity to the present*. London: Fontana.

Radcliffe, M. (2000). Doctors and nurses: New game, same result. *British Medical Journal, 320*(7241), 1085. doi:10.1136/bmj.320.7241.1085

Risse, G. B. (1999). *Mending bodies, saving souls: A history of hospitals*. Oxford: Oxford University Press.

Roter, D. (2000). The enduring and evolving nature of the patient-physician relationship. *Patient Education and Counselling, 39*, 5–15.

Seymour, J. E. (2000). Negotiating natural death in intensive care. *Social Science & Medicine, 51*, 1241–1252.

Stein, L. I. (1967). The doctor-nurse game. *Archives of General Psychiatry, 16*(1967), 699–703.

Stewart, M. A. (1995). Effective physician-patient communication and health care outcome: A review. *Canadian Medical Association Journal, 152*(9), 1423–1433.

Szasz, T. S., & Hollender, M. H. (1987 [1956]). A contribution to the philosophy of medicine: The basic models of the doctor-patient relationships. In J. D. Stoeckle (Ed.), *Encounters between patients and doctors* (pp. 165–177). Cambridge, MA: MIT Press.

Thompson, D. R., & Stewart, S. (2007). Handmaiden or right-hand man: Is the relationship between doctors and nurses still therapeutic? *International Journal of Cardiology, 118*(2007), 139–140.

Ubel, P. (2012). *Critical decisions*. Melbourne: The Text Publishing Company.

Wanless, D. (2004). *Securing good health for the whole population: Population health trends*. London: UK Treasury.

Wicks, D. (1999). *Nurses and doctors at work: Rethinking professional boundaries*. Sydney: Allen & Unwin.

Wilson-Barnett, J. (1986). Ethical dilemmas in nursing. *Journal of Medical Ethics, 12*(3), 123–135.

Notes

1 Parts of this chapter draw on material published in a report, *Patient–clinician communication: An overview of relevant research and policy literatures* (2013). The report was commissioned by the Australian Commission on Safety and Quality in Health Care and prepared by University of Technology, Sydney, Centre for Health Communication.

2 Data from ARC-Linkage Grant LP0775435: Emergency Communication: Addressing the challenges in healthcare discourses and practices. Ethics approval identification number: UTS-HREC 2008–201A. Legend: P = patient Garth; N1 = triage nurse; N2 – second triage nurse; N3 = staff nurse; D1 = junior doctor; [ ] = explanatory text; (much) = best guess

Part 2

Communicating quality and safety across service and clinical domains

3

Communicating with the patient in primary care settings

Jill Thistlethwaite and George Ridgway

Learning objectives

This chapter will enable you to:
- demonstrate an understanding of the context in which a primary care consultation takes place;
- demonstrate an understanding of the nature and structure of a consultation in primary care;
- demonstrate an awareness that consultations have biomedical, social and psychological components, with the relevance of each varying depending on the patient's and doctor's agenda;
- define paternalism, the patient-centred approach and shared decision-making;
- recognise a GP's role and responsibilities towards a patient;
- demonstrate an understanding of the importance of shared communication between health professionals;
- recognise how consultations may be affected by cost and the health service.

Key terms

Biopsychosocial model
General practice
Patient-centred
Risk communication
Shared decision-making

Overview

Primary care settings are locations in the community where patients seek medical care. They are usually general practices or community clinics. In these practices and clinics, the consultation between the clinician – often a doctor – and the patient is the most central kind of communication.

Primary care and primary health care have slightly different meanings. Primary care is health care provided at the initial point of contact with a healthcare professional in the community. In Australia this will be predominantly a general practitioner (GP) but in some locations, such as in rural and remote areas, it may be a nurse practitioner, remote area nurse, pharmacist or allied health professional. Primary health care is a broader term. It has been defined by the World Health Organization as including curative treatment by the first healthcare professional contacted, as well as promotional, preventative and rehabilitative services provided by multidisciplinary teams of healthcare professionals working together collaboratively (WHO, 1978). Its ultimate goal is better health for all.

The Royal Australian College of General Practitioners (RACGP) states that GPs play a central role in healthcare delivery in Australia. It defines general practice (also known as family medicine) as providing person-centred, continuing, comprehensive and coordinated whole person health care to individuals and families in their communities (RACGP, n.d.). GPs are frequently the first health professionals contacted when a person has a health-related problem. They work with other health and social care professionals as appropriate and when necessary, and refer patients to other medical specialists for secondary and hospital-based care.

In this chapter we consider the nature and purposes of the consultation between a GP and a patient, and the communication strategies involved on both sides. We also discuss how the interaction is affected by the wider health service and the remuneration involved. The emphasis in this chapter will be on the clinician sharing information with the patient, and with other GPs and health professionals involved in the care of the patient.

Research into communication between patients and GPs has shown that, in the last few decades, GPs have increasingly moved from a paternalistic style of consultation to a more **patient-centred** approach. GP consultations are often complex as they involve interactions with patients who may present with 'undifferentiated problems' that do not have or may not lead to a specific diagnosis *and that may remain unexplained and ambiguous.*

> **patient-centred**
> putting the needs of the patient at the centre of processes and priorities.

Communication in this setting is further complicated by the fact that GPs are generalists. That is, they focus on health promotion and disease prevention, as well as diagnosis and treatment of patients of all ages, ethnicities and social status. Nowadays, they frequently work in teams (the primary care team) and many have specialist interests in certain areas of practice.

Introduction

One of the distinguishing features of consultations in **general practice** is that the patient may bring any problem or query to the doctor. Thus we say that such inter-actions involve patients with undifferentiated problems or complaints. The wording here is from the traditional bio-medical model in which a patient has a 'presenting complaint' and the doctor then takes a 'history of the presenting complaint' (HOPC). The first part of a consultation usually involves the GP gathering information and the second part involves the GP sharing information about the possible diagnosis and the management plan. The plan may include investigations and treatment. The GP may also take the opportunity, if there is time, to talk about health promotion and disease prevention. Such activities may include check-ing if the patient is up to date with immunisations and health screening, if a recent blood pressure reading has been recorded, and discussing risk factors for cardiovascu-lar disease and cancer. GPs frequently refer patients to other healthcare professionals such as hospital specialists (for example, a medical doctor), allied health profession-als (for example, a physiotherapist) and mental health professionals (for example, a psychologist). Patients referred for certain conditions and for team-based care under Medicare arrangements are eligible for a reduction in the usual fees charged by some healthcare practitioners. It is important for shared care arrangements that relevant information is exchanged between all the professionals involved with the permission of the patient.

> **general practice**
> that area of medicine that is available to us in the community when we have minor ailments, or ailments whose nature and severity are as yet unclear and need the attention of a general practitioner (GP). GPs work in primary care.

Components of a general practice consultation: information-gathering

Information is gathered about the following:
- the presenting complaint;
- the history of the presenting complaint (for example, when and how the symptoms started, how severe, where, and so on);
- previous medical history (particularly if the GP has no previous medical records – physical and psychological);
- medication history (past and present medications including over-the-counter and prescribed);
- family medical history;
- social history (including employment, smoking, alcohol use, illicit drug use, exercise, and so on).

Of course, not all consultations begin with a 'presenting complaint' or a set of symptoms. The patient may have a very specific agenda such as a sexual health check, a prescription renewal or a screening procedure (for example, a cervical 'Pap' smear test). Patients may also use one problem as a way of initiating a consultation on something entirely different once rapport has been established.

There is a danger with the traditional history-taking that the patient is bombarded with a set of closed questions requiring only a 'yes/no' or minimal response – for example, 'Have you had blood in your urine?'; 'How often do you get up at night to go to the toilet?' Such a bombardment of questions may reduce the opportunity for the patient to speak about their specific concern. The doctor should use a mix of open and closed questions. For example, the GP may start with a very open invitation: 'Tell me about the pain'. The doctor can monitor the effect of such questions and whether they encourage the patient to tell the story in the patient's own words. The doctor may need to follow this up with more focused questions to gain a better understanding of the symptom and its effect on the patient.

There are three models of communication, each distinguished by the degree of patient involvement. The biomedical approach to patient problems involves the application of science to clinical medicine. It aligns with a doctor-centred or paternalistic model of communication. Here, the disease and not the patient is the focus, and the aim is a physical diagnosis and potential cure frequently through issuing a prescription. The patient is not involved in the process after the initial 'complaint'. The GP adopts a 'fatherly' ('paternal') manner and provides for the patient's perceived needs without giving them any responsibility.

By contrast, the **biopsychosocial model** takes into account not only physical symptoms but also the patient's psychological and social factors: the patients' understanding of their problem and their emotional response to that problem (Pendleton et al., 2003).

> **biopsychosocial model**
> a model that extends the medical model from focusing purely on patients' biological problems to also paying attention to their psychological and social problems.

Then we have the patient-centred model, in which the patient's agenda (involving both explicit and initially hidden components) is paramount. The GP explores the patients' ideas about what is wrong, their concerns about their symptoms and possible diagnoses, the effect of the problem on their daily life, and their expectations of coming to the doctor – what they hope to achieve in the consultation (Stewart et al., 2013). Each approach may benefit a particular patient and their complaint, and may be more or less suitable given the time available for the consultation.

Consultations with a GP in Australia may last from under five minutes to over half an hour. The length and complexity of a consultation determines how much a GP is paid. Medicare reimburses doctors for their time. If the Medicare fee is the same as the fee charged by the practice to the patient (that is, the practice 'bulk bills'), then there is no gap fee for the patient to pay. However, GPs may charge patients above the Medicare price and thus the patient is 'out of pocket' depending on the gap.

Practice example 3.1

The consultation described below is based on a real-life example. John Baxter (JB), a 35-year-old accountant, has booked a 15-minute appointment with Dr Malik (GP). JB has been to the surgery before, but this is the first time he has seen this particular doctor. When he enters the consulting room he appears well and in no discomfort. The GP had a quick look at his computerised medical record before he came in – JB has been seen previously for travel advice and vaccinations, and last year for a mild viral illness.

GP: What can I do for you today?

JB: I've been getting a pain in my chest for the last few days doctor.

GP: Tell me about the pain. Can you show me where you get it?

The GP proceeds to ask standard questions about the history of the pain, for example, how often it occurs, how long it lasts, whether anything seems to bring it on, what JB has taken for it, what other symptoms are associated with the pain, and so on. This takes about four minutes. He also asks if JB smokes (no), what exercise he does (goes to gym three times a week), and whether he has a family history of chest or heart problems (his uncle had a heart attack when he was 70 years old but recovered).

GP: It certainly sounds as if the problem is muscular, probably due to the extra work you have been doing in the gym lately. I will just take your blood pressure and listen to your chest and heart.

The GP carries out a short examination.

GP: Well, everything seems to be fine. Your blood pressure is excellent and you look in good shape. Just cut back on the weights when you go to the gym, take some paracetamol and come back to see me in a week or so if you are no better.

JB: Oh OK, thanks doctor.

He gets up from his seat and starts to leave, then stops.

JB: It couldn't be anything more serious could it?

GP: Well, I don't think you need to worry about a heart problem. The pain doesn't sound cardiac at all.

JB: Good.

GP: You still seem concerned. Is there anything that is particularly worrying you about the pain? What do you think it might be?

JB: Well, you see, a colleague of mine has just been diagnosed with lung cancer and he went to his doctor with chest pain, and now he has to have radiation and stuff. He's only 10 years older than me and hasn't smoked since he was in his 20s. I used to smoke a bit when I was at uni. So it just made me think I shouldn't ignore this.

Analysis and reflection

The consultation between John Baxter and Dr Malik illustrates a number of points about the nature of such interactions. In this case Dr Malik has access to John's previous medical records, though these may not be complete. In Australia people are able to consult at any general practice surgery at which they can obtain an appointment. Thus, records, which are frequently computerised, may be held on several different computer systems over the course of a patient's life. At the present time computers are not linked between practices. Nor are hospital records accessible in the community, though this may change in future once the electronic patient record (EPR) held centrally becomes more widely used.

Patients may request that their records be transferred from one practice to another if they move house, for example, but it is rare for any one GP to be able to see a full medical history. Letters following hospital admissions and clinic visits should be sent to the referring GP, but these are not always timely or received by the correct person. This can lead to fragmented care if important medical events are not accessible at the time of a consultation. It also means that each GP or practice may have to ask similar questions such as family history, with the repetition annoying the patient.

Moreover, we all know that past events in our lives can be forgotten or our memories become distorted over time. Patients may not remember the exact details of their past medical histories or what drugs they have taken (or even the names of their current medication). Thus, in this scenario Dr Malik cannot assume that he has all the details about John Baxter's medical history. In fact, he has no idea what John may be consulting about.

In general practice one of the challenges for doctors is that patients may present with any type of problem: undifferentiated problems or complaints. The GP may just have had a very difficult and emotional consultation with a person, such as breaking bad news, and then the next patient may request a sexual health check. The GP should be able to change communication style in response to each patient's problem and needs, and give undivided attention to the person being seen.

Let us return to the consultation seen above. As John Baxter enters the consulting room, the doctor will be forming an impression: does John look ill, is he in discomfort, is he anxious? Dr Malik begins with an open invitation to John to present his reason for consulting. As the pair have not met before Dr Malik might have considered introducing himself, but he has probably assumed that the receptionist has informed John of his name. John states his problem: a 'pain in the chest'. Chest pain is a common symptom and it can have many causes from the serious (for example, heart attack) to the self-limiting (for example, pulled muscle). Dr Malik will already be considering the possible diagnoses in this case. He will take into account the patient's age and history (if available). He will also be making an assessment of John's physical status. Having decided that John is not acutely ill, he uses another open invitation or question to elicit more details about the pain, and then focuses down into a standard 'pain history', followed by an appropriate examination.

For Dr Malik the consultation appears to be going well. He has excluded serious causes for chest pain and suggested a management plan. However, the patient has another agenda; he is not reassured by the doctor's conclusion. John's query about whether the pain may have a more serious medical cause or 'aetiology' is interpreted by Dr Malik as a concern about cardiac problems.

In Dr Malik's experience, patients often worry they are having a heart attack if they have chest pain. John, though, has another anxiety. He is able to express his concern about his colleague's diagnosis. However some patients may not have been able to share their worries without an explicit invitation to do so. If Dr Malik had adopted a patient-centred approach, he would have asked John earlier in the consultation, while gathering information, about his ideas and concerns about the pain. He would still have to exclude other causes, but he could specifically allay the anxiety about lung cancer. If John had not raised the question about cancer he would have left the consultation with his anxiety unresolved and, perhaps, sought another opinion elsewhere.

Implications for practice

The 'first half of the consultation'

Conducting consultations in a patient-centred manner has long been shown to improve healthcare outcomes (Stewart et al., 2013). Certainly a patient's anxiety is reduced if a health professional explores the patient's understanding of the problem and any ideas and concerns about its cause and diagnosis (Evans et al., 1987). The patient-centred approach involves considering patients as 'experts' in relation to their own health. In a classic study titled 'Meetings with experts' (Tuckett et al., 1985), in which the experts are the patient *and* the doctor, the authors defined a successful consultation as one in which a shared understanding was reached.

When a person makes a GP appointment they have an agenda that they wish to be dealt with. This may be a diagnosis of a new symptom, or it may involve a repeat prescription or advice about a continuing problem or lifestyle issue. The patient's opening remarks, in response to the doctor's invitation, are the only part of the consultation over which they have much control (Neighbour, 1987). Some patients rehearse what they are going to say before they enter the consulting room. Many are anxious and indeed this is a potent cause of 'white coat hypertension': a person's blood pressure is raised above their usual reading when they consult a doctor (Pickering et al., 1988).

To minimise the chance of inducing 'white coat hypertension' in their patients, GPs are advised during their training not to interrupt a patient during their opening remarks. Studies have shown that people are unlikely to speak for more than 30 seconds without prompts, but many doctors ask questions before the patient has finished speaking, and may miss important cues about the agenda (Rabinowitz et al., 2004).

As noted, patients often have a 'hidden agenda' as well as their more overt one. This is another reason for the GP needing to consider the possibility that the patient's real motive for consulting is not mentioned straight away (McKinley & Middleton, 1999). The hidden agenda may be revealed when discussing ideas and concerns, but it is advisable for doctors to ask before closing a consultation: 'Is there anything else I can help you with today?' Sometimes the patient brings up their additional agenda only when they are about to leave – the 'doorknob' comment (Weston, Brown & McWilliam, 2002). The danger is then that the doctor disregards the comment due to time pressures and the patient leaves with an unresolved problem.

There is also a risk, however, that overzealous doctors, particularly inexperienced GPs, try to uncover a hidden agenda in every consultation (Thistlethwaite & Morris, 2006). Sometimes consultations are straightforward. It is also possible the patient has a second concern but one which they are not yet ready to raise in the first consultation.

Finally, some patients may not be used to doctors who adopt a patient-centred approach. Many, particularly older patients who are used to paternalistic GPs, may feel they are wasting a doctor's time with their concerns, especially if they perceive them to be not medical (Bensing, 1991). Many people are unable to share their own ideas and may not be used to discussing their health problems. However, patients with psychosocial problems have been shown to appreciate the patient-centred approach (Little et al., 2001).

The 'second half of the consultation'

The second half of a consultation in general practice is frequently concerned with information sharing and management plans. After the GP has gathered information, doctors have to decide how much information to share with patients about their diagnosis, prognosis and treatment options. A patient-centred approach in the first half of the consultation may change into a paternalistic approach in the second half. In fact the patient-centred approach should also include the patient and the doctor finding common ground regarding management (Stewart et al., 2013). Management includes lifestyle changes, such as advice about smoking and weight reduction, as well as options regarding pharmacological treatments, referrals, surgery and so on.

Many health professionals still talk of patient 'compliance' – the patient needs to comply with the management plan otherwise they are labelled 'non-compliant'. A vast amount of research has shown that many patients do not 'comply' with their prescribed treatments, with average adherence rates for patients with diabetes being between 36% and 93% across various studies (Cramer, 2004). There are many reasons for this, most of which are due to poor communication in the consultation, patients not being involved in decision-making, their different interpretations of risk, and the complexity of the treatment regimen (Claxton, Cramer & Pierce, 2001). Cost may also be a factor in those countries where there are no 'free' prescriptions.

Patients have been shown to want the following information from their GPs: clear information about what is wrong; a realistic idea of prognosis; what they can do to help themselves (that is, self-care); sources of help; what to tell their family; and how to prevent further illness or worsening of their condition (Coulter, Entwistle & Gilbert, 1999). In addition, in relation to any recommended medicines they want to know what the medication does and what it's for; possible and common side effects; dos and don'ts such as whether they can take other medication and whether they can still drink alcohol; and how to take it (Dickinson & Raynor, 2003).

Theoretical links

The process of information sharing and the dialogue between patient and professional in regards to management is called **shared decision-making**. The process has the following characteristics: both the patient and the doctor (in this case) are involved; both parties share information; both work together to agree on preferences for treatment; and both reach an agreement on the treatment to start (Charles, Gafni & Whelan, 1997). In addition it is important for the patient and doctor to discuss their values: 'values-based practice aims to support balanced decision-making within a framework of shared values, based on a premise of mutual respect' (Fulford, Peile & Carroll, 2012, p. 24).

> **shared decision-making**
> the interaction process between the healthcare practitioner and the patient who come together to devise treatment plans. Shared decision-making becomes possible when there is mutual listening and shared dialogue.

Shared decision-making also requires the doctor to be able to translate technical information and jargon on options, risks and benefits into clear and unbiased language (Towle, Godolphin & Richardson, 1997). The GP's expertise as a generalist is based on a broad knowledge base. The information GPs share with patients and the options they present will be guided by evidence (that is, evidence-based practice) as well as their own experience of clinical practice. In a study of the use of explicit evidence by doctors, GPs were found to be influenced by brief reading of the medical literature, interaction with their peers, opinion leaders, patients (patient choice and previous patient responses to treatment), pharmaceutical representatives, and their own early training (Gabbay & Le May, 2004). Peer interaction occurs with GP partners and local networks, such as Medicare Locals, which were set up by the Australian government in 2011 to plan, deliver and fund extra health services to communities.

A difficult part of information sharing is enabling patients to understand *risk*: the risk of a disease, the risk of treatment such as medication and surgery, risks arising from non-treatment, and risks to other people if certain conditions such as infectious diseases do go untreated. **Risk communication** should be an open dialogue (a two-way conversation) leading to better understanding and thus better decisions about clinical management (Edwards et al., 2000). People respond to information about risk in different ways and are influenced by how much they trust the giver of the information; the relevance of the risk to their everyday life; how the information fits in with their existing knowledge, beliefs and experience;

> **risk communication**
> discussions that healthcare practitioners and patients have about the risks that may be inherent in particular treatments and care decisions.

and the importance of any decision they are making (Alaszewski & Horlick-Jones, 2003). The language of risk can be ambiguous and misinterpreted: 'common' and 'rare' mean different things to different people. The use of quantitative data such as numerical odds, numbers-needed-to-treat and sensitivity/specificity figures are not easily explained or understood. The community risk scale (Calman & Royston, 1997) combines standardised terms with familiar descriptions. For example, a risk of 1 in 10000 has a magnitude of 6, is equivalent to one case in a small town, and the risk of having a road vehicle accident (in the UK).

Conclusion

GPs play a central role in primary healthcare delivery in Australia, providing a person-centred, continuing, comprehensive service to patients of all ages, ethnicities and social status, in which communication strategies are as important as history-taking and diagnosis. A distinguishing feature of general practice consultations is that the patient may bring any problem or query to the doctor. Consequently, it is important that relevant information is exchanged between all the professionals involved with the permission of the patient. There are three models of communication distinguished by the degree of patient involvement. While the expert GP can change communication style in response to the patient's problem a patient-centred approach leading to 'shared decision-making' improves healthcare outcomes.

Practice example 3.2

The following is an example of a common management decision-making process in the general practice setting. Leonora Rossetti (LR), a 56-year-old school receptionist consults her GP, Dr Frances Gould (FG), for follow-up of her previously raised blood pressure (BP). She has had several readings over the last three months with FG and the practice nurse, and the average reading has been about 160/105 (where the acceptable level would be below 140/90). FG has arranged various investigations to assess LR's health risk due to this persistent hypertension (raised blood pressure), and the aim of this consultation is to discuss whether LR should start treatment to lower the BP.

FG: Good afternoon, Leonora. Thank you for coming back. How are you today?

LR: Not too bad, doctor. It's the school holidays so I have a few days off.

FG: Well, as you know, your blood pressure has stayed high and we need to consider what to do about lowering it. We've discussed the risks of high blood pressure and how to control it. So today I would like to talk about starting you on treatment.

LR: Well, doctor, I would really like to avoid that if at all possible. I'm worried about side effects. Is there another way to bring it down?

continued ›

Practice example 3.2 continued ›

FG: Have you managed to increase the amount of exercise you are doing? Have you managed to lose any weight?

LR: I've been trying doctor but it's really hard to find the time. I have cut down on my salt like you suggested and I've cut out fried food and take-aways.

FG: I really think it's time to try some tablets. They are only once a day and you shouldn't have any problems with them. Some people get a cough but that's not common.

LR: Are you sure that's necessary, doctor? Could I try and lose some weight and then have it checked again?

FG: Here's a prescription. I really think this would be the best idea, particularly as your mother had a stroke last year. We really should try to prevent that happening to you.

Reflective questions

1. How do you think this consultation went from the perspective of the GP? And from the perspective of the patient?

2. How likely do you think it is that Leonora will take her tablets every day? Give reasons for your answer.

3. Think of a time you or someone you know has been given a prescription for medication. Did you/they take all the medication as prescribed? Why/why not?

4. What could the doctor do to increase the likelihood that Leonora will take her pills? What communication strategies could GPs employ to involve patients in decision-making about management plans?

5. Consider a time you consulted a GP. What did you think went well, and why? What might have been done differently, and why? Did you feel you had time to discuss any anxieties with the doctor?

6. What is the difference between open and closed questions? When should each type be used? Consider a conversation with a friend and reflect on how you use questions, pauses and listening to share information.

7. What do you feel will be the outcome if a patient is unable to share their hidden agenda with the doctor? Why is this important?

Further reading

Hoffman, T. C., Légaré, F., Simmons, M.B., McNamara, K., McCaffery, K., Trevena, L. et al. (2014). Shared decision making: What do clinicians need to know and why should they bother? *Medical Journal of Australia*, 201, 35–39.

This article is a summary of the rationale for and processes involved in shared decision-making, with clinical examples. It is a good introduction to the topic.

Silverman, J., Kurtz, S., & Draper. J. (2013). *Skills for communicating with patients.* (3rd ed.) Abingdon: Radcliffe Medical Press.

This is one of the principal texts about communication skills for patient care. It is relevant for all health professionals and takes an evidence-guided approach.

Thistlethwaite, J. E. (2012). *Values-based interprofessional collaborative practice.* Cambridge: Cambridge University Press.

Personal and professional values influence how health professionals interact with patients/clients and each other. This book, with many clinical scenarios mainly based in primary care settings, defines values and explores how health professionals work together and with patients.

References

Alaszewski, A., & Horlick-Jones, T. (2003). How can doctors communicate information about risk more effectively? *British Medical Journal, 327,* 728–731.

Bensing, J. (1991). Doctor-patient communication and the quality of care. *Social Science and Medicine, 32,* 1301–1310.

Calman, K. C., & Royston, G. (1997). Personal paper: Risk language and dialects. *British Medical Journal, 316*(7139), 1242.

Charles, C., Gafni, A., & Whelan, T. (1997). Shared decision-making in the medical encounter: What does it mean? (or it takes two to tango). *Social Science and Medicine, 44,* 681–692.

Claxton, A. J., Cramer, J., & Pierce, C. (2001). A systematic review of the associations between dose regimens and medication compliance. *Clinical Therapeutics, 23,* 1296–1310.

Coulter, A., Entwistle, V., & Gilbert, D. (1999). Sharing decisions with patients: Is the information good enough? *BMJ, 31,* 318–322.

Cramer, J. (2004). A systematic review of adherence with medications for diabetes. *Diabetes Care, 27,* 1218–1224.

Dickinson, D., & Raynor, D. K. T. (2003). Ask the patients – they may want to know more. *British Medical Journal, 327*(7419), 861.

Edwards, A. G. K., Hood, K., Matthews, E. J., Russell, D., Russell, I. T., Barker, J. et al. (2000). The effectiveness of one-to-one risk communication interventions in health care: A systematic review. *Medical Decision Making, 20,* 290–297.

Evans, B. J., Kiellerup, F. D., Stanley, R. O. et al. (1987). A communication skills programme for increasing patients' satisfaction with general practice consultations. *British Journal of Medical Psychology, 60,* 373–378.

Fulford, K. W. M., Peile, E., & Carroll, H. (2012). *Essential values-based practice. Clinical stories linking science with people.* Cambridge: Cambridge University Press.

Gabbay, J., & Le May, A. (2004). Evidence based guidelines or collectively constructed 'mindlines'? Ethnographic study of knowledge management in primary care. *British Medical Journal, 329,* 1488–1492.

Little, P., Everitt, H., Williamson, I. Warner, G., Moore, M., Gould, C. et al. (2001). Preferences of patients for patient centred approach to consultation in primary care: Observational study. *British Medical Journal, 322,* 468–472.

McKinley, R. K., & Middleton, J. E. (1999). What do patients want from doctors? Content analysis of written patient agendas for the consultation. *British Journal of General Practice, 328*, 796–800.

Neighbour, R. (1987). *The inner consultation.* Lancaster: MTP Press.

Pendleton, D., Schofield, T., Tate, P., & Havelock, P. (2003). *The new consultation. Developing doctor-patient communication.* Oxford: Oxford University Press.

Pickering, T. G., James, G., Boddie, C., Harshfield, G. A., Blank, S., & Laragh, J. H. (1988). How common is white coat hypertension? *JAMA, 259*, 225–228.

Rabinowitz, I., Luzzatti, R., Tamir, A., & Reis, S. (2004). Length of patient's monologue, rate of completion, and relation to other components of the clinical encounter: Observational intervention study in primary care. *British Medical Journal, 328*, 501–502.

RACGP. (n.d.). What is general practice? Retrieved April 2014 from http://www.racgp.org.au/becomingagp/what-is-a-gp/what-is-general-practice/

Stewart, M., Brown, J. B., Weston, W. W., McWhinney, I. R., McWilliam, C. L., & Freeman, T. R. (2013). *Patient-centered medicine* (3rd ed.). Abingdon: Radcliffe Medical Press.

Thistlethwaite, J. E., & Morris, P. (2006). *The patient-doctor consultation in primary care. Theory and practice.* London: Royal College of General Practitioners.

Towle, A., Godolphin, W., & Richardson, A. (1997). *Competencies for informed shared decision making (ISDM). Report on interviews with physicians, patients and patient educators and focus group meetings with patients.* Vancouver: University of British Columbia.

Tuckett, D., Boulton, M., Olson, C., & Williams, A. (1985). *Meetings with experts. An Approach to sharing ideas in medical consultations.* London: Tavistock Publications.

Weston, W.W., Brown, J. B., & McWilliam, C. L. (2002). Being realistic. In J. B. Brown, M. Stewart & W. W. Weston (Eds.), *Challenges and solutions in patient-centered care. A case book.* Abingdon: Radcliffe Medical Press.

World Health Organization (WHO). (1978). *Primary health care.* Geneva: Author.

4

Communicating across rural and metropolitan healthcare settings

Donella Piper, Vicki Parker and Jane Gray

Learning objectives

This chapter will enable you to:
- define the concept of 'rurality' and understand what 'rurality' means in the context of the Australian healthcare system;
- describe the generalist nature of rural health practice;
- understand the specific challenges faced in service delivery including:
  - workforce issues relating to recruitment, retention and training;
  - coordination of care across long distances and different types of facilities;
  - access to specialty services and the need to tailor models of care to the rural context;
- reflect on rural health services' close ties to their communities and what this means for community expectations of health services and the way in which rural health professionals manage close personal and professional relationships;
- consider the role of communication in overcoming health inequity and disadvantage experienced by people in rural communities.

Key terms

Clinical networks
Generalist practitioners
Rurality
Telehealth

Overview

The purpose of this chapter is twofold. First, it provides you with an understanding of what **rurality** means in the context of the Australian healthcare system. Second, it highlights, via practical examples, some of the main communication issues relating to patient safety faced by rural health service providers and patients.

> **rurality**
> physical proximity, or remoteness from, to metropolitan settings. Regional geographical areas in closest proximity to metropolitan areas are often referred to as rural areas. Remote geographical areas are those the furthest away from metropolitan settings.

One of the main communication issues is the coordination of care across long distances. Coordination of care across long distances involves different types of facilities and health professionals having to share information. Coordination of care across long distances is necessary because rural patients access a variety of services, and these services need not be co-located. For this reason, services need to network about care delivery: communicate with one another about how to deliver care to rural patients in ways that create continuity and maintain access.

> **telehealth**
> the use of information and communication technology to provide healthcare services to people who are at a distance from the healthcare service. Telehealth is used to transmit different kinds of information, reducing the need for people to travel.

Practice example 4.1 presents a case study of one rural patient's journey through the health system. It highlights the vulnerability of patients in rural areas. Practice example 4.2 demonstrates access issues often faced by rural patients. It asks you to reflect on how new and emerging **telehealth** and information technology initiatives are seeking to address some of these communication challenges.

Introduction

Those providing health care to rural patients face a number of challenges depending on the degree of 'rurality' involved. 'Rurality' is defined according to the Australian Standard Geographical Classification – Remoteness Areas system (ASGC-RA). The ASGC-RA is explained as 'a geographic classification system that was introduced on 1 July 2010. It was developed by the Australian Bureau of Statistics (ABS). The ASGC-RA allows quantitative comparisons between 'city' and 'country' Australia' (ABS, 2010 cited in Commonwealth of Australia, 2012, p. 6). According to the ABS, 'as at June 2009, 68.6% of the population resided in Australia's major cities. Of the total population, 29.1% resided in regional areas and just 2.3% lived in remote or very remote Australia' (ABS, 2010 cited in Commonwealth of Australia, 2012, p. 5).

The *National Strategic Framework for Rural and Remote Health* states:

> The RA categories are defined in terms of the physical distance of a location from the nearest urban centre based on population size. The five RA categories under the ASGC system are:

- RA1 – Major Cities of Australia;
- RA2 – Inner Regional Australia (rural);
- RA3 – Outer Regional Australia (rural);
- RA4 – Remote Australia (remote), and
- RA5 – Very Remote Australia (remote). (Commonwealth of Australia, 2012, p. 6)

According to the *National Strategic Framework for Rural and Remote Health* 'the terms "rural" and "remote" are used to encompass all areas outside Australia's major cities. This includes areas that are classified as inner and outer regional (RA2 and RA3) and remote or very remote (RA4 and RA5)' (Commonwealth of Australia 2012, p. 5). The different categories are set out in Figure 4.1.

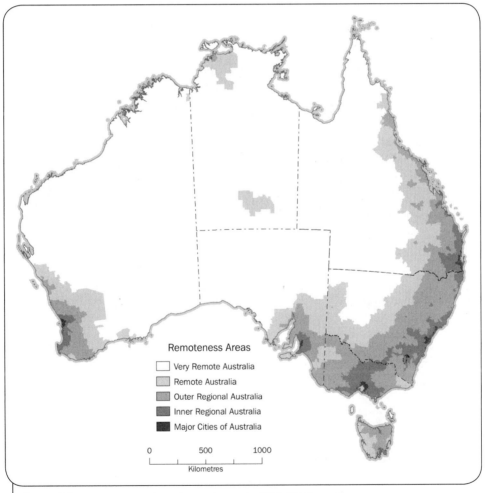

Figure 4.1 Remoteness area boundaries of Australia (ABS, 2011)

As Figure 4.1 demonstrates, the largest remoteness category is 'very remote' or RA5 – over 5.5 million square kilometres (72.5% of the Australian land area). Next in size is the 'remote' (RA4) category at 1.02 million square kilometres (13.2%); and finally the 'outer regional' (RA3) and 'inner regional' (RA2) categories cover 10.8% and 3.2% of Australia's land area, respectively (Commonwealth of Australia, 2012, p. 5). Approximately seven million people, about one-third of Australia's total population – live outside major cities (Commonwealth of Australia, 2012, p. 5). According to the Australian Institute of Health and Welfare:

> [t]he relationship of remoteness to health is particularly important for Indigenous Australians, as they are more likely to live outside metropolitan areas than non-Indigenous Australians. In 2011, just over one-third of Indigenous Australians lived in Major cities (34.8%), compared with over 70% of non-Indigenous Australians. Only 1.7% of non-Indigenous Australians lived in Remote or Very remote areas, compared with about one-fifth of Indigenous Australians (7.7% in Remote and 13.7% in Very remote areas). Indigenous Australians represent 16% and 45% of all people living in Remote and Very remote areas respectively. (AIHW, 2014, 7.7)

The population distribution for each remoteness area is set out in Table 4.1.

Table 4.1 Estimated resident population by remoteness

	Estimated resident population (2009)	Percentage of total population
Major cities	15 068 655	68.63
Inner regional	4 325 467	19.70
Outer regional	2 062 966	9.40
Remote	324 031	1.48
Very remote	174 137	0.79
Total	**21 955 256**	**100.00**

Source: Adapted from ABS (2010). *Regional Population Growth, Australia, 2008–09* cited in Commonwealth of Australia (2012)

The Australian Government Department of Health Doctor Connect website (http://www.doctorconnect.gov.au/internet/otd/publishing.nsf/Content/locator, retrieved October 20, 2014) enables individuals to insert a town or street address name to identify the correct RA classification for that location.

....

The challenges facing rural and remote health care

When it comes to the health of a population, remoteness, or rurality, has several consequences. The Australian Institute of Health and Welfare's (AIHW) report, *Australia's Health 2014*, states for example that 'Australians in regional and remote areas tend to have shorter lives and higher rates of disease and injury than people in major cities' (AIHW, 2014, 5.6). The main reasons for the difference are a lack of 'educational and employment opportunities, income, and access to goods and services' (AIHW, 2014, 5.6). Further reasons include rural patients' need for more long distance travel, access to fresh foods, and access to health services (Commonwealth of Australia, 2012).

Another consequence of rurality is increased disease risk factors and increased levels of illness (Commonwealth of Australia, 2012). In addition, death rates increase with remoteness (AIHW, 2014). One of the reasons for the increased disease factors and levels of illness is the higher rate of poverty experienced by residents of rural, regional and remote areas compared to those in metropolitan areas. In their report, entitled *A Snapshot of Poverty in Rural and Regional Australia*, the National Rural Health Alliance (NRHA) and the Australian Council of Social Services (ACOSS) state: 'Allowing for the costs of housing, poverty is slightly worse in rural, regional and remote areas (13.1 per cent "outside capital cities") than in capital cities (12.6 per cent). When housing costs (which are higher in capital cities) are not taken into account, that divide becomes starker.' (NRHA & ACOSS, 2013, p. 3).

The *National Strategic Framework for Rural and Remote Health* (Commonwealth of Australia, 2012) summarises the consequences of rurality as follows:

> [h]igher mortality rates and lower life expectancy; higher road injury and fatality rates; higher reported rates of high blood pressure, diabetes, and obesity; higher death rates from chronic disease; higher prevalence of mental health problems; higher rates of alcohol abuse and smoking; poorer dental health; higher incidence of poor antenatal and postnatal health; and higher incidence of babies born with low birth weight to mothers in very remote areas. (Commonwealth of Australia, 2012, p. 13)

Service delivery in rural and remote areas is very different to that in the city (Commonwealth of Australia, 2012). Some of the reasons for this are the increased costs incurred in providing health services in remote locations due in part to the lack of existing infrastructure that can be utilised and the lack of trained and skilled workers. In addition there is greater dependence on primary healthcare providers such as general practitioners (GPs). While there is a higher use of emergency departments in rural areas, these emergency departments are usually serviced by visiting medical officers (VMOs), who are often GPs. Facilities are smaller, yet they must provide a broader range of services such as aged and community care to a more geographically dispersed population (AIHW, 2014).

In addition, prevailing service models and models of care are often better suited to metropolitan settings than to rural and remote settings. The reason for this, according to the *National Strategic Framework for Rural and Remote Health* (Commonwealth of Australia, 2012), is that most health service education and planning take place in metropolitan settings, with little regard for the differences that rurality brings. Despite a number of more recent incentive programs and rural clinical placements:

> traditional training approaches and funding mechanisms have led to the uneven distribution of healthcare professionals across the country. This can be seen in the disparity in the number of healthcare professionals between metropolitan and the most remote parts of the country. For example, in 2006 very remote areas had:
>
> • 58 generalist medical practitioners per 100 000 population (compared to 196 per 100 000 in capital cities);

- 589 registered nurses per 100 000 population (compared to 978 per 100 000 in major cities); and;
- 64 allied health workers per 100 000 population (compared to 354 per 100 000 in major cities). (Commonwealth of Australia, 2012, p. 9)

This uneven distribution of the health workforce, together with workforce shortages, often results in heavy workloads for rural clinicians. As a consequence of limited resources and time, rural health professionals often become **generalist practitioners** with broad knowledge and flexible work practices. According to McNeil et al. (2014) there exists the expectation that rural health practitioners 'will provide a wider range of services [than their metropolitan counterparts]. Flexibility in role bounda- ries and overlapping knowledge and skills' is therefore nec- essary between health professionals (McNeil, Mitchell & Parker, 2014, p. 2).

> **generalist practitioners**
> a health professional (particularly a rural one) who runs a practice that requires a wide skill set and specific skills in the assessment and coordination of care across a broad range of age groups and health problems.

Given these complexities, careful communication and ongoing cooperation between rural health professionals and with the community is essential in order to meet the health needs of rural communities. This means that rural clinicians are often closely associated with non-health agencies and community groups that provide social services. Being members of a small community, health professionals are often well known to their patients. This may pose a number of challenges in relation to personal and professional boundaries around issues such as confidentiality and incident management, for example.

The *National Strategic Framework for Rural and Remote Health* states there are:

> further complexities for planning, managing and delivering public hospital services in rural and remote locations as they:
> - are generally smaller than metropolitan centres;
> - have high fixed costs of operation;
> - are less able to achieve the economies of scale experienced in large hospitals; and
> - are often the default service provider in the absence of private sector options, adequate primary health and aged care services provision. (Commonwealth of Australia, 2012, p. 11)

Furthermore:

> [P]eople in rural and remote areas needing to access health services are often influenced by:
> - travel distance to relevant health services, including the availability of transport and the cost of travel;
> - uncertainty about how to use and access services, including the availability of emergency care and retrieval services;
> - cultural and language barriers; and
> - poorer understanding of health issues and how to access health services. (Commonwealth of Australia, 2012, p. 29)

There can be cultural and language barriers (particularly for Aboriginal and Torres Strait Islander peoples and for people from culturally and linguistically diverse backgrounds) and poorer understanding of health issues, or poor health literacy (Commonwealth of Australia, 2012, p. 30).

Past experience also has an influence on whether or not people access care. Lack of support for travel from rural and remote areas to metropolitan centres for specialist care is often viewed by patients as difficult to coordinate and disruptive to family and professional life. Accordingly, such appointments may be delayed or cancelled. This can mean that people prefer to live with their condition rather than access treatment far from home (Commonwealth of Australia, 2012, p. 30).

These challenges create specific communication issues for patient safety. Practice example 4.1 highlights the challenges and vulnerability faced by patients who live in rural communities. Practice example 4.2 highlights the challenges of access to specialty services. The second example will also touch on the changes brought about by new and emerging telehealth initiatives.

Practice example 4.1 _ Mrs Edith Burgess' story

Mrs Edith Burgess, aged 69, lives with her husband in a small rural community in central New South Wales. Following a visit to the dentist who was concerned about a lesion in her mouth, she went along to see her GP, who gave her a referral to a specialist in a larger centre about 150 kilometres from where she lives. This specialist indicated he felt there was nothing to be concerned about and suggested a follow-up appointment in six months' time. During the six months the lesion became more uncomfortable and was making it difficult for Edith to chew. Edith was visiting a relative on the coast and that relative suggested she go along to see her GP, who promptly referred her to the Head and Neck Cancer Clinic at the city's Cancer Centre. The lesion was found to be cancerous, requiring urgent extensive surgery and follow-up radiotherapy once the wound had healed.

Having the surgery meant that Edith spent two weeks away from home and her family. The shock of diagnosis and preparation for surgery were emotionally and physically difficult. Her husband, Barry, couldn't leave the farm due to the need to care for animals. It was hard for him to be kept informed about what was happening and hard for Edith to be without him. She felt disconnected from home and her usual support networks.

After recovering from surgery Edith moved back home to the farm. Every three weeks she was required to travel three and a half hours down and back to the Specialist Cancer Services for treatments. She said: 'They must have thought I was half an hour away because they'd ring up on the day and say, "Come in at 3:30 p.m. today". I ended up going back down and staying there until the treatments were finished.' She tried to book accommodation that was available onsite at the Cancer Centre, but it was not always available, in which case she stayed at the nearest hotel.

continued ›

Practice example 4.1 continued ›

In the city she was cared for by a multidisciplinary team of health professionals. When she returned home she was still in need of support from a dietician and speech pathologist; this required a car journey of one and a half hours each way. The services available locally were limited. From time to time physiotherapy services were available at the local Multi-Purpose Health Centre. However, this centre had difficulty recruiting staff and often staff, particularly those with young families, didn't stay long.

Her local GP was very supportive, but did not understand the full nature of her surgery or the complex nature of her needs. He complained that he had not been notified of her admission to hospital nor had he received any information following discharge. Her children and the children of the GP had grown up together, attended the same schools and often visited each other. Follow-up care was provided by appointment with the specialist services; this once again required a full day of travel. Edith often felt depressed about her situation and worried about how she and Barry would manage if she became dependent or died. She did not feel comfortable raising these issues with her GP or with Barry for fear of raising his concerns.

Analysis and reflection

Practice example 4.1 highlights the vulnerability of rural patients. Part of this vulnerability stems from the challenge of access to specialty care and of needing care to be coordinated over long distances. In relation to access, the story demonstrates the generalist nature of healthcare services in rural areas, characterised by small numbers of some health professions and the absence of others. Like many rural patients, the local and regional clinicians and hospitals could not treat Edith's condition and she needed to access specialist services.

Another aspect of the vulnerability was the feeling of isolation experienced by Edith. Edith's case highlights the problems that arise through being isolated from support structures and services. The case highlights frequent disruptions to care and added financial burden due to transportation issues, and geographic distances due to rural patients having to travel and at times relocate in order to access specialist services.

There are two critical kinds of communication that become evident here:

1. *Proactive communication*: This communication routinely and proactively connects health and social care services such that delays in treatment remain limited, and harm from fragmented care is obviated. This communication is pre-structured; it consists of negotiated agreements linking the rural, community, GP and metropolitan services involved in the care of rural patients. Such inter-service agreements ensure these patients' treatments remain continuous or, if the treatments cannot be continuous, patients are accompanied with effective explanations about what will happen next, why, and where (see Chapter 12).

2. *Retrospective communication*: This communication retrospectively identifies and rectifies care fragmentation and care disconnection that patients are suffering or have suffered. This communication is restorative; it is oriented towards 'hearing' the rural patient, and the issues they express about their care, especially where there is poor communication between hospital- and specialist-based services, or between primary care and community services in rural community, in order to rectify discontinuities.

Reflective questions

1. What are the factors that may lead to delay in rural people seeking health care?
2. What communication could be put in place to support Mrs and Mr Burgess?
3. Identify the actual and potential communication deficits that have resulted in the situation described above. Why do they occur?
4. What are the consequences of those deficits for Edith and other patients like her?
5. Consider the impact of living in a rural community for the health-service needs of different population groups, in particular older people, those with chronic diseases or cancer, and families with young children.
6. Consider what it is like for health professionals to work in rural areas, without easy access to resources and support networks. What communication processes and practices could improve the situation?
7. What two-way dialogue between rural and metropolitan services should occur and how? What structural processes could be implemented to ensure consistent and sustainable two-way communication?
8. Consider the communication implications for patients and health professionals who live and work together within small communities.

Implications for practice

Three kinds of strategies have been put in place to address the issues raised by Edith's story:

1. improved access to specialist services via a networked system;
2. improved care coordination within this networked system; and ·
3. programs aimed at increasing the number and/or skills of health professionals in rural areas.

In order to facilitate access to specialist services, hospitals are grouped together into local health districts (in New South Wales) or local hospital networks (in other states and territories) (AIHW, 2014). These districts or networks are described by the AIHW (2014, section 2.1) as:

> small groups of local hospitals, or an individual hospital, linking services within a region or through specialist networks across a state or territory … A total of 136 local hospital

districts and networks have been established across all states and territories. Of these, 123 are geographically based networks and 13 are state or territory-wide networks that deliver specialised hospital services across various networks and districts.

Figure 4.2 sets out the rural and regional New South Wales local health districts. There are seven rural local health districts.

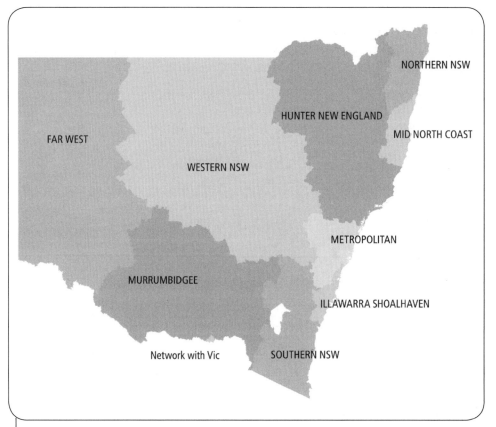

Figure 4.2 Map of New South Wales rural and regional local health districts (http://www.health.nsw. gov.au/lhd/pages/default.aspx)

All local health districts or networks span a number of small community hospitals, district hospitals, rural referral hospitals, and sometimes a tertiary referral (metropolitan) hospital. These services are often geographically dispersed and offer different services. Generally, the smaller hospitals offer less specialist services. In addition, there are **clinical networks** connecting rural clinicians to one another and to those working in metropolitan settings. The aim of clinical networks is to ensure emphasis on services and patients through engendering cooperation across sites, focusing on clinical issues and creating a dynamic system and supportive and innovative practice community. In New South

clinical networks
networks that link clinicians working in similar field of practice across services and geographic locations.

Wales, for example, the rural health network is supported through the Agency for Clinical Innovation, a branch of the New South Wales Ministry of Health.

While Edith was able to provide private transport to access specialist services within her local health district, not all rural patients have the resources to do this. In recognition of this, all Australian states and territories operate a Patient Assisted Travel Scheme (PATS) and other transport assistance. As described on the Australian Government Rural and Regional Health website:

> [T]hese schemes provide a subsidy to assist with travel, escort and accommodation expenses incurred when rural and remote Australians travel over 100 kilometres to access specialised healthcare which is not available within a specified distance from their place of residence. (http://www.ruralhealthaustralia.gov.au/internet/rha/Publishing.nsf/Content/home, retrieved January 25, 2015)

Some of the larger hospitals have their own share-accommodation for rural patients; however, in some jurisdictions, unfortunately, this accommodation is gradually being closed down (Samera, 2013).

But these resources alone are not sufficient to guarantee that all districts (or networks) are linked through structured proactive communication, and that their links are checked through retrospective (restorative) communication. Accordingly, a number of state departments of health have developed 'care coordination' policies, manuals and programs. These policies, manuals and programs serve to improve all patients' journeys through the districts (or networks), particularly the journeys of rural and remote patients.

For example the NSW Health care coordination reference manual advocates 'the development of local protocols [to] assist in the transfer of care for patients returning home from metropolitan services to rural and remote areas' (NSW Health, 2011, p. 6). (These protocols are an example of proactive communication.) Other practical steps put in place include:

- assessing the availability of access to pharmaceutical services (for example, a patient who lives at a great distance from such a service may be able to obtain amounts of a drug different to usual to limit travel to the service);
- transferring rural and remote patients back to the originating hospital or, if this is not possible, to a clinically appropriate hospital closer to the patient's home;
- ensuring a range of transport options to and from the patients' home;
- considering the time, distance and dislocation involved for carers who are required to attend with patients and/or transport patients to and from acute health services (NSW Health, 2011);
- prioritising support for services that are bulk-billed or free of charge in order to remove the economic hurdles that rural and Indigenous patients often face;
- delivering culturally appropriate services to reduce cultural barriers that are otherwise experienced by many Indigenous patients; and
- supporting clinical upskilling sessions that are provided by visiting health practitioners to strengthen the capacity of local health services and practitioners to manage patients' ongoing care.

To address the problem of the low numbers of some health professions who want to work in rural and remote areas, other solutions have been proposed. One is mandatory rural placement for junior doctors (Rowe, Campbell & Hargrave, 2014). While requiring adequate levels of senior support and supervision, and incurring significant costs to rural GP practices (Laurence et al., 2014), mandatory rural placement is an effective means of creating interest among junior doctors to practise in rural areas.

In addition, 'outreach clinics' have also been established. This means that specialists travel to rural and remote areas to provide services. The Rural Doctors Network (RDN), for example, describes itself as 'funded by the Australian Government Department of Health (DoH) to administer the delivery of medical outreach services to rural and remote Aboriginal communities in New South Wales (NSW) and the Australian Capital Territory (ACT)' (Rural Doctors Network, n.d.).

The High Risk Maternal Foetal Outreach Clinic in Moree, located in the Hunter New England local health district, provides an example of a Medical Specialst Outreach Assistance Program (MSOAP), funded by the federal government (NSW Agency for Clinical Innovation, 2014a). This program involves specialists travelling to Moree to provide obstetric services to high-risk patients. This means that a high level of communication between practitioners, services and patients is required to coordinate and provide the outreach services. A team from the John Hunter Hospital in Newcastle (described on the NSW Agency for Clinical Innovation website <http://www.aci.health.nsw.gov.au/ie/projects/hrm-moree> as consisting of a maternal foetal medicine specialist; obstetrics and gynaecology senior registrar; clinical midwifery consultant; neonatal ICU nurse specialist and an Aboriginal maternal and infant health service manager (NSW Agency for Clinical Innovation, 2014a)), must communicate with a local team (described on the NSW Agency for Clinical Innovation website as consisting of a midwife; Aboriginal health education officer; ultra sound sonographer and a social worker (NSW Agency for Clinical Innovation, 2014a)). Members of the local team liaise with the patient to devise a birth plan and coordinate appointments and referrals with the specialist team (NSW Agency for Clinical Innovation, 2014a). Aside from the obvious logistics and communication issues associated with liaising between provider sites and teams, the project has been seen as providing a benefit in terms of communicating education and shared knowledge between the providers. While outreach services are provided by practitioners visiting rural and remote sites, they are increasingly provided via telehealth (see Chapter 16).

An example of another solution aimed at addressing rural workforce issues is the Murrumbidgee local health district Enhanced Scope of Practice model of care project (NSW Agency for Clinical Innovation, 2014b). The aim of this project was to develop the rural nursing workforce within the Murrumbidgee local health district to ensure that patients using emergency departments in small communities where a medical officer was not present were able to access appropriate treatment, provided by a registered nurse acting in an advanced capacity, rather than being transferred to a larger facility (NSW Agency for Clinical Innovation, 2014b). While this project was not focused on communicating between facilities about the care of rural patients, it highlights the important role communication plays in improving access to services for rural patients. The enhanced scope of practice project utilised different communication modalities to deliver education and training to upskill nurses. These included interactive online learning and videoconference education sessions conducted with a larger base hospital within the local health district. The enhanced scope of practice model was found to improve access and patient satisfaction (NSW Agency for Clinical Innovation, 2014b). More details about the project are available on the Agency for Clinical Innovation website (NSW Agency for Clinical Innovation, 2014b).

Australian state governments are becoming increasingly committed to creating continuity of care for rural and remote patients. This is evident through recent initiatives such as the Integrated Care Program in New South Wales, through which the state government awarded large amounts of funding to non-metropolitan districts (networks) for projects promoting care integration. While the benefits of this program are a long way from being realised, much more attention is now paid by governments to the plights of patients whose care is fragmented as a result of geographic distance or a lack of resources, or both.

Theoretical links

The issues experienced by Edith in the first practice example are not unique. Brundisini and colleagues (2013) reviewed literature published in Australia, Europe, New Zealand and North America. The review focused on what the authors describes as 'the advantages and disadvantages rural patients with chronic diseases face when accessing both rural and distant care' (Brundisini et al., 2013, p. 1). Despite the focus on patients with chronic diseases, some of the results may also be applicable to acute patients.

Overall the researchers found that 'people who live in a rural area may feel more vulnerable – that is, more easily harmed by their health problems or experiences with the health care system' (Brundisini et al., 2013, p. 1). The review identified three themes in patients' experiences, described by the researchers as 'geography, availability of health care professionals, and rural culture' (Brundisini et al., 2013, p. 1). The researchers identified that geography may make patients vulnerable to 'referral games':

> Patients may … feel powerless in 'referral games' between rural and urban providers. People with low education or without others to help them may find navigating care more difficult. (Brundisini et al., 2013, p. 1)

The second challenge identified is that rural and remote patients may prefer to receive treatment from local clinicians: '[P]atients like seeing clinicians who have known them for a long time, and like how familiar clinicians treat them as a whole person.' (Brundisini et al., 2013, p. 1). Third, rurality may incline patients to become more self-reliant, and shirk formal services:

> [P]atients may feel like outsiders in city hospitals or clinics. As well, in rural communities, people may share a feeling of self-reliance and community belonging. This may make them more eager to take care of themselves and each other, and less willing to seek distant care. (Brundisini et al., 2013, p. 1)

The theoretical implications of these issues for how health professionals communicate centre on the following issues: how they can overcome the 'tyranny of distance' between themselves and the patient; how they can maintain continuity of care with patients whose care is enacted across different services that may be geographically dispersed and therefore involving very different people; and how they can establish and maintain trust with patients whom they may not encounter very frequently face to face.

Clearly, these challenges place an extra burden on how all those involved in the care for rural and remote patients communicate with one another. Clear inter-service agreements about how rural and remote patients are transferred between the services are critical. Increasingly, these challenges are tackled with the help of e-health resources capable of connecting people across time and space (see Chapter 16).

Conclusion

Achieving effective communication across rural and metropolitan contexts is a complex process. Effective communication links to the particular circumstances and needs of rural and remote communities. That said, rural clinicians need to work within the limitations of the resources available to them and to be aware of when, how and whom to refer to when necessary. Metropolitan clinicians, particularly those in tertiary referral centres, need to be aware of the needs of the rural communities and to provide access and support when required. Communication between the two needs to be respectful of the knowledge and skills within each jurisdiction and the vulnerability of rural patients. The sharing of information, resources and responsibility will ensure safety and reduce inequities for rural patients.

Practice example 4.2   **A patient with a spinal fracture**

This example summarises the story of a patient who suffered a spinal injury in a rural area. It highlights the access and transport issues faced by rural patients seeking specialist care. The patient's story is as follows.

continued ›

Practice example 4.2 continued ›   A 28-year-old male competing in a motocross racing event was injured when falling off his motorbike in a rural area. The patient was transported to a metropolitan tertiary trauma referral centre in line with New South Wales Ambulance trauma protocols. He was diagnosed with a fracture of his L2 vertebra and was deemed suitable for management in a thoracic lumbar sacral orthosis (TLSO). As a part of prescription of this brace the patient was required to be fitted with the TLSO in a lying position, and was asked not to sit up without the TLSO in place. He had an uneventful admission and was discharged home after three days.

Three days after discharge the patient's mother contacted the tertiary referral centre, indicating that the brace was broken and was not working correctly. Advice was provided that the patient would need to call an ambulance and request transport to a hospital for investigation and repair of the brace. The patient was transported to the closest facility, a small hospital. The staff there were not able to assist the patient as no one was skilled or confident in fitting or managing TLSOs. After several phone calls from the rural facility to the tertiary centre everyone agreed that the only solution was for the patient to be transported to the tertiary referral centre for management. This would involve bypassing two larger and closer hospitals, which were also not considered capable of assisting the patient. After being informed of a wait of several hours for transport and likely overnight admission before transport would become available, the patient and family made a decision to tape the brace together (and accept the risks associated with this) and to drive the three hours to the tertiary referral centre.

Upon arrival at the tertiary facility a 20-minute consultation at the facility was able to rectify the issue and repair the brace. The issue was the trivial loosening of a small support post in the brace; this would have been easily correctable at any facility if appropriate training, communication methods and support had been available.

Reflective questions

1. Why can't more neurosurgeons and physiotherapists be employed at small community and district hospitals to combat the problems encountered in practice example 4.2?
2. How do you think the transport issues encountered in this scenario might be improved?
3. Why do you think staff in the community and rural referral hospital were not able to figure out the problem with the brace?
4. Imagine you are working in the emergency department at a small rural hospital when a patient with a spinal injury arrives. What would you need to know to care for the patient? How would you feel about treating them?
5. Research the digital radiology system known as the Picture Archiving Computer System (PACS). How could PACS have assisted the patient in practice example 4.2? How could other telehealth initiatives or other communication strategies be utilised to prevent this type of situation arising again?

Further reading

Bourke, L., Waite, C., & Wright, J. (2014). Mentoring as a retention strategy to sustain the rural and remote health workforce. *Australian Journal of Rural Health 22*(1) 2–7.
The article proposes mentoring as a successful workforce retention strategy in rural and remote health services. It reports on the facilitators and barriers to mentoring in rural and remote areas.

Paliadelis, P. S., Parmenter, G., Parker, V., Giles, M., & Higgins, I. (2012). The challenges confronting clinicians in rural acute care settings: A participatory research project. *Rural and Remote Health, 12*. http://www.rrh.org.au/articles/subviewaust.asp?ArticleID=2017.
Rural clinicians experience challenges that are both similar and different to metropolitan clinicians. The article highlights the unique challenges experienced by rural clinicians as well as the innovative solutions implemented by them.

Parker, V., McNeill, K., Mitchell, R., Higgins, I., Paliadelis, P., Giles, M., & Parmenter, G. (2013). How health professionals conceive and construct interprofessional practice in rural settings: A qualitative study. *BMC Health Services Research, 13*, 500. doi:10.1186/1472-6963-13-500
This study finds that there are several unique factors that affect interprofessional practice (IPP) in rural areas, including recognition of the benefits of IPP, funding to support IPP, proximity to services, and workforce resources.

Rowe, C., Campbell, I., & Hargrave, L. (2014). Rural experience for junior doctors: Is it time to make it mandatory? *Australian Journal of Rural Health, 22*(2), 63–67.
This research determines whether rural practice terms for junior doctors result in increased interest in rural practice and whether these terms improve learning experiences, clinical skills and insight into difficulties of rural practice.

Russell, D., Humphreys, J., Ward, B., Chisholm, M., Buykx, P., McGrail, M. et al. (2013). Helping policy-makers address rural health access problems. *Australian Journal of Rural Health, 21*(2), 61–71.
This paper presents a framework that assists policy-makers to evaluate how well policy targets access to health services in rural and remote areas. The authors argue that in order for policies to be effective they need to incorporate the access issues experienced by rural and remote Australians.

Web resources

Australian Government Department of Health, *Doctor connect*: http://www.doctorconnect. gov.au/internet/otd/publishing.nsf/Content/locator
Australian Government Department of Health, *Telehealth*:
http://www.health.gov.au/internet/main/publishing.nsf/Content/e-health-telehealth
Australian Journal of Rural Health: http://ruralhealth.org.au/ajrh
Australian Rural Health Education Network: http://www.arhen.org.au
Health Education and Training Institute (HETI), *Rural and Remote*: http://www.heti.nsw.gov. au/rural-and-remote

NSW Health, *Rural Health*: http://www.health.nsw.gov.au/rural/pages/default.aspx
Rural Health Research Gateway (US): http://www.ruralhealthresearch.org

References

Australian Bureau of Statistics (ABS). (2010). *Regional population growth, Australia, 2008–09.*
    Cat no: 3218.0. Retrieved from http://www.abs.gov.au/ausstats

—— . (2011). *2011 Australian statistical geography standard: Remoteness structure*, map,
    Cat. no: 1270.0.55.005. Retrieved from February 5, 2015 from http://www.ausstats.
    abs.gov.au/ausstats/subscriber.nsf/0/A277D01B6AF25F64CA257B03000D7EED/$F
    ile/1270055005_july%202011.pdf

Australian Institute of Health and Welfare (AIHW). (2014). *Australia's Health 2014*. Australia's
    Health Series no. 14. Cat. no. AUS 178. Canberra: Author.

Brundisini, F., Giacomini, M., DeJean, D., Vanstone, M., Winsor, S., & Smith, A. (2013). Chronic
    disease patients' experiences with accessing health care in rural and remote areas: A
    systematic review and qualitative meta-synthesis. *Ont Health Technol Assess Ser, 13*(15),1–
    33. Retrieved January 29, 2015 from http://www.hqontario.ca/en/documents/eds/2013/
    full-report-OCDM-rural-health-care.pdf

Commonwealth of Australia. (2012). *National Strategic Framework for Rural and Remote
    Health.* Retrieved January 29, 2015 from http://www.ruralhealthaustralia.gov.au/internet/
    rha/publishing.nsf/Content/NSFRRH-homepage

Laurence, C., Coombs, M., Bell, J., & Black, L. (2014). Financial costs for teaching in rural and
    urban Australian general practices: Is there a difference? *Aust J Rural Health, 22*(2), 68–74.

McNeil, K., Mitchell, R., & Parker, V. (2014). The paradoxical effects of workforce shortages on
    rural interprofessional practice. *Scand J Caring Sci.* doi:10.1111/scs.12129

National Rural Health Alliance (NRHA), & Australian Council of Social Services (ACOSS).
    (2013). *Joint report: A snapshot of poverty in rural and regional Australia.* Retrieved from
    http://ruralhealth.org.au/documents/publicseminars/2013_Sep/Joint-report.pdf

NSW Agency for Clinical Innovation. (2014a). High risk maternal foetal outreach clinic in
    Moree. Retrieved January 25, 2015 from http://www.aci.health.nsw.gov.au/ie/projects/
    hrm-moree.

—— . (2014b). Murrumbidgee local health district enhanced scope of practice model of care.
    Retrieved January 25, 2015 from http://www.aci.health.nsw.gov.au/ie/projects/enhanced-
    scope-of-practice

NSW Health. (2011). *Care coordination: From admission to transfer of care in NSW public
    hospitals – reference manual.* North Sydney: NSW Health, Centre for Health Advancement.

Rowe, C., Campbell, I., & Hargrave, L. (2014). Rural experience for junior doctors: Is it time to
    make it mandatory? *Aust J Rural Health, 22*(2), 63–67.

Rural Doctors Network. (n.d.). Health outreach services. Retrieved January 25, 2015 from
    http://www.nswrdn.com.au/site/outreach

Samera, L. (2014). Rural patients travel for health care. *MJA, 201*(10), 566. doi:10.5694/
    mja14.01195

5

Communicating in emergency care

Marie Manidis

Learning objectives

This chapter[1] will enable you to:
- define key factors that impact on ED communication;
- describe typical kinds of communication between ED clinicians and patients;
- explain how to communicate with ED patients without making ED care appear fragmented and lacking in logic;
- determine information needs, and respond to emotional as well as clinical cues.

Key terms

Disposition
History-taking
Interprofessional communication
Triage

Overview

This chapter delves into the specific communication challenges and practices of practitioners in emergency departments (EDs). The chapter alerts you to how communication is structured and affected by the rapidity of ED care and the limited time that patients spend in the ED, the space layout of EDs, the equipment used in the ED, and the different disciplinary tasks and responsibilities of ED practitioners. The chapter examines how these factors can conspire to *fragment* knowledge about patients. That is, ED work requires repeated questioning and checking by practitioners as they care for their patients.

The chapter further addresses how emergency care clinicians communicate with patients and how they communicate with colleagues. Thus, emergency care clinicians talk to a diverse range of patients who are often seriously ill or injured often without comprehensive information to assist the making of decisions. As well, emergency care clinicians talk to a range of practitioners with different training backgrounds and care perspectives. To draw these issues out, the chapter presents vignettes of actual encounters in the ED between clinicians and patients. In doing so, the chapter identifies some key learning and reflection items for you.

Introduction

The ED has a variety of purposes: acute medical assessment and treatment involving multidisciplinary healthcare practices, as well as tertiary training and liaising with referral sites, with some services linked to community health facilities. Many EDs in city locations are part of tertiary referral hospitals,[2] and are seen and used as training sites for junior doctors and nurses.

ED clinicians include many part-time and full-time healthcare workers, including social workers, physiotherapists, diabetes educators, dieticians, occupational therapists, pharmacists, radiographers and radiation scientists, sonographers, and so on. This wide variety of staff is compounded by other factors, such as the emergency focus of the care provided, the training requirements of junior clinicians, staff shortages, constant interruptions to care tasks (Coiera et al., 2002), and frequent shift changeovers, as well as interprofessional and interdepartmental rivalries (Nugus, 2009). A key way of managing this complexity is through face-to-face talking, including at clinical handovers, a key communication activity in the ED.

Clinical handover is a process involving the passing on of information and responsibility to the next clinician. Formal clinical handovers are conducted at shift changes, when a staff member leaves the ED (for lunch, a toilet break, and so on), when the patient arrives by ambulance, or when a patient is handed over to a ward. Handovers are usually verbal, and should be accompanied by the patient's notes or written documentation (Australian Commission on Safety and Quality in Health Care, 2010). There are also multiple other instances when practitioners hand over to colleagues informally, or when they just discuss patient-related issues 'in passing'.

Recent research has focused on the vulnerabilities of the formal handover process (Cohen & Hilligoss, 2010). Some studies have suggested improvements to the way that doctors and nurses do handovers by asking more questions, clarifying issues, and generally making the handover more interactive or 'dialogic' (Ye et al., 2007). Other studies have shown that those engaged in handovers may be able to standardise their communication to suit their own contexts (Iedema & Ball, 2010). A major report in 2008 in New South Wales suggested locating handovers at patients' bedsides with nurses and doctors present to facilitate both their own and patients' involvement (Garling, 2008).

Other more recent research suggests that the handover might be considered as one aspect only in negotiating patient information and care responsibility. In practice, practitioners communicate almost constantly about their patients and responsibilities (Manidis, 2013; Manidis, Iedema & Scheeres, 2012). Among other things, this communication involves asking the patient again and again why they are there, whether they are allergic to anything or in pain, and so on. These repetitions may become tiring for the patient and suggest a lack of care continuity and an absence of team collaboration. Unfortunately, this repetitiveness is necessary and integral to how ED clinicians do their work and keep up with changing circumstances.

Practice example 5.1[3]

N4:	G'day [to D1].
D1:	G'day Elizabeth, my name's Fred.
P:	Elizabeth.
D1:	I'm one of the doctors.
P:	Alan [N4's name], Fred, I'm learning.
N4:	You are.
D1:	What's been going on?
P:	Ooh oh everything.
D1:	OK.
P:	Ah.
D1:	In particular?
P:	Well, the oxygen drop is was what Dr D was worried about. And, oh, coughing and I have been a smoker, I'm not denying it. But ever since [chuckles] I had the Vibramycin[4] ...
D1:	Yeah.
P:	... I've ... it seems to have got rid of everything in the nose and my mouth and my lungs, coughing stuff up, but I'm not having – not coughing enough up. I can't seem ...
D1:	OK
P:	To get it up, so. There's something obviously – I need a bomb under me.
D1:	Sure. Besides the trouble with the breathing, like not being able to get your breath, what are the other problems? Sort of have you got no energy, have you had temperatures?
P:	No.
D1:	Sweats?
P:	Ah, well the last couple of nights I've had night sweats.
D1:	OK.
P:	Very sweaty.

continued ›

Practice example 5.1 continued ›

D1:　Yup.

P:　And, um, I've been too tired to get out of bed and I was nearly gonna get out and have a shower, then I thought 'no, I'll get a chill'.

D1:　OK.

N4:　Ssh.

N4 tells D1 to be quiet and also holds up his hand as he does the ECG reading.

Later in the consultation D1 has trouble getting Elizabeth's cannula in and he arranges for a more senior clinician to do this for him. This break in the **history-taking** means that by the time he returns to Elizabeth much later on he needs to go over her history again as he admits he has 'probably' forgotten what she told him earlier. He also admits to being confused about her symptoms because he has another patient on the day with a similar condition to hers.

D1:　But did you say that – I'm just trying – I'm getting my patients mixed up – you – you feel like there's more in there than what you're able to get up …

After this, D1 takes up the conversation again completing the history-taking by asking what medications Elizabeth is on, etc. D1 tells Elizabeth he will proceed with a chest X-ray, have a look at her chest, take some blood and do a few other tests. He informs her he will also ask her to do a spirometry test which she is very reluctant to do.

Analysis and reflection

During Elizabeth's stay in the ED, five nurses and two doctors (one junior) care for her. Nurse Peter (N2) is the third clinician Elizabeth engages with, having already spent time with Nurse 1, the **triage** nurse, and the paramedics. Elizabeth will still need to talk to several other practitioners, including five more nurses, two doctors, one registrar and several radiography staff before she leaves the ED.

The structure of how ED clinicians engage with Elizabeth appears similar to that of the common patient consultation (Roter, 2000). However, a key difference between the common consultation and the ED consultation is that in the ED patients engage with multiple practitioners, often in rapid succession. This means that ED consultations (if that is the right term), instead of taking place in a quiet office and with the benefit of additional equipment – a computer, phone, printer, and so forth – take place in a very busy environment where colleagues are dispersed and constantly moving

history-taking
the process of questioning and observation that a practitioner undertakes to establish what has happened to, or what is wrong with a patient.

triage
the process of assessing and sorting patients' illnesses and/or injuries in terms of acuity and urgency, usually undertaken by a nurse at the front desk of an emergency department. The triage category indicates the urgency of the patient's need for medical and nursing care.

(collecting or replacing equipment, rotating between patients), and where noise – loud voices, beepers and overhead announcements – continually interrupt conversations.

As N2 leaves Elizabeth to collect an armband, we note that this is typical of what happens in an ED consultation. When he returns to her bedside, however, he repeats his earlier questions almost exactly as he asked them before, signalling (unintentionally) to Elizabeth that he approaches her not as a person, but instead acts out 'protocol-based' routine to information-gathering. Finally, when N2 addresses Elizabeth as 'Lizzie', this suggests quite a high level of familiarity, which may not have been appropriate.

Reflective questions

1. Why do you think N2 asks Elizabeth's date of birth and full name (twice over) even though they are already written on the medical record?
2. Can you think of a way N2 might check these details differently, especially the way he repeats his questions verbatim (in full)?
3. What effect would the shortened version of Elizabeth's name have on her?
4. Would this affect you if you (or someone you know well) were the patient?
5. What clinical protocols are evident in this practice example?
6. In the conversation transcript, how could N4 and D1 have communicated more effectively with each other?
7. How will D1's questions to Elizabeth assist him to understand Elizabeth's condition better than what is in her triage notes or in the GP's letter, or what the triage nurse has told him in a handover?
8. How could D1 speak to Elizabeth and show her that he understands Elizabeth has already spent well over an hour in the ED and has told the triage nurse and N2 what her symptoms are?
9. How does D1 take Elizabeth's existing knowledge into account when he communicates with her? When he returns later to her in the consultation, how could he have avoided telling Elizabeth that he was confused about her symptoms and had forgotten her history?

Implications for practice

In the above exchange, as in many others, Elizabeth's practitioners are interrupted in what they are doing (Coiera et al., 2002; Manidis, 2013). To add to this, her clinicians face a number of other challenges. In Elizabeth's case, D1's challenges include confusion between her symptoms and another patient's, and an inability to insert a cannula. N2's challenges are missing equipment (the armband) and his novice status. For all clinicians, communicating in the ED environment can be very complex.

Despite this complexity, it is critical that clinicians forge continuity of care for the patient. Continuity of care is generally understood as the key to safe and high-quality care. Practice example 5.1 illustrates that continuity of care should not be thought of as just created through clinical handover. Instead, continuity arises from a combination of (1) a clinical handover (as a first stage), (2) effective **interprofessional communication**, and (3) iterative questioning of the patient to ensure the patient's situation has not changed significantly, and the same knowledge still obtains (Manidis, Iedema & Scheeres, 2012).

> **interprofessional communication**
> how professionals from different professional backgrounds communicate with one another.

What is further important from Elizabeth's example above is that when patients like her are re-questioned, nurses and doctors should make clear to their patients why they are repeatedly asking the same questions. For example, N2 could have explained *why* he was asking Elizabeth for her name and date of birth again. *He* knew why he was doing it, but Elizabeth didn't. For her, the repeated questions were most likely confusing and even alienating. The nurse's focus therefore was on his protocols and not on what Elizabeth might be experiencing as the patient. Similarly, having to re-ask her history, D1's focus is on checking his facts *anew with Elizabeth* rather than before he gets to her. On the one hand, asking her again reminds him of her case details, but he does so by saying he has 'probably forgotten half of it'. His requestioning puts an additional burden on Elizabeth, who has to answer the same questions once more, and signals poor continuity of care to her as D1 is not making links to earlier responses she has given.

Theoretical links

As noted earlier, talking is the quickest and most reliable way of communicating critical patient information in the ED, given the complexity of patients and the speed of care developments (Ayatollahi, Bath & Goodacre, 2013; Eisenberg et al., 2005; Manidis, 2013; Nugus, 2007). Work in the ED requires fast thinking, frequent checking, and constant vigilance by ED practitioners. ED models of care tend to be designed as though care consists of a staged and linear flow of activities (as envisaged in Figure 5.1).

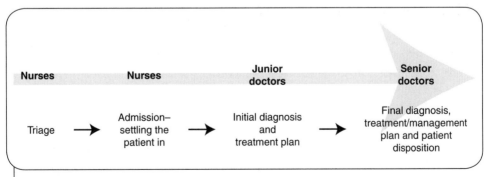

Figure 5.1 The stages of care in the ED (Manidis, 2013, p. 93) based on McGregor et al. (2010)

In practice, however, these stages overlap significantly as clinicians are constantly having to re-establish the most up-to-date state of affairs. What confounds this effort at re-establishing what is current are the high number of rotating and novice staff, staff shortages, frequently missing equipment, and staff and patient mobility. For these reasons, each new clinician's visit to the patient's bedside tends to begin as a new encounter: they often cover old ground, seek the same information, such as whether or not the patient has allergies, or whether they are in pain. Some nurses or doctors refer to earlier discussions with other practitioners or with the patient themselves, but many also forget what has gone before (Manidis, 2013).

This repetitive communication work and the frequent errors that thereby can and do occur confirm that patients play a significant role in their own care. They correct clinicians' use of their names, they repeat symptoms, and they even inform clinicians about what their colleagues (and even they themselves) have already done for the patient! Patients, however, cannot and should not always be relied on to be lucid, consistent, or well enough to ensure their own safety and continuity of care.

Conclusion

As a novice ED practitioner, particularly as a junior doctor or a junior staff nurse, you will need to learn rapidly how to manage the challenges of working with very sick and injured patients and with diverse disciplinary colleagues. Communicating with patients (repetitively if necessary) and learning to rely on colleagues and team members are your best resources for keeping patients safe in what is a noisy, distracting and often confusing work environment (Eisenberg et al., 2005; Nugus, 2007). Expert clinicians are able to gather, remember and relocate information in this chaotic environment. They are able to weave together caring for multiple patients, speaking to multiple colleagues, and keeping people safe in spite of the constantly shifting circumstances that perturb what they know and do. Most importantly they understand the need to cooperate with their colleagues.

Practice example 5.2[5]

Here we examine what happens to Jerry,[6] a 67-year-old palliative care patient with metastasised cancer in his leg, originating from kidney cancer. Jill, Jerry's wife, a former nurse, accompanies him to the ED. We find out during the consultation that Jill has been carefully recording a detailed history of Jerry's entire, very serious illness for a number of years.

When he first arrives in the ED, the paramedics need to move Jerry onto his bed. The triage nurse establishes that Jerry feels pain only on movement but feels none while he is lying still. The paramedic explains to Jerry how they will move him over on to the

continued ›

Practice example 5.2 continued ›

bed, but soon they decide they need *another pair of hands* and they call off the floor Nurse Janita (N2), who agrees to help. She is busy and has to quickly complete another task. As N2 enters the room to assist in moving Jerry, she brushes aside attempts by the paramedics to alert her to the likelihood of causing Jerry pain if he is not moved very carefully.

P: [Jerry yells out in pain]
Z1:   Yeah.
Z2:   Very painful yeah so [...]
N2:   Sorry darling, um.
Z2:   We'll make sure that it goes with you.
P: No, don't you move that leg.
N: What are we – what are we looking after you fallen (over) or what?
Z2:   No no he's got CA of the bone.
N2:   Oh, OK.
Z2:   And he's had a rod put in, it's quite painful.
P: You're about to grab that and just jerk it,
N2:   I'm – I'm – I.
P: And I'm going to scream if you do.

The paramedics end up explaining Jerry's fragility to N2 *post facto* and Jerry himself resorts to threats of screaming if she tries to move his leg again. Her visit to his bedside is one of many – scheduled and unscheduled – that take place throughout his consultation. Jerry's doctors and nurses visit (and revisit) his bedside on 39 separate occasions – Doctor Surita (D1) undertakes six visits and the nurses 22. On many occasions, gaps in knowledge about Jerry, such as illustrated above, are evident. Handover details, even discussions with Jerry (such as when he tells them his preferred name) are later forgotten, confused, ignored, (mis)understood and/or utilised idiosyncratically. Managing the network of care requires recognising the complexity of the multiple clinicians and artefacts involved in Jerry's care, as shown in Figure 5.2, and accordingly communicating proactively with colleagues.

This complexity goes beyond the here and now of Jerry's consultation, reaching to his GP, his previous hospital, his palliative care team and so on. Figure 5.2 illustrates that during the consultation itself, there are more interactions between D1 and one staff nurse, and there are also several handovers between them, the triage nurse, the radiographer and the orderlies. When nurses or doctors take a break, when shifts change, when Jerry's notes are relocated or delayed from his previous hospital, when his nurses and doctors are interrupted or when they are called away by other emergencies, the remaining clinicians must work hard to check Jerry's progress and what has been done, or what has happened to him in the interim. As stated earlier, Jerry's nurses and the junior doctor tend to

continued ›

Practice example 5.2 continued ›

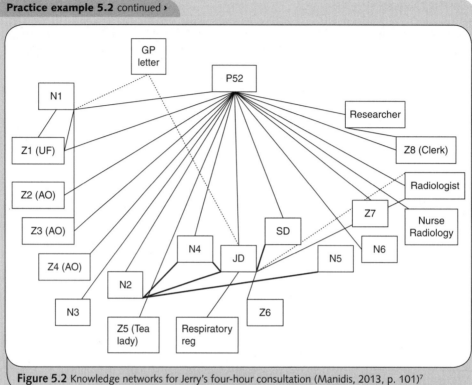

Figure 5.2 Knowledge networks for Jerry's four-hour consultation (Manidis, 2013, p. 101)[7]

consequently rely heavily on Jerry (and Jill), rather than on the notes, handovers and each other, to refresh what they need to know.

Reflective questions

1. What aspects of the time pressures in ED care are revealed in practice example 5.2?
2. What could Nurse Janita (N2) have done differently to avoid hurting Jerry?
3. How difficult would it have been for Jerry to intervene in his own care – telling Nurse Janita (N2): 'No don't you move that leg … You're about to grab that and just jerk it … And I'm going to scream if you do'?
4. Describe your own or a family member's visit to an ED. What changes to the communication, if any, would you propose?

Further reading

Apker, J., Mallak, L., & Gibson, S. (2007). Communicating in the 'gray zone': Perceptions about emergency physician-hospitalist handoffs and patient safety. *Academic Emergency Medicine, 14*(10), 884–894.

This study investigates the communication practices and issues of clinical handover in EDs by interviewing ED practitioners. Handoffs are identified as problematic with insufficient information, incomplete data and omissions that can have adverse impacts on patient safety and outcomes.

Athlin, A. M., von Thiele Schwarz, U., & Farrohknia, N. (2013). Effects of multidisciplinary teamwork on lead times and patient flow in the emergency department: A longitudinal interventional cohort study. *Scandinavian Journal of Trauma, Resuscitation and Emergency Medicine, 21*, 76. doi:10.1186/1757-7241-21-76

This reports a Swedish study undertaken on the assumption that overcrowding in EDs and non-effective working routines create longer waiting times for emergency care. When the study was undertaken, teamwork was seen as the solution to these issues.

Ayatollahi, H., Bath, P. A., & Goodacre, S. (2013). Information needs of clinicians and non-clinicians in the emergency department: A qualitative study. *Health Information and Libraries Journal, 30*(3), 191–200.

This study seeks to identify the information needs of ED staff and investigate where they obtained their information. The study identifies that patient information is the most important information they require and verbal communication is most frequently used. The researchers conclude that technology could not be considered as a simple solution to information needs in the ED.

Fairbanks, R. J., Bisantz, A. M., & Sunm, M. (2007). Emergency department communication: Links and patterns. *Annals of Emergency Medicine, 50*(4), 396–406.

This article reports on research in paediatric and adult acute care, showing that practitioners enage in approximately 42 communication events per hour with a third of these being interruptions. The authors conclude that face-to-face communication is the predominant mode of communication in the ED.

Web resources

Australasian College for Emergency Medicine (ACEM): http://www.acem.org.au
Australian Commission for Safety and Quality in Healthcare: http://www.safetyandquality.gov. au/search/Clinical+handover
Australian Institute of Health and Welfare. (2013). *Australian hospital statistics 2013–13: Emergency department care*, Canberra: Author. http://www.aihw.gov.au/workarea/ downloadasset.aspx?id=60129544764
Emergency Medicine Australasia: http://www.acem.org.au/Standards-Publications/EMA.aspx

References

Australian Commission on Safety and Quality in Health Care. (2010). *Reporting for safety: Use of hospital data to monitor and improve patient safety: Windows into safety and quality.* Sydney: Author.
Ayatollahi, H., Bath, P. A., & Goodacre, S. (2013). Information needs of clinicians and non-clinicians in the emergency department: A qualitative study. *Health Information and Libraries Journal, 30*(3), 191–200.

Cohen, M. D., & Hilligoss, P. B. (2010). The published literature on handoffs in hospitals: Deficiencies identified in an extensive review. *Quality and Safety in Health Care, 19*(6), 493–497.

Coiera, E. W., Jayasuriya, R. A., Hardy, J., Bannan, A., & Thorpe, M. E. C. (2002). Communication loads on clinical staff in the emergency department. *Medical Journal of Australia, 176*(9), 415–418.

Eisenberg, E. M., Murphy, A. G., Sutcliffe, K., Wears, R., Schenkel, S., Perry, S., & Vanderhoef, M. (2005). Communication in emergency medicine: Implications for patient safety. *Communication Monographs, 72*(4), 390–413.

Garling, P. (2008). *Final report of the Special Commission of Inquiry: Acute care in NSW public hospitals, 2008 – Overview.* NSW Department of Health. Retrieved from http://www.lawlink.nsw.gov.au/lawlink/Special_Projects/ll_splprojects.nsf/pages/acsi_index

Iedema, R., & Ball, C. (2010). *NSW ambulance emergency department handover project report.* Sydney: NSW Health & University of Technology, Centre for Health Communication.

Iedema, R., & Manidis, M. (2013). *Patient-clinician communication: An overview of relevant research and policy literatures.* Sydney: Australian Commission on Safety and Quality in Health Care and University of Technology, Centre for Health Communication.

Manidis, M. (2013). Practising knowing in emergency departments: Tracing the disciplinary and institutional complexities of working, learning and knowing in modern emergency departments. Unpublished doctoral thesis, University of Technology, Sydney.

Manidis, M., Iedema, R., & Scheeres, H. (2012). Information Transfer in ERs. *Focus on Patient Safety, 15,* 2–4, 6.

Nugus, P. (2007) The organisational world of emergency clinicians. Unpublished doctoral thesis, University of New South Wales, Sydney.

——. (2009). Selling patients. *British Medical Journal, 339,* b5201.

Roter, D. (2000). The enduring and evolving nature of the patient-physician relationship. *Patient Education and Counselling, 39,* 5–15.

Ye, K., Taylor, D.M., Knott, J. C., Dent, A., & MacBean, C. E. (2007). Handover in the emergency department: Deficiencies and adverse effects. *Emergency Medicine Australia, 19,* 433–441.

Notes

1 Parts of this chapter draw on material published in a report, *Patient–clinician communication: An overview of relevant research and policy literatures* (2013). The report was commissioned by the Australian Commission on Safety and Quality in Health Care and prepared by University of Technology, Sydney, Centre for Health Communication.

2 Hospitals linked to universities and therefore to the training of doctors, nurses and other allied health workers

3 Patient dialogue reproduced from Iedema and Manidis's 2013 commission report, *Patient–clinician communication: An overview of relevant research and policy literatures.*

4 Brand name for an antibiotic

5 Patient dialogue reproduced from Manidis's 2013 doctoral thesis, 'Practising knowing in emergency departments: Tracing the disciplinary and institutional complexities of working, learning and knowing in modern emergency departments'.

6 Not his real name

7 Legend: N1–N6 = staff nurses; Z1–Z8 = non-clinical and paramedic staff (e.g. AO = ambulance officer); JD = junior doctor; SD = senior doctor

Communicating in intensive care

K.J. Farley, Gerard J. Fennessy and Daryl Jones

Learning objectives

This chapter will enable you to:
- communicate when your patients are critically ill;
- convey bad news to families, and discuss death and dying;
- negotiate plans under difficult circumstances with patients and families;
- navigate relationships with members of the multidisciplinary healthcare team.

Key terms

Acceptance
Critically ill
Depression
Empathy
Family meetings
Grief
Intensive care
Multidisciplinary healthcare team

Overview

This chapter introduces you to how to communicate when patients are **critically ill**. The chapter addresses how communication in the intensive care unit (ICU) frequently includes conveying bad news to families, and discussing death and dying, and outlines how to run a successful ICU

> **critically ill**
> in such a state of health as to need ongoing medical and nursing attention, and likely to rely on medical technologies.

family meeting or 'family conference'. It describes difficulties in using family members as surrogate decision-makers, and explains how the emotions described by the Kübler-Ross model of **grief** affect families of critically ill patients.

As ICU patients are frequently too ill to communicate, ICU treatment involves making many clinical decisions without direct communication with the patients themselves. As these decisions often have to be made within significant time constraints, it is important to have a method to accurately and sensitively communicate with patients (if possible), their families, and other healthcare professionals.

grief
the sorrowful feelings experienced when our loved ones suffer or die.

family meetings
meetings between clinicians and family members of the patient. These meetings take place when the patient is not able (due to being unconscious or delirious) to contribute to discussions about the patient's future care plans.

multidisciplinary healthcare team
a team that is made up of members whose professional backgrounds are different – for example, a team made up of doctors from different specialties, or a team consisting of a nurse, allied health professional, doctor and social worker.

Family meetings can be made more effective by simple measures, including arranging the physical environment, adopting a structured communication approach to counterbalance the at times unpredictable aspects of difficult discussions, inviting the right people, minimising interruptions, and using silence and time judiciously to ensure everyone remains 'on the same page'.

Having a critically ill family member in the ICU is highly stressful and difficult, even when the patient survives. Families commonly experience several stages of grief, as described by Kübler-Ross (Kübler-Ross, 1969). These stages tend to shape the ways in which family members communicate, their ability to comprehend or retain information given to them, and the communication styles to which they respond best.

Communication with patients and staff is a core skill for everyone who works in the ICU. Every day, there are various challenges, not least because ICU patients are always very ill. These challenges range from negotiating plans under difficult circumstances with patients and families, to the less obvious but equally important challenge of navigating relationships with members of the **multidisciplinary healthcare team**.

The ICU is a highly emotionally charged environment, primed for miscommunication. However, with careful planning and a structured approach, conflict can generally be avoided. The practice example cases contained in this chapter outline common ICU communication themes by giving instances of good and poor communication in the context of care of the critically ill.

We describe a standardised approach to family meetings to manage the practical and emotional dimensions of difficult discussions. We also discuss the framing of grief experienced by family members in terms of the Kübler-Ross model. Finally, we outline a number of ways to avoid family and patient discussion going poorly.

Family meetings and using the family as surrogates

The process of discussing the situation and options available to critically ill patients usually involves meetings with families. Such meetings can be informal or formal, and may be

continued ›

continued ›

few or many. Where possible it is important to communicate progress and treatment options to the patient but, as patients are frequently unable to communicate, this may not be possible. It is then necessary to conduct discussions with family members who act as surrogate decision-makers for the patient. Using a family member as a surrogate decision-maker may be extraordinarily difficult for families. This is particularly true when they are unsure of the patient's treatment preferences, or when they may harbour guilt or anger over the patient's illness situation (Curtis & Rubenfeld, 2001).

Introduction

By its very nature, the ICU is a place where patients are often very ill, and may die or develop severe disability. For patients and families alike, being admitted to ICU is literally life changing. In order to deliver the best care, and to avoid potentially negative experiences, clear and effective communication should be a high priority for ICU clinicians. Communication is a learned skill and one in which we should be mentored (Iedema et al., 2004).

Communication between patients and staff in ICU is a core part of the job of all healthcare professionals working in this area. On a daily basis, ICU staff encounter communication challenges, including both doctor–nurse–patient–family relationships and communication with healthcare professionals from other disciplines who have their patients admitted to ICU.

The nature and severity of illnesses and the types of treatments provided in the ICU make communication in this environment different from communication in other medical environments. In ICU, clinicians face patients' limited ability to communicate, they are in a busy physical environment, there is the urgency of ICU care, and there is a lot of involvement from other specialties and disciplines from outside the ICU.

Patients' limited ability to communicate

Due to many factors, including severity of illness, delirium, sedating medications or breathing tubes, the patient is unlikely to be able to meaningfully participate in conversations or decision-making regarding their health or treatment choices. Communication therefore frequently involves surrogate decision-makers and may not directly involve the patient at all. For the same reasons, the patient may never have the opportunity to express their wishes or treatment goals. Decisions must be made by others, guided by assumed knowledge of 'what the patient would have wanted', and what is medically appropriate.

Busy physical environment

The ICU is an environment characterised by noise, light and activity 24 hours a day. Cubicles may be separated only by curtains, reducing privacy and allowing nearby conversations to be heard easily. The ICU staff may also have multiple competing demands on their time, including family meetings, assessing new patients, urgent procedures and unexpected emergencies. The ICU is thus not conducive to calm and private communication, and a deliberate effort needs to be made to try to alleviate this.

Urgency of care

In the setting where there is frequent rapid deterioration in the patient's clinical state (for example, bleeding requiring an operation), life-changing decisions must be taken very rapidly, with little time for comprehensive communication with families or outside staff.

Multidisciplinary involvement

In the ICU there are often a larger number of interested parties to any decision or conversation than would be usual in the general ward setting. These may include ICU medical and nursing staff, 'patient unit' medical staff (that is, medical staff from specialties where the patient might have been originally admitted, before becoming so ill as to require transition into the ICU), allied health staff, social workers, and family members who may wish to be involved in serious decision-making. 'Multi-party negotiations' require different communication techniques from the 'two-way' communication between the parent unit and the patient in the general wards or outpatient clinics.

depression
a doubting of self-worth, and experiencing feelings of dejection and despondency.

acceptance
resigning yourself to an outcome, situation or decision.

All of these factors – patients' limited ability to communicate, busy physical environment, the urgency of care, and multidisciplinary involvement – mean that consideration and attention to every aspect of communication is needed to avoid misunderstandings, conflict, and potentially poorer outcomes for patients. This can be achieved by careful planning of family meetings, helping grieving families by understanding the Kübler-Ross grief stages, and addressing the potential for staff miscommunication both within and outside the ICU.

Kübler-Ross model of grief as it applies to families

The five stages of grief proposed by Kübler-Ross are denial, anger, bargaining, **depression** and **acceptance** (Kübler-Ross, 1969). These affect families as well as patients, and strategies can be developed to guide the family through their grieving process. Although the stages are not meant to be an exhaustive list of emotions, they may encompass the main grief journey experienced by most family members during and after a catastrophic illness. Importantly, the stages may not be sequential and in fact may not be experienced by all people. There is dispute as to whether these stages apply to families of loved ones (Freidman & James, 2008), but it is a useful framework to begin our understanding of grief.

The practice example cases contained in this chapter outline common issues faced by clinicians working in ICU, with instances of good and poor communication, in the context of care of the critically ill.

Practice example 6.1

You are called to the emergency department to see Mr Bill James, a 78-year-old man with multiple co-morbidities who now has a perforated bowel. Even in a healthy person this condition is associated with considerable morbidity, but with his extensive medical history there are only limited options available. The surgical and anaesthetic teams are reluctant to operate as they feel this would be futile. Mr James is too unwell to participate in the meeting, so you decide to discuss the treatment options and appropriateness of **intensive care** support with his wife and daughter.

> **intensive care**
> an area of the hospital where patients who are critically ill are treated, and therefore needing ongoing attention and often several technologies to keep them alive.

Doctor: Hi, my name is Dr Francis. I am one of the doctors from the intensive care team, and this is Brendan, one of the nurses caring for Mr James. Before we start, is it possible to go round and introduce yourselves?

Wife: Hi I'm Eileen, Bill's wife.

Daughter: And I'm Lucy, Bill's my dad.

Doctor: Thanks for that, Eileen and Lucy. As I mentioned, I am one of the doctors from intensive care. We have been asked to see Bill, because as you probably realise, he is very unwell.

Wife: Thank you. Yes, we realise that he is really sick. I am really concerned about him. We can't even understand what he is saying to us right now.

continued ›

Doctor: Yes, we are very worried about him too. Do you think you could tell me a little about Bill and about what you understand of his current situation?

Wife: Well, he's been unwell for some time with the diabetes, and he was in hospital last month with a heart attack. He's only been home a week, and then he got so sick last night. He had really bad stomach pain. I didn't know what to do.

[Pause]

Doctor: (nodding) You did the right thing by bringing him in.

Daughter: Since his first heart attack two years ago, he really hasn't been happy with his life. He can't go out into the garden, he can't take his dog out.

Wife: Yes, he's really not satisfied with what his life is like these days. It's so sad because he used to be so active, and now he can't do anything that he loves. He's had enough.

[Wife begins crying, consoled by daughter, two minutes' silence]

Doctor: I'm sorry he is so unwell. You obviously care for him a great deal.

[Pause, two minutes]

Daughter: So what's going to happen with him now?

Doctor: Well, as I mentioned before, Bill is incredibly ill. From the scans and the blood tests, it appears that he has a hole in his bowel, and this is leaking poo into his abdomen. Unfortunately, because of this, his kidneys have shut down and his heart is needing a lot of medication to keep his blood pressure up.

Wife: Are they wanting to do an operation for the bowel?

Doctor: At this stage, there are very limited treatment options, and I need to talk to you about them. More importantly, we need to discuss what Bill would want under these circumstances.

Wife: I don't want him to go through another operation. He wouldn't want that. He couldn't face the recovery.

Daughter: Yes, I know it sounds terrible, it sounds like we don't love him, but we just don't want him to suffer. He wouldn't want surgery.

[Pause]

Doctor: No. And I can assure you we do not want him to suffer either.

Wife: Please just keep him comfortable. Please make sure he is not in pain.

Doctor: I can assure you he will not suffer. From our conversation, it is clear to me that you understand what Bill's wishes would be. It is clear that he would not want an operation, and the surgeons and I feel that an operation is not the

continued ›

Practice example 6.1 continued ›

> best thing for him. We won't do any operation. We will keep Bill comfortable with as much pain relief as he needs, and make sure he is not suffering at the end of his life.

Wife: (sobbing) Thank you.

[Pause]

Doctor: Do you have any questions or concerns about what we have spoken about?

Analysis and reflection

Practice example 6.1 is an example of a well-planned family meeting, in a difficult and challenging scenario, with an outcome that is patient-centred and acceptable to all parties.

The doctor has been clearly appraised beforehand of the clinical situation, and has consulted with the nursing staff and the surgical and anaesthetic teams about what options would be medically suitable for Bill. He begins by introducing himself, and his role and the other members of the team, before asking for the names and roles of the family members. This shows interest in the family, and thus in the patient.

He then puts forward the proposition that the patient is very sick, and listens attentively to the responses of the family. This allows him to gauge how much understanding the family has about the current situation, and gives them the opportunity to express their views.

He validates their understanding, and then expresses a desire to find out about Bill's life and wishes. From here, the family have an opportunity to give a narrative of the situation they have faced together over the past few weeks, including his recent deterioration in his quality of life and his dissatisfaction with this.

There are periods of deliberate silence (see Chapter 15) to give the family time to grieve and comprehend the gravity of Bill's situation. Once the option of an operation is raised, the family are able to express his wishes with certainty. The doctor is then able to affirm that supporting Bill's wishes is a common goal, and goes further by explicitly stating that comfort is a priority as Bill is at the end of his life. This scenario is helped considerably by the fact that the family have a clear appreciation of Bill's quality of life and what his choices for treatment would be.

Implications for practice

This is a challenging scenario that involves many layers of communication and many potential areas for miscommunication. Talking to family members as surrogates for the

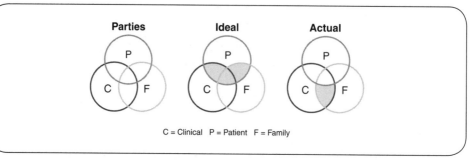

Figure 6.1 Venn diagrams showing ideal versus actual clinical decision-making – when the patient is unable to communicate. (Image credit: Gerard J. Fennessy and Jon X. Chew)

patient is a common way medical treatment decisions are made for patients sick enough to need ICU care, and this may apply at times to other areas of medicine (refer to Figure 6.1).

Relying on family members to be surrogate decision-makers places all parties in a potentially difficult situation. The family may or may not know the patient's treatment choices, or agree between themselves on preferences for care. They may feel distressed by the burden on decision-making or be influenced by religious or personal beliefs that may be at odds with the patient's wishes.

Further, the clinical teams are usually in the early stages of new therapeutic relationships with the patient (as the patient is likely to have been transferred from another specialty). The team needs to make decisions, balancing their medical knowledge, expected prognosis, their interpretations of the 'pre-morbid states' (Bill's illness history), and the patient's prior expressed wishes. Frequently, and unfortunately, the patient has no direct say in their treatment.

Using a structured approach can facilitate most family meetings, although this needs to be flexible enough to adapt to specifics of the family and their way of dealing with what usually is a catastrophic and grief-stricken period of their lives. It is critically important to pay attention to the layout of the meeting room (Figure 6.2).

A key step in any family meeting is to have a pre-meeting with relevant medical parties to clarify the known facts, agree on the messages that will be conveyed, and establish what treatments are suitable to be offered to the patient. This should be followed by the family meeting itself, and then a post-meeting debrief and wrap-up (refer to Table 6.1).

The meeting should start with personal introductions, as it is essential to understand the roles each party is playing and their importance in the decision-making process. Writing down the significant family members' names and roles gives the family acknowledgment of your commitment to engage with them, and ensures you are able to remember this important information.

The next step is to frame the meeting, so that the family understands what the purpose of the meeting is. Although many families will have an appreciation of the gravity of the information about to be conveyed, this is not always the case. A 'warning shot'

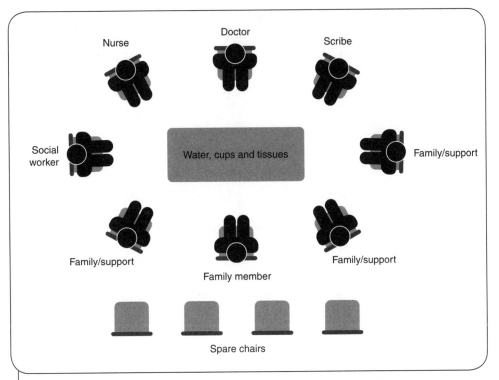

Figure 6.2 Suggested layout and participants for family meetings in ICU, providing an open communication style with room for family members and support people. (Image credit: Gerard J. Fennessy and Jon X. Chew)

indicating that very bad news is about to be delivered may be helpful. Occasionally, the family will bring their own agenda – or agendas! – to the meeting. It is important that everyone's issues are addressed, or that another meeting is scheduled if they are unable to be fully addressed at the time.

Families often go through stages of grief, as described by Kübler-Ross. These include denial, anger, bargaining, depression and acceptance. These may not be sequential, or experienced by everyone, and family members may move through the stages at variable rates such that each family member might be experiencing different stages. There is no formulaic approach to dealing with these stages – they are each situation-specific, and it may be helpful to seek advice from a senior colleague or experienced professional (such as a social worker) if difficulties arise. Recognising the stage of grief each family member is experiencing may help to navigate through some of the more difficult discussions, particularly those involving different views on how to proceed.

Irrespective of family members' stage of grief and differences of opinion, general strategies for good communication in a family meeting include:

- using clear and unambiguous language (for example, saying 'lung cancer' rather than 'a shadow on the lung', or saying 'I think she may die tonight' rather than 'the treatment is not working just yet');

Table 6.1 Family meetings – suggested structure

Stage	Purpose
Pre-meeting	Gather relevant staff (including bedside nurse and/or charge nurse, support people, other medical teams).
	Provide staff with an overview of purpose of meeting, and assess if there are any potential staff issues or family issues beforehand.
Meeting: Introduction	Introductions of people present.
	Overview of the context in which the meeting is being held.
Meeting: Exploration	Find out about the patient and their background.
	Establish the family's understanding of events that have led up to the current illness.
Meeting: Explanations	Explain in lay terms the medical events that have led to the current clinical illness.
	Discuss the potential options that are available, and help direct the family through their grief.
Meeting: Conclusion	Check with the family that they understand what the clinical situation is.
	Reinforce the proposed plan, and check their understanding and acceptance.
	Close the meeting, and consider a plan for further meetings.
Post-meeting	Staff debrief.
	Initiate a plan for any issues brought up during the meeting.
	Document the meeting and decisions.

- allowing enough time for the family to process information – this may require multiple short family meetings separated by hours or even days, rather than one long and complex session where a lot of information is given at once;
- allowing periods of silence, so the family can process what is happening, and feel they have the time to express that which may be difficult to say;
- giving the family frequent opportunities to ask questions or seek clarification;
- acknowledging how the family is feeling and offering support where possible.

Infrequently, there are situations where, despite the use of time, multiple meetings and clear unambiguous language, families or patients will still be in conflict with medical staff. Such situations are some of the most challenging in medicine. There is no perfect way to deal with these situations, and a formulaic approach may indeed be counterproductive. Seek senior assistance as soon as possible in these situations.

It is important to remember that the family has known the patient for the whole of their lives and is intimately entwined with them as a human being. Although medical staff are overwhelmingly non-maleficent, it is sometimes difficult for families to trust that you are an advocate for the patient, rather than an advocate for the unit, the staff, the health system as a whole, and the resources allocated to the ICU. Your relationship with that family may last hours, days or weeks, and there may be repeated admissions, and even 'iatrogenic' (hospital-caused) problems (such as infections and medication errors).

Given the stressful nature of critical illnesses and the fact that one in five patients die in an ICU, it is not surprising that conflict with family sometimes occurs. Indeed, it is surprising it does not happen more often.

In addition to communicating with patients and their relatives, ICU clinicians also need to communicate frequently with other members of the interprofessional team. Nursing staff have a crucial role in the care of patients and their families in the ICU, as they spend a lot of time directly with the family. It is important to ensure there is unified communication with the family to maintain their confidence in the treatments offered.

When there are differing opinions within or between professions – as there will be – it is important that these are addressed in an open, non-threatening way, preferably away from the bedside and family (see Chapter 20). Although many aspects of ICU treatment are ultimately the responsibility of the medical staff, experienced nursing and allied staff are a valuable source of guidance and information on which a clinician can base ongoing communication with the family and other staff.

Visiting teams – clinicians from other specialties – are a helpful resource in communicating with patients and their relatives. Their communication should align with that of ICU staff, because inconsistent information can be deeply problematic for families. Confusion or conflict may arise if the team has strong views on continuing treatment, or if they are represented mostly by junior staff who, in the eyes of the family, lack adequate authority. This may be compounded if there is a lack of active dialogue with the ICU clinicians, if they convey mixed messages to the family, or if they are inexperienced in dealing with grieving families.

Such problems can be minimised by ensuring that any communication is both documented in the patient's file and verbally handed over to the ICU medical staff. In addition, if major treatment decisions are going to be discussed, communication with senior members of the treating team should be undertaken.

Theoretical links

Intensive care has obliged medical professionals to engage with what Roy Porter calls 'the rituals of death':

> With new monitoring machinery, quasi-surgical interventions and the growth of respirators and all the other technology associated with the intensive care unit – the hospital became the place, not where the patient came to die, but where the apparently terminal patient might almost miraculously be *rescued* from death. Doctors thereby assumed control over the rituals of death: what was left of the 'good death' of the religious *ars moriendi* yielded to the priests in white coats.
> (Porter, 1999, pp. 692–693)

Early descriptions of intensive care portrayed doctors as conceiving of patients' diseases as purely technical problems (Zussman, 1992). For their part, nurses tended to be described as wedged between the 'iron authority' of doctors and the deep uncertainty of patients' fates (Cronqvist et al., 2001). More recently, we have begun to acknowledge that the realities of ICU practice and communication are more complex than this. Nevertheless, the growing technical capability of the ICU has meant that ICU professionals are now expected to navigate through the complex maze of patients' needs, families' feelings and cultural expectations, other specialties' views of what is appropriate treatment, and organisational resource constraints (Seymour, 2001).

Here, communication can be deeply challenging. Not surprisingly, working in intensive care can at times be distressing for doctors and nurses alike (Mok, Lee & Wong, 2002). Nurses may report feelings of helplessness, inadequacy and depression from identifying too closely with patients' suffering (McKerron, 1991). For their part, doctors may experience distress when faced with being unable to rescue a patient, and having to communicate with the family about dying (Feldstein & Gemma, 1995). For these reasons, careful preparation for intensive care practice and communication is critical (Fins & Solomon, 2001).

At times, ICU clinicians may be reluctant to communicate their own experiences of working in an ICU (Costello, 2001). Communicating about one's experiences is important however to ensure emotional growth, or when skills to manage the sensitivities of others and of the self need to be developed (Hillman, 2010).

empathy
a mental state whereby a person, experiencing compassion, shows they are affected by another person's suffering, and takes steps to alleviate that person's suffering.

Besides self-reflection, there are three core evidence-based communication skills for ICU professionals (Schaefer & Block, 2009; Scheunemann et al., 2011). They are **empathy**, prognosis discussion, and shared decision-making. Empathic communication – that is, identifying and responding to emotions – is crucial, and can be summarised by the VALUE mnemonic (Table 6.2).

Table 6.2 VALUE mnemonic for empathic communication

V	Value family statements
A	Acknowledge emotions
L	Listen
U	Understand the patient as a person
E	Elicit questions

Prognostic information needs to be delivered skilfully, involving an alignment of team and family understandings of prognosis with excellent communication skills on both sides. The family should be asked if they are ready to discuss prognosis and, once permission is given, the family's understanding of this should be checked.

Forewarning of family members, particularly with an expected time frame, prepares them to face the possibility of death. Shared decision-making is a process whereby the decisions about the patient's treatment are shared by the surrogates and the medical team, where the physician is guided by the knowledge and wishes of the patient and family. This can turn into a complex process, as while it is imperative that family values and wishes are taken into account, it must be ensured that the burden of medical decision-making is not passed over to the family. Expert advice is recommended.

Other evidence-based strategies for improving communication in the ICU include provision of written information on bereavement, structured family meetings, particularly using the VALUE mnemonic (Table 6.2), as well as ethics and palliative care consultations, which may reduce the burden of grief on family members (Lautrette et al., 2007; Scheunemann et al., 2011).

Conclusion

There are many opportunities for communication and miscommunication in the ICU. There are numerous factors that contribute, including a highly pressurised work environment, unpredictability of patient outcome and progress, unexpected changes in patient conditions, and patients' frequent inability to communicate their preferences about health and treatment choices.

It is easy to become desensitised to the stages of grief experienced by families when their relatives are critically ill. Communication and negotiation can be improved by recognising the different stages of grief experienced by family members, and by reflecting on their impact on yourself as practitioner. More often than not, the use of time is the most useful tool in assisting families to understand what is commonly a life-changing event in their lives, and therefore not without impact on the professionals themselves.

Finally, it is imperative that open and honest communication with staff both within the ICU and outside the ICU is fostered and maintained. Here, it is critical that professionals are able to discuss their views, impressions and feelings, without having to fear them being dismissed by their colleagues.

Practice example 6.2

You are the bedside nurse looking after a 63-year-old man, Mr Brendan Smith, who has had a cardiac arrest and remains deeply unconscious with a severe hypoxic brain injury. At the bedside are the patient's sister, brother and two children – his wife has just stepped out to go to the toilet. The doctor walks in and you witness the following conversation.

Doctor: Hi, Mrs Smith (looks at the sister), my name is Jane; I am one of the intensive care doctors. Can you tell me what you know about how your husband is going? He's not doing very well at all, is he? Did you know he had a big heart attack – in fact his heart stopped and he was brought back to life by the ambulance officers?

Sister: Actually I'm Sarah, his sister, no, I haven't heard much about …

continued ›

Practice example 6.2 continued ›

[Interrupts]

Doctor: Well, things aren't going well for your husband at all, I have to tell you. He has a severe hypoxic brain injury resulting from his VF arrest and (phone rings) – sorry, I just need to take this call –

[2 minutes later the doctor walks back in]

Doctor: So where were we? That's right, I was just saying that there's nothing else we can do for Mr Jones and we need to take the breathing tube out and let him pass on naturally.

[Patient's wife walks in]

Wife: What did you say? Who are you anyway? Did you say you're going to let my husband die? He's been here for a week. Why haven't you made him better yet? [Starts shouting] This hospital is terrible. If he was somewhere else with better doctors he'd be better by now! He was perfectly healthy before he came here!

Doctor: Well, actually I am a very good doctor. I won the prize at medical school and no one else has ever complained about me before. I think you are being very unfair as we've never even met before!

Reflective questions

General

1. What do you think the doctor did well in this interaction?
2. What do you think could have been done better?
3. How important are introductions and names in the ICU?
4. What sort of things can you do to facilitate remembering these?
5. Is there a role for ground rules during these meetings?
6. Should you have a pre-meeting meeting with the staff prior to the actual meeting?

Jargon and euphemisms

1. What do you think about the medical jargon this doctor has used?
2. What words could have been used instead?
3. The doctor used the term 'pass on' as a euphemism for 'die'. What other euphemisms are often used to indicate death or dying?
4. What are the pros and cons of using these terms?

Location and distractions

1. What is the ideal location and who should be present for a family meeting such as this one?
2. What steps can be taken to minimise distractions in family meetings?

3. What should a healthcare worker, who has multiple responsibilities in the ICU, do with their on-call phone during a family meeting?

Stages of grief

1. What stage of Kübler-Ross grief do you think this patient's wife is in?
2. How could the doctor have handled the wife's emotions better?
3. What are the stages of grief that people commonly go through?
4. Is this a normal way to cope with familial illness in the ICU?

Interprofessional communication

1. What feedback could the nurse provide to the doctor to improve their communication skills for the next family meeting they are involved in?
2. How and when would you give this feedback?
3. What are the potential barriers to nursing staff approaching doctors?
4. Does the traditional hierarchical structure of medicine impede open communication?
5. If so, how can organisations break down the hierarchical structure to enable every staff member to express their views?
6. What is the role of leaders in ICU to facilitate interprofessional communication?

Further reading

Kübler-Ross, E. (1969). *On death and dying*. New York: Macmillan.
This book forms the basis of the common theory and understanding of grief, death and dying, and the stages of grief that most people go through. Although not universally accepted, it provides a useful framework for understanding the process of grief – denial anger, bargaining, depression and acceptance – in order to help understand the mental frame patients and their families may be in.

Laurtrette, A., Darmon, M., Megarbane, B., Joly, L. M., Chevret, S., Adrie, C. et al. (2007). A communication strategy and brochure for relatives of patients dying in the ICU. *New England Journal of Medicine, 356*, 469–478.
This article looks at the value of using a proactive communication strategy, such as providing written information on death and dying and allowing longer time for families to talk with the medical staff about their loved one's illness. It shows that family members who receive the interventions are less likely to suffer post-traumatic stress disorder and depression.

Web resources

DonateLife Australia: http://www.donatelife.gov.au/home
International Society of Advance Care Planning and End of Life Care (ACPEL): http://www.acpelsociety.com

References

Costello, J. (2001). Nursing older dying patients: Findings from an ethnographic study of death and dying in elderly care wards. *Journal of Advanced Nursing, 35*(1), 59–68.

Cronqvist, A., Theorell, T., Burns, T., & Lutzen, K. (2001). Dissonant imperatives in nursing: A conceptualization of stress in intensive care in Sweden. *Intensive and Critical Care Nursing, 17*, 228–236.

Curtis, J .R., & Rubenfeld, G. D. (2001). *Managing death in the intensive care unit*. Oxford: Oxford University Press.

Feldstein, M., & Gemma, P. (1995). Oncology nurses and chronic compounded grief. *Cancer Nursing, 18*(3), 228–236.

Fins, J. J., & Solomon, M. Z. (2001). Communication in intensive care settings: The challenge of futility disputes. *Critical Care Medicine, 29*(2), N10–N15.

Friedman, R, & James, J. W. (2008). The myth of the stages of dying, death and grief. *Skeptic Magazine, 14*(2), 37–41.

Hillman, K. (2010). *Vital signs: Stories from intensive care*. Sydney: NewSouth Publishing.

Iedema, R., Sorensen, R., Braithwaite, J., & Turnbull, E. (2004). Speaking about dying in the intensive care unit, and its implications for multi-disciplinary end-of-life care. *Communication and Medicine, 1*(1), 85–96.

Kübler-Ross, E. (1969). *On death and dying*. New York: Macmillan.

Laurtrette, A., Darmon, M., Megarbane, B., Joly, L. M., Chevret, S., Adrie, C., et al. (2007). A communication strategy and brochure for relatives of patients dying in the ICU. *New England Journal of Medicine, 356*, 469–478.

McKerron, L. C. (1991). Dealing with stress of caring for the dying in intensive care units: An overview. *Intensive Care Nursing, 7*, 219–222.

Mok, E., Lee, W., & Wong, F. (2002). The issue of death and dying: Employing problem-based learning in nursing education. *Nurse Education Today, 22*, 319–329.

Porter, R. (1999). *The greatest benefit to mankind: A medical history of humanity from antiquity to the present*. London: Fontana.

Schaefer, K. G., & Block, S. D. (2009). Physician communication with families in the ICU: Evidence based strategies for improvement, *Current Opinion in Critical Care, 15*, 569–577.

Scheunemann, L. P., McDevitt, M., Carson, S. S., & Hanson, L. C. (2011). Randomised, controlled trials of interventions to improve communication in intensive care, a systematic review. *Chest, 139*(3), 543–554.

Seymour, J. E. (2001). *Critical moments: Death and dying in intensive care*. Buckingham: Open University Press.

Zussman, R. (1992). *Intensive care: Medical ethics and the medical profession*. Chicago: University of Chicago Press.

7

Communicating about end-of-life care

Aileen Collier

Learning objectives

This chapter will enable you to:

- discuss the characteristics of good communication from the perspective of dying patients and their families;
- describe why effective communication is essential to good end-of-life care;
- identify contemporary issues relating to communicating about the end of life;
- describe the key challenges inherent in communicating about care at the end of life;
- reflect on personal experiences and/or fears that might have an impact on the way you communicate with patients and families and your colleagues about care at the end of life.

Key terms

Death anxiety
Emotional labour
End-of-life care

Overview

This chapter addresses the ways in which health practitioners communicate with patients and families and each other about end-of-life care. It offers a critical look at how dying patients are 'positioned' by how they are communicated with and about in the healthcare organisation. The chapter also asks what this positioning means for how and where they are likely to die. The chapter presents examples of what happens in practice and offers resources for enabling health practitioners to overcome the limits of existing approaches to end-of-life communication.

Like few other aspects of health care, **end-of-life care** brings how we communicate with dying patients and with each other as health practitioners into sharp focus. In the domain of end-of-life care, effective communication is critical because it is really the only means we have to tackle the complexities, uncertainties, and differences in understanding and expectation that vex us towards the end of life.

> **end-of-life care**
> care provided when a person and their family are living with a life-limiting illness and its effects.

A focus on end-of-life communication is important for other reasons too. First, the biggest number of users of Western healthcare services are people with chronic diseases (75%), and most present with more than one disease: they have 'multiple co-morbidities'. Many of these patients die from their chronic illnesses; this means that their care is hugely complex: they may need to draw on the expertise of more than one service or specialty at the same time. In addition, most of these patients (around 70%) will die in a healthcare institution (Seale, 2000). This means that, unless they are looked after at home by relatives, people with a life-limiting illness will spend most of their last days in an acute care hospital, not in a hospice (a service that specialises in care for the dying) or under the care of specialist palliative care services (Palliative Care Australia, 2010, p. 14).

Introduction

Many healthcare professionals, academics and policy-makers agree that Western healthcare systems are not sensitive to the needs of dying patients and their families. The reasons for this are many and varied. In this chapter we begin by exploring some of the factors (organisational, educational, and personal) that contribute to creating these unmet needs. Assisted by practice examples, we look at patients' and families' experiences of end-of-life care and the impact poor communication can have on people's safety. The practice examples help us to identify communication strategies that might help patients and families to feel safer while under our care.

Let us first consider some of the factors that have a negative influence on communication at the end of life.

Organisational factors

Western healthcare systems tend to focus on treating a person's disease and curing it, rather than caring for the person as a person. Of course, cure is important, but as healthcare professionals we need to integrate curing with caring. The overarching concerns of the healthcare system, however, are often centred on hospital efficiency (budgets). Systems and services are under pressure to prioritise budgets and targets, making it very difficult for healthcare professionals to care in the way that they would choose (Benner, Hooper & Kyriakididis, 1999). What is more concerning, however, is that the health-care priority setting is not always sensitive to the needs and wants of patients and their families. This is the case even when these needs and wants emphasise simpler care and cheaper solutions. Only recently have the priorities of patients and consumers begun to be taken into account (Coulter, 2011).

By and large, hospital care tends to be organised around the priorities of 'disease'-focused medical specialties. This way of structuring health care may meet the needs of a person with a single disease or medical problem, but it does not meet the needs of people with multiple morbidities. As noted above, most users of our healthcare system are people with multiple morbidities (Barnett et al., 2012). Given that, the 'single-disease' focus of most healthcare services is not in synchronicity with the needs of the majority of patients. The single-disease focus means that most healthcare services and medical specialties operate in relative isolation from one another, and lack systematic approaches to collaboration and cooperation. This produces fragmentation of health care in general, and in end-of-life care in particular (Australian Commission for Safety and Quality in Healthcare, 2013; Curtis & Shannon, 2006; Ferrell, 2006; Sorensen & Iedema, 2007).

Compounding the single-disease structure of the healthcare system is that our hos-pital buildings are usually built with a focus on accommodating and reinforcing that single-disease structure of specialty clinical interventions. In reality, patients and families are rarely asked to contribute to the design of new hospital buildings; this serves to perpetuate the status quo in healthcare architecture and interior design. One excep-tion and an example that you may wish to follow up on is that of the children's hospital in Brisbane. The design and development of this new hospital involved children and their families from the outset and is centred on caring for the whole family (Queensland Government, 2014).

For the most part, however, this single-disease approach to health service structure and architectural and interior design means that hospitals are very foreign worlds for patients and families. This is particularly true for dying patients whose care is out of step with most of the acute care that goes on in hospitals. Thus, hospitals are full of threatening medical symbols for those whose disease is chronic and their life limited: white walls everywhere, corridors and consultation rooms full of machines and tech-nology, and people in white coats in a hurry (Radley & Taylor, 2003). Another problem with many healthcare environments is finding suitably private spaces where we can have end-of-life conversations. Too often, and sadly, such conversations are conducted in busy wards or in corridors. Along with finding themselves in a strange and threat-ening environment, patients and families are also under significant stress due to their suffering, impending loss, and grief. Despite all of this, we as healthcare professionals often expect ourselves and others to make reasoned and rational end-of-life decisions (Hillman & Chen, 2009).

Furthermore, it is not unusual for older people to be moved frequently between home, nursing homes and hospitals; and within the hospital from ward to ward where juggling of acute beds to meet demand takes precedence over the comfort of those receiving end-of-life care. Being moved around beds, rooms or institutions can be extremely stressful for patients generally, and for dying patients it can be traumatic (Burge et al., 2006). In addition, being in hospital means being disconnected from home and from what is most familiar (Evans et al., 2006). As a result, patients often feel unsafe in hospitals and care institutions generally.

Clinical factors

There are four critical problems associated with what clinicians know (or don't know) about patients who are dying. The first is that many healthcare professionals have difficulty in diagnosing dying as such (Christakis, 1999). That is, it remains immensely challenging to predict the approach and speed of death. The phrase 'diagnosing dying' presumes that diagnosis is possible, but diagnosing dying is in fact very challenging. Many studies have sought to devise checklists but researchers have had to acknowledge that the onset of dying is a complex and unpredictable phenomenon, near enough impossible to subject to an algorithm.

The second is that, even when death is known to be imminent, clinicians have difficulty openly acknowledging that patients are dying. These two problems conspire to create situations where clinicians continue to treat rather than take alternative or 'palliative' action, even with the knowledge that death is imminent (Sullivan et al., 2007). Continued treatment manifests in unnecessary investigations and 'heroic' medical interventions (interventions that do not offer much hope) being the default choice of healthcare professionals right up to the moment of death (Middlewood, Gardner & Gardner, 2001; SUPPORT, 1995).

A third worrying aspect of all this is that only 47% of physicians has been found to actually know that their patients would have preferred to avoid resuscitation or CPR (SUPPORT, 1995). A surprising 46% of all 'do not resuscitate' (DNR) orders (medical clinicians having formally decided and noted the patient should not be resuscitated) were written less than two days before patients' death.

The fourth issue is that family members have reported moderate to severe pain affecting 50% of conscious patients who died in the hospital. This means that the priorities of treating clinicians are out of step with the needs of their patients. To die in pain, particularly when already being cared for in a healthcare environment, should not be necessary.

The SUPPORT study was designed to solve the challenge of identifying dying and caring better for dying patients. Critically, the intervention phase of the SUPPORT study failed to produce any significant improvement in quality of care. The investigators acknowledged that their aims had been unrealistic. For one, dying was found to be too complex a phenomenon to be fully 'tamed' by medical or clinical science. But even those practitioners who were assisted to achieve a more effective identification of dying did not alter their communication with critical stakeholders, and they avoided dying as a prognosis (SUPPORT, 1995).

Educational factors

Junior doctors and nurses are rarely prepared for their first experiences of death. Early experiences of death and dying can stay with healthcare professionals and influence future practices (Cooper & Barnett, 2005; Sorensen & Iedema, 2009). Many healthcare professionals often feel ill prepared to care for people at the end of their lives (Gibbins, McCoubrie & Forbes, 2011). Policy-makers and universities are trying to improve this situation. For example, the Australian government has funded national projects such as the Palliative Care Curriculum for Undergraduates (PCC4U) to encourage the integration of palliative care education in undergraduate and relevant postgraduate health curricula (Queensland University of Technology in collaboration with Queensland Government, Flinders University & Curtin University of Technology, 2014). A tension remains, however: junior clinician education (in medicine, nursing and allied health) tends to avoid dealing with the full implications of the clinical factors discussed immediately above. Health professional education therefore tends to fall short when it comes to training novices for the clinical uncertainties and communication complexities surrounding dying.

Personal factors

Doctors, nurses and allied health professionals are continually exposed to disease and death. Some authors posit that, along with fear of their own death (**death anxiety**), this constant exposure may be an important reason why healthcare professionals find it difficult to communicate with dying people and their families (Kasket, 2006; Peters et al., 2013). Healthcare professionals' perceived need to alter feelings in order to maintain an outward façade for patients and families has been termed **emotional labour**: the hard work health professionals need to do to not become overly emotional. This emotional labour can result in professional caregivers becoming emotionally disconnected from their own feelings, and from the feelings of those around them (Brotheridge & Grandey, 2002). In turn, this can lead to healthcare professionals using defensive and asocial behaviours, resulting from their detachment and denial of their own feelings towards dying people and their families (Solomon, Greenberg & Pyszczynski, 2000).

> **death anxiety**
> the fears that we experience in the face of death.
>
> **emotional labour**
> the emotional work many people do in formal work situations. This work centres on mitigating their feelings towards others. Often this labour is about appearing more friendly and patient than people might be in informal situations in everyday life.

So how do these factors influence patients' and families' experiences of end-of-life care? Let's turn now to practice example 7.1.

Practice example 7.1

Below is the first excerpt from an interview conducted with a patient James and his daughter, Tracey. James was an inpatient in the oncology ward of a large metropolitan hospital where he had been for several months prior to the interview. He was discharged to his home prior to being admitted to the local palliative care unit where he died several weeks after the interview.

Tracey: They can't cure him.

James: They [doctors] can't cure me, they know that. I think they [doctors] are just using me as a 'guinea pig' and especially after the way they [doctors] spoke the other day.

Interviewer: What was it about the way of speaking that made you feel like that?

James: I think it's the attitude of the doctors. They're up there instead of down there … [non-verbally uses his hand to express height difference] … Their [doctors'] heads are higher than … they're not listening to you! You're saying stuff to them, it's going over their [doctors'] head. They're not even putting it in the book [case-notes and/or other documentation]. The nurse comes back and tells you: 'I'm sorry I can't do anything, there's nothing in the book.'

Tracey: Hmm, quite a few times that's happened. Last Thursday, that's the first day he [James] got the diarrhoea and he informed them [clinicians] and I was on my way in [to the hospital].

James: Yeah.

Tracey: Somewhere between 10 a.m. and 11 o'clock, I got him in here [to the hospital]. 1:30 p.m. I spoke to the nurse, the male nurse and everything, and he was all apologetic. He [the nurse] couldn't do anything until something was written down in the book [clinical documents] and he said that he's paged the doctor and they're [the nursing staff] still waiting on him [the doctor] to come up. It hit 4:30 in the afternoon and I needed to start making my way home and still no doctor had been up and he's [James] got diarrhoea, sweating profusely, severe cramps, pain everywhere! Yeah communication, like they [clinicians] need to improve communication, like between doctors and doctors they're shocking …

James: Yeah.

Tracey: [The communication] Between doctors and nurses is bad but the doctors between doctors are absolutely shocking

James: You tell them something, the nurse passes and says, 'Aw I need to get permission from this person and that person', but they don't seem to get the thing across …

Tracey: … the information across properly.

James: They [the nursing staff] put it down, half the time I don't think the doctors read it, just look at it and glance and piss off, that's it.

Reflective questions

1. What did you learn from reading this part of the transcript and what insights about communication and end-of-life care did it provide? What is it about how practitioners communicate with James that makes him feel like 'a guinea pig'?

2. James tells us: 'I think it's the attitude of the doctors. They're up there instead of down there … [non-verbally uses his hand to express height difference] … Their heads are higher than … they're not listening to you.' What do you think James means by this?

3. What do you think are the personal and professional qualities that patients and families expect of practitioners?

4. What kind of defensive behaviours have you seen healthcare professionals adopt?

Analysis and reflection

In the transcript above, James and Tracey convey shortcomings in communication at several levels. First, at the level of patient–practitioner communication, James expresses how he is left feeling like a 'guinea pig' as a result of the kind of interactions he has had with the medical team. In other words, he feels as though he is something to be experimented on and conveys how he feels objectified as a disease stage. Further, James feels his concerns are left unheard by the way that practitioners position themselves 'above' him, both because of how they position themselves in relation to him by standing over him, and by talking in technical language. Third, at the level of team communication, James suffers poor symptom management as a result of a lack of systematic communication among different disciplines and among medical specialists.

What may be 'normal' communication in the view of healthcare professionals in fact has significant ramifications for James and his family. These ramifications include inadequate pain and symptom management, as well as emotional distress to which the clinicians fail to attend. Critically for James and Tracey, these incidents occur as a result of ineffective communication both at the point of healthcare workers' interactions with them as consumers, and at the level of team communication. In short, James and Tracey's account encapsulates what unsafe care means for patients and families. Their account provides us with some clues as to how unsafe care arises.

Implications for practice

Patients with life-limiting illnesses need to be able to communicate effectively with healthcare professionals. Importantly, James and Tracey do not put unsafe care down to one event or incident. Rather, their experience of unsafe care is a result of an unfolding series of events. For James and Tracey inadequate interpersonal communication is both an adverse event and leads to further adverse events, such as unmet symptom needs. Furthermore, patients like James have knowledge and expertise about their own illnesses and needs, and practitioners need to take these into account if they are to meet the safety expectations of today's patients (Hor et al., 2013).

What tends to be forgotten in today's health care is that patients like James want to be recognised as unique individuals and understood in the context of their own unique lives and values (Cherlin et al., 2004; Kuhler, 2002; Masson, 2002; Steinhauser et al., 2000; Steinhauser et al., 2014). In addition, dying patients have a need to reciprocate and contribute to others by way of knowledge, time or gifts and a wish to participate in the same interactions that are important throughout all of life (Steinhauser et al., 2000). These needs and expectations are just as important in the context of healthcare relationships.

Likewise, family members like Tracey express a desire for loved ones to be treated as individuals. They want to be 'known' by practitioners just as patients do (Masson, 2002; Steinhauser et al., 2014). Families look to practitioners to keep them informed of signs of deterioration and impending death (Steinhauser et al., 2014). Families also expect healthcare professionals to make it possible and easy to 'visit and be present with the patient' – not impossible and hard (Cherlin et al., 2004, p. 114). Family members want practitioners to care for them as a family and not to abandon them (Cherlin et al., 2004).

At the heart of being able to respond to people like James and Tracey, then, are the qualities of wisdom and humility as well as clinical expertise. That is, what matters in circumstances where patients are dying are behaviours, responses and communication that respect people's own norms and values. Usually, what this means is that the healthcare professional treats the patient and the family in the way they would expect to be treated themselves (Healy, 2007).

In order for James and Tracey to be the central focus – rather than James's leukaemia and its treatment – the clinical care team needs to take note of, and be driven by, James' needs at any particular point in time. Team members need to be able to respond to James and Tracey in a flexible way – not bound by a particular specialty, discipline or level of seniority. This kind of response requires the team to adopt shared responsibility for the patient, not a rigid hierarchical, over-regulated and bureaucratised structure. Such 'dynamic' teams exhibit flexibility and adaptability. Within dynamic teams, the most appropriate individual team member is able to respond and take the lead at any particular moment in time, depending on what the patient needs (Davison & Hyland, 2003; Iedema et al., 2005).

So what does all of this really mean in terms of how you might respond to people like James and Tracey? Healthcare professionals frequently ask 'What can I say?' and/ or 'What do I do?' Novice practitioners can find communication models and communication tools helpful in this regard. Yet we know that standard expressions are often of limited value in a specific interactional context and in response to individual situations (see Chapter 19). The use of scripted answers may constrain how clinicians respond to patients and their families. In other words, when communicating with dying patients and their families it is not so much what you say or do that matters, but how you *are with them* (Dobkin, 2011).

Theoretical links

In this chapter, we conceptualise communication not as separate from treatment or care, but as integral to care and treatment. Separation of technical skills and communication as care can lead to disregard for communication as the domain of particular experts such as psychologists or social workers (Liben, 2011). In this thinking, communication is often diminished to a 'soft extra' (Milton, 2008). Practical and technical needs matter to patients and families, but these needs are not divorced from interpersonal needs. A paradigm shift is needed so that communication becomes integral to care and the safety of patients and families, rather than viewing care of the 'person', 'psyche' or 'spirit' as 'soft extras' supplied if, and only when, there are available resources or adequate time. As already noted in earlier chapters (Chapter 1) communication is closely linked to producing both indirect and direct health outcomes (Street et al., 2009).

Second, SUPPORT study investigators concluded some time after the study that they had perhaps overemphasised the rational decision-making process and underestimated the human aspects of suffering and death (Benner, Hooper & Kyriakididis, 1999). In other words, response to the richness and mystery of the unfolding situation of dying cannot be reduced to reason, technology and logical decision-making. Hence, humanity is required alongside clinical technical competence for patient safety at the end of life.

This humanity is just as important for you as a healthcare professional. Such humanity manifests as reciprocity; reciprocity means that you respond to the other as you would want the other to respond to you were you in their position. Reciprocity is just as important for healthcare workers as it is for patients and families (Sobel, 2008). Any encounter, no matter how momentary, can communicate to patients or families whether they are safe or not. That is, the kind of communication that patients and families expect does not necessarily demand additional time. As James and Tracey describe: 'They [healthcare practitioners] [should] talk to him [James] while they are doing it [the nursing or medical intervention or task]'.

Through feeling connected with professionals (and other healthcare workers including non-professional staff such as the receptionist), patients and families like James and Tracey may also feel connected to the 'bigger healthcare system'. These connections require healthcare professionals to be open to patient and family expertise in relationships of trust, and to reciprocate their interpersonal needs.

Conclusion

In this chapter, we have provided an opportunity for you to consider the impact on dying patients and their families of communication that is suboptimal. You will have noted that good end-of-life care is critically dependent on good communication, because technology and science are not adequate for predicting or dealing fully with the process of dying. Practitioners of all disciplines have a responsibility at personal, professional, team and organisational levels to attend to communication at the end of life. Practice example 7.2 provides an opportunity for you to further reflect on what good communication means for people like James and Tracey.

Practice example 7.2

The following extract takes up James and Tracey's narrative again.

Tracey: But the communication. The amount of times we've said to them [clinicians] too that his [James's] state of mind is not the best at the moment. Like he had seizures and stuff like that; he had bleeding of the brain. Well of course he knows he's got leukaemia, he knows he's going to die and everything but can they ring us first and let us know? We left all our numbers.

James: Yeah, they hadn't rang.

Tracey: Yeah and they [healthcare workers] told us, 'Yeah go home and get some rest and everything'. So we [family] said, 'Alright'. We left our numbers and everything and said, 'If anything happens [to James] can you please ring us?'

James: But they didn't ring.

Tracey: We rang about 7:30 in the morning and the nurse just turned around and said, 'Aw he's only had about 10 seizures, but he's fine.'

James: [Laughs]

Tracey: And we were like, 'If any of that [seizures or deterioration] started up again you were supposed to ring us.' Because at that stage we were told it [death] could be any minute; that the next seizure could kill him. Not even a phone call.

Interviewer: So what would it take for you to be safe in this environment?

James: To go home and just have a nurse come to the house I think would be a better situation. Because it works on your mind; if you want to stay alive you need to put your mind to something that you want to do. Well I

continued ›

	wanted to go home and then they [the doctors] nearly killed me themselves just three weeks ago. I had a meeting to go to. I worked it out with them, told them everything, they said, 'Yeah, you'll be able to go to it.' But then they [the doctors] cancelled me. It looked like they were going to cancel this one but we [the family] said, 'Stuff them, we're going anyway.'
Tracey:	Yeah, this was on Sunday. Mum, it was the anniversary of Mum's death and they keep pumping this whole antibiotic in; another two weeks, another two weeks.
James:	Yeah.
Tracey:	And like when he was having the seizures and having the bleeds and everything and we were told, 'It [the death] won't be long.' And we said to them, 'Well, he's DNR, he doesn't want to be resuscitated. What's the antibiotics actually doing for him?' Because we wanted to stop it, if that was just prolonging his life and I kept worrying is that just prolonging his life?
James:	I think they just treat us as like a guinea pig.
Tracey:	And you know so we wanted to stop everything and then we were told [by the medical team], 'No, the antibiotics are actually helping manage the pain' and stuff like that and we said, 'Well if that's the case, we'll continue with the antibiotics.'
James:	But they're [antibiotics] not, they [antibiotics] weren't doing anything.
Tracey:	Well, it [the treatment] wasn't. The antibiotics were actually just confusing his body.
James:	But there is one or two of nursing staff, the new ones; the trainees and they're terrific.
Interviewer:	What is it that makes them terrific, James?
James:	I think it's an attitude.
Tracey:	And I think it's that they take the time to actually,…
James:	Sit down and talk to you and listen to you for a few minutes.
Tracey:	But even, if they, you know, communicate while they're doing it [the clinical task] or they use his name.
James:	Yeah.
Tracey:	And introduce themselves.
Interviewer:	So you are saying that there are some positive communication qualities?
Tracey:	There are positive qualities like …
James:	Oh yeah.
Tracey:	Some of the doctors and everything as soon as something is going to happen or change they'll let us know and they'll explain it properly to us

continued ›

Practice example 7.2 continued ›

	and then you get other doctor it's like they're talking to you but not talking with you [uses gestures to indicate talking 'at' rather than talking 'with'] and explaining things properly. Like if I went to medical school and got a degree, I would probably be able to understand them, but I didn't.
James:	Yeah, I think that's what a lot of the doctors forget; that we're only patients. We don't have medical degrees. We don't understand all that type of stuff that they're talking about.
Tracey:	That's it and then you get certain cases like we've been through so many highs and lows with Dad and like the really lows; there's some days we come in here and it's like we're absolutely brain dead.

Reflective questions

1. What are the key communication issues at stake in the description above?
2. What do you think James and Tracey consider as effective team communication?
3. What are the effects of team communication on the care of James and Tracey?
4. What strategies might you adopt to avert the resuscitation scenario described above?
5. How would you go about having a discussion about goals of care with James and Tracey now?
6. You are an outside consultant invited by the clinical team looking after James and Tracey to provide advice about team communication. What changes would you propose and how would you recommend they be implemented?

Reflective questions

Please read both practice examples again.

1. What feelings were you aware of as you read James' and Tracey's narrative?
2. What narratives of your own, both personal and professional, if any, resonated with James' and Tracey's narrative?
3. Reflect on your interactions with patients, families and colleagues about end-of-life care over the past few months; how might your experiences, values and beliefs about death and dying influence the way that you care for people like James?
4. Read the guidelines by Clayton et al. in the 'Further reading' section of this chapter. How might these guidelines assist you to respond to James and Tracey? In light of what you have learnt in this and other chapters, discuss with a peer what the limitations of these guidelines might be.
5. What are your own responsibilities and those of your organisation to enhance communication at the end of life?

Further reading

Benner, P., Kerchner, S., Corless, I. & Davies, B. (2003). Attending death as a human passage: Core nursing principles for end of life care. *American Journal of Critical Care, 12*(6), 558–561.

This paper emphasises death as 'biographical' rather than 'physiological'. In doing so, it places relational connections as a central tenet of providing individualised end-of-life care.

Chochinov, H. M. (2004). Dignity and the eye of the beholder. *Journal of Clinical Oncology, 22*(7), 1336–1340.

This paper explores dying patients' perceptions of their sense of dignity and hope. The characteristics and quality of encounters patients have with practitioners are discussed through the lens of how these encounters can augment or diminish patient's sense of dignity.

Clayton, J. M., Hancock, K. M, Butow, P., Tattershall, M. N. H. & Currow, D. C. (2007). Clinical practice guidelines for communicating prognosis and end-of-life issues with adults in the advanced stages of a life-limiting illness, and their caregivers. *MJA, 186*(12 (supplement)), 77–108.

This is a helpful set of guidelines developed by experts in the field to assist clinicians to discuss end-of-life issues with patient and their families .

Kearney, M. (2000). *A place of healing: Working with suffering in living and dying.* Oxford: Oxford University Press.

This book, written by a palliative care physician, challenges the conventional notion of 'detached concern' – the idea that practitioners should be simultaneously detached or objective and compassionate concerning clinical encounters (Lief & Fox, 1963). Michael Kearney argues instead for a healthcare approach that integrates conventional Western medicine with the ancient approach termed 'Asklepian healing', involving a collaborative approach between patient and practitioner to reach the healing potential of both parties.

Ragan, S. L., Wittenburg-Lyles, E. M., Goldsmith, J. & Sanchez-Reilly, S. (2008). *Communication as comfort: Multiple voices in palliative care.* New York and London: Routledge.

This book explores the complexities of communication through the multiple voices of patients, families and professional caregivers.

Web resources

Advance Care Planning Australia: http://www.advancecareplanning.org.au
CareSearch: http://www.caresearch.com.au/caresearch/tabid/1471/Default.aspx
Healthtalk: http://www.healthtalkonline.org/Dying_and_bereavement/Living_with_Dying/Topic/1188/

References

Australian Commission for Safety and Quality in Healthcare (ACSQH). (2013). Safety and quality of end-of-life care in acute hospitals: A background paper. Sydney: Author.

Barnett, K., Mercer, S. W, Norbury, M., Watt, G., Wyke, S., & Guthrie, B. (2012). Epidemiology of multimorbidity and implications for healthcare, research and medical education: A cross-sectional study. *Lancet, 380*, 7–9.

Benner, P, Hooper, D., & Kyriakididis, P. (1999). *Clinical wisdom and interventions in critical care: A thinking in action approach.* Philadelphia: WB Saunders Company.

Brotheridge, C., & Grandey, A. (2002). Emotional labour and burnout: Comparing two perspectives on people work. *Journal of Vocational Behaviour, 60*, 17–39.

Burge, F. I., Lawson, B., Critchley, P., & Maxwell, D. (2006). Transitions in care during the end of life: Changes experienced following enrolment in a comprehensive palliative care program. *BioMed Central Palliative Care, 4*(3).

Cherlin, E., Schulman-Green, D., McCorkle, R., Johnsom-Hurzeler, R., & Bradley, E. (2004). Family perceptions of clinicians' outstanding practices in end-of-life-care. *Journal of Palliative Care, 20*(2), 113–116.

Christakis, N. A. (1999). *Death foretold: Prophecy and prognosis in medical care.* Chicago and London: University of Chicago Press.

Cooper, J., & Barnett, M. (2005). Aspects of caring for dying patients which cause anxiety to first year student nurses. *International Journal of Palliative Nursing, 11*(8), 423–430.

Coulter, A. (2011). *Engaging patients in healthcare.* Milton Keynes: Open University Press.

Curtis, J. R., & Shannon, S. E. (2006). Transcending the silos: Toward an interdisciplinary approach to end-of-life care in the ICU. *Intensive Care Medicine, 32*, 15–17.

Davison, G., & Hyland, P. (2003). Palliative care: An environment that promotes continuous improvement, learning and innovation. In E. Geisler, K. Krabbendam & R. Schuring (Eds.), *Technology, healthcare and management in the hospital of the future* (pp. 105–123). Westport: Praeger Publishers.

Dobkin, P. (2011). Mindfulness and whole person care. In T. Hutchison (Ed.), *Whole person care: A new paradigm for the 21st century* (pp. 69–82). New York: Springer.

Evans, W. G., Cutson, T. M., Steinhauser, K. E., & Tulsky, J. A. (2006). Is there no place like home? Caregivers recall reasons for and experience upon transfer from home hospice to inpatient facilities. *Journal of Pallative Medicine, 9*(1), 100–110.

Ferrell, B.R. (2006). Understanding the moral distress of nurses witnessing medically futile care. *Oncology Nursing Forum, 33*(5), 922–930.

Gibbins, J., McCoubrie, R., & Forbes, K. (2011). Why are newly qualified doctors unprepared to care for patients at the end of life? *Medical Education, 45*, 389–399.

Healy, B. (2007). Medicine, the art. *U.S. News and World Report*, p. 86.

Hillman, K., & Chen, J. (2009). *Conflict resolution in end of life treatment decisions.* Sydney: Sax Institute.

Hor, S., Godbold, N., Collier, A., & Iedema, R. (2013). Finding the patient in patient safety. *health: An Interdisciplinary Journal for the Social Study of Health, Illness and Medicine*, 1–17. doi:10.1177/1363459312472082

Iedema, R., Sorensen, R., Braithwaite, J., Flabouris, A., & Turnbull, L. (2005). The teleo-affective limits of end-of-life-care in the intensive care unit. *Social Science and Medicine, 60*, 845–857.

Kasket, E. (2006). Death and the doctor. *Existential Analysis 17*(1), 137–150.

Kuhler, D. (2002). *What dying people want: Practical wisdom for the end of life.* Cambridge: Perseus Book Group.

Liben, S. (2011). Empathy, compassion and the goals of medicine. In: T. A., Hutchison (Ed.), *Whole person care: A new paradigm for the 21st century* (pp. 59–82). New York: Springer.

Lief, H. I., & Fox, R. C. (1963). Training for 'detached concern' in medical students. In H. I. Lief, V. F. Lief, & N. R. Lief (Eds.), *The psychological basis of medical practice* (pp. 12–35). New York: Harper & Row.

Masson, J. D. (2002). Non-professional perceptions of 'good death': A study of the views of hospice care patients and relatives of deceased hospice care patients. *Mortality, 7*(2), 191–209.

Middlewood, S., Gardner, G., & Gardner, A. (2001). Dying in hospital: Medical failure or natural outcome? *Journal of Pain and Symptom Management, 22*(6), 1035–1104.

Milton, C. L. (2008). Boundaries: Ethical implications for what it means to be therapeutic in the nurse-person relationship. *Nursing Science Quarterly, 21*(1), 18–21.

Palliative Care Australia. (2010). *Health system reform and care at the end of life: A guidance document.* Canberra: Author.

Peters, L., Cant, R., Payne, S., O'Connor, M., McDermott, F., Hood, K. et al. (2013). How death anxiety impacts nurses' caring for patients at the end of life: A review of literature. *The Open Nursing Journal, 7*, 14–21.

Queensland Government. (2014). *Lady Cilento children's hospital: Delivering the best care for our kids.* Brisbane: Queensland Health.

Queensland University of Technology in collaboration with Queensland Government, Flinders University, & Curtin University of Technology. (2014). Palliative care curriculum for undergraduates (pcc4u). Retrieved March 12, 2015 from http://www.pcc4u.org

Radley, A., & Taylor, D. (2003). Images of recovery: A photo-elicitation study on the hospital ward. *Qualitative Health Research, 13*(1), 77–99.

Seale, C. (2000). Changing patterns of death and dying. *Social Science and Medicine, 51*, 917–930.

Sobel, R. (2008). Beyond empathy. *Perspectives in Biology and Medicine, 51*(3), 471–478.

Solomon, S., Greenberg, J, & Pysczynski, T. (2000). Pride and prejudice: Fear of death and social behaviour. *Current Directions in Pyschological Science, 9*(6), 200–204.

Sorensen, R., & Iedema, R. (2007). Advocacy at end-of-life research design: An ethnographic study of an ICU. *International Journal of Nursing Studies, 44*, 1343–1353.

—— (2009). Emotional labour: Clinicians' attitudes to death and dying. *Journal of Health Organisation and Management, 23*(1), 5–22.

Steinhauser, K. E., Christakis, N. A., Clipp, E. C., McNeilly, M., McIntyre, L. M., & Tulsky, J. A. (2000). Factors considered important at the end of life by patients, family, physicians and other care providers. *Journal of American Medical Association, 284*, 2476–2482.

Steinhauser, K. E., Voils, C. I., Bosworth, H., & Tulsky, J. A. (2014). What constitutes quality of family experience at the end of life? Perspectives from family members of patients who died in the hospital. *Palliative and Supportive Care*. doi:10.1017/S1478951514000807

Street, R. L., Mackoul, G., Arora, N. K., & Epstein, R. M. (2009). How does communication heal? Pathways linking clinician-patient communication to health outcomes. *Patient Education and Counselling, 74*, 295–301.

Sullivan, A. M., Lakoma, M. D., Matsyuama, R. K., Rosenblatt, L., Arnold, R. M., & Block, S. D. (2007). Diagnosing and discussing imminent death in the hospital: A secondary analysis of physician interviews. *Journal of Palliative Medicine, 10*(4), 882–893.

SUPPORT. (1995). A controlled trial to improve care for seriously ill hospitalised patients. *JAMA, 274*, 1591–1598.

8

Communicating in surgery

Elizabeth Manias

Learning objectives

This chapter will enable you to:
- recognise that sentinel events in surgery, which involve incidents and accidents of a catastrophic nature, are linked to communication failures as a main cause;
- identify key guidelines and policies that have been developed to support health professionals to provide exemplary communication in surgery;
- explain that the main challenges affecting effective communication in surgery are the different environments that patients are required to move through, the extensive productivity and efficiency requirements that need to be addressed in surgery, and the different health professional disciplines involved in providing surgical care.

Key terms

Checklist
Communication
Consent
Postoperative care
Preoperative care
Surgical Safety Checklist
Time out

Overview

This chapter addresses communication issues arising in and around surgery. After being admitted to hospital for surgery, patients move along what is called 'the perioperative pathway'. This pathway is comprised of preoperative, intraoperative and

communication
the process of people engaging in the exchange of knowledge, information, feelings and meanings. Communication can encompass spoken and written language, bodily gestures and meanings invested in things outside of the human body such as visual displays and architectural designs.

preoperative care
care in the time before a patient enters the operating room.

postoperative care
care in the time that the patient leaves the post-anaesthetic care unit and is directed to the surgical ward for recovery from surgery.

checklist
a list such as a 'to-do list' containing critical steps or items that need to be taken into account before initiating work processes. The checklist counteracts the shortcomings of human memory and inadequate attention to detail.

perioperative pathway
the patients' care immediately before, during and immediately following surgery by a group consisting of the surgeons, anaesthetists, nurses, operating room technicians, and other health professionals.

Surgical Safety Checklist
a list of activities devised by the World Health Organization; the checklist should be completed three times: before induction of anaesthesia, before skin incision by the surgeon, and before the patient leaves the operating room.

postoperative care domains. **Preoperative care** involves medical assessment before surgery. Intraoperative care is the surgery itself. **Postoperative care** involves handover to the surgery ward and monitoring of the patient to ensure they recover fully from the surgery.

Communication failure can happen in any one of these situations, potentially leading to adverse outcomes. The chapter considers how communication failure can occur, and the strategies that can be implemented to improve communication. Some of these strategies focus on ensuring appropriate planning and preparation of surgical care before patients enter the operating room, including utilising a surgical **checklist** before the surgery starts, anticipating and avoiding complex communication situations right along the whole **perioperative pathway**, and conducting relevant and accurate handovers at strategic points.

Introduction

Communicating well in and around surgery is crucial for patient safety. The settings where communication takes place involve more than just the operating room or theatre. They comprise the preoperative environment, prior to when patients enter the operating room, the intraoperative environment, including the holding bay, operating room and post-anaesthetic care unit, and the postoperative environment, involving the surgical ward. Collectively, these settings are called the perioperative pathway (Braaf et al., 2012). To comprehensively address communication that supports surgery, it is necessary to consider patient care activities that occur across the whole perioperative pathway and not just those activities that take place within the operating room. The necessity of focusing on the whole perioperative pathway has also been acknowledged by the World Health Organization, through its **Surgical Safety Checklist** (World Health Organization, 2009a) and its 'Safe Surgery Saves Lives' initiative (World Health Organization, 2009b).

Approximately 234 million major surgeries are performed worldwide each year (Elder, 2014; Weiser et al., 2008). If surgery is not carried out safely, the potential for catastrophic consequences is high. Sentinel events, which are serious situations that occur independently of a patient's condition, are not uncommon in Australian hospitals. Recent figures for 2012–13 show that retaining of instruments or other materials left in the body following surgery, leading to repeated procedures, was the second most common type of sentinel event. Surgical procedures involving the wrong patient or the wrong body part, causing death or permanent loss in function, was the fifth most common type of sentinel event (Department of Health, 2014). Common contributing factors associated with sentinel events relate to procedures and guidelines, human resource and staffing issues, and communication problems (Department of Health, 2014).

Due to the potentially serious nature of adverse events associated with surgery, key bodies have devised many initiatives to assist policy-makers, hospital managers and health professionals to improve surgical care to patients. These initiatives include the Surgical Safety Checklist devised by the World Health Organization (World Health Organization, 2009a) (Figure 8.1). The intent of the checklist is to help health professionals consider safety as pertaining to the whole perioperative pathway, and to create improved communication among the various healthcare disciplines involved. This checklist is not intended to be a regulatory tool, but rather a tool to identify areas where communication may fail, causing serious surgical incidents, including deaths and complications.

In recognising the value and importance of the Surgical Safety Checklist, a number of professional associations in Australia, such as the Royal Australasian College of Surgeons, in consultation with the Australian and New Zealand College of Anaesthetists and the Australian College of Operating Room Nurses, have modified the checklist to suit the Australian and New Zealand context (Royal Australasian College of Surgeons et al., 2009) (Figure 8.2). Checklists such as these act as supportive tools for health professionals and are not regulatory documents.

Other resources pertinent to communication in surgery include ones made available by the Australian Commission on Safety and Quality in Health Care (2012), in its National Safety and Quality Health Service Standards. These standards need to be used by all Australian healthcare organisations for them to be formally accredited for their various healthcare activities. The standards of particular relevance to communicating in surgery include Standard 2, Partnering with Consumers; Standard 5, Patient Identification and Procedure Matching; and Standard 6, Clinical Handover. The challenge for health professionals is to reflect critically on how these standards apply to their own practice and how these standards can be actively used to improve communication with other healthcare disciplines and with patients, with the ultimate aim of facilitating patient safety. Patient identification ensures that the correct person is undergoing the surgical procedure to be performed. Correct identification is also associated with making sure the right surgical site is used and surgical procedure is carried out. Procedure matching is the process by which the surgical team identifies the correct procedure to be performed on a particular patient. This process involves identifying the correct operation site and side.

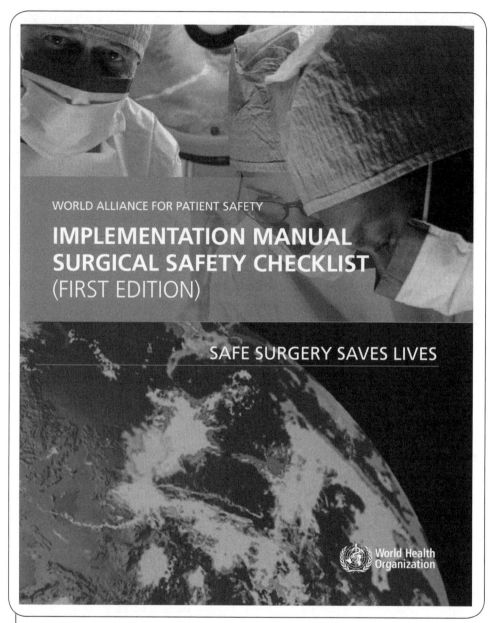

Figure 8.1 *Implementation Manual: Surgical Safety Checklist* of the World Health Organization

It is important to consider what is good and what is ineffective communication in surgery to be able to propose improvements in practice. Communication failure is defined as a problem in the content of the communication encounter, in the audience involved in the communication encounter, in the occasion of the communication encounter, or in the purpose of the communication encounter (Lingard et al., 2004). Extensive work has been undertaken on the prevalence of communication failures in the perioperative

Surgical Safety Checklist (Australia and New Zealand)

Before induction of anaesthesia ▸ ▸ ▸ ▸ ▸ Before skin incision ▸ ▸ ▸ ▸ ▸ ▸ ▸ ▸ ▸ ▸ Before patient leaves operating room

SIGN IN

☐ **PATIENT HAS CONFIRMED**
- IDENTITY
- SITE
- PROCEDURE
- CONSENT

☐ **SITE MARKED/NOT APPLICABLE**

☐ **ANAESTHESIA SAFETY CHECK COMPLETED**

☐ **PULSE OXIMETER ON PATIENT AND FUNCTIONING**

DOES PATIENT HAVE A :

KNOWN ALLERGY?
☐ NO
☐ YES

DIFFICULT AIRWAY/ASPIRATION RISK?
☐ NO
☐ YES, AND EQUIPMENT/ASSISTANCE AVAILABLE

RISK OF >500ML BLOOD LOSS (7ML/KG IN CHILDREN)?
☐ NO
☐ YES, AND ADEQUATE INTRAVENOUS ACCESS AND FLUIDS PLANNED

PROSTHESIS/SPECIAL EQUIPMENT:

IF PROSTHESIS (OR SPECIAL EQUIPMENT) IS TO BE USED IN THEATRE, HAS IT BEEN CHECKED AND CONFIRMED?
☐ YES
☐ NOT APPLICABLE

TIME OUT

☐ **CONFIRM ALL TEAM MEMBERS HAVE INTRODUCED THEMSELVES BY NAME AND ROLE**

☐ **SURGEON, ANAESTHESIA PROFESSIONAL AND NURSE VERBALLY CONFIRM**
- PATIENT
- SITE
- PROCEDURE

ANTICIPATED CRITICAL EVENTS

☐ **SURGEON REVIEWS:** WHAT ARE THE CRITICAL OR UNEXPECTED STEPS, OPERATIVE DURATION, ANTICIPATED BLOOD LOSS?

☐ **ANAESTHESIA TEAM REVIEWS:** ARE THERE ANY PATIENT-SPECIFIC CONCERNS?

☐ **NURSING TEAM REVIEWS:** HAS STERILITY (INCLUDING INDICATOR RESULTS) BEEN CONFIRMED? ARE THERE EQUIPMENT ISSUES OR ANY CONCERNS?

HAS ANTIBIOTIC PROPHYLAXIS BEEN GIVEN WITHIN THE LAST 60 MINUTES?
☐ YES
☐ NOT APPLICABLE

HAS THROMBOPROPHYLAXIS BEEN ORDERED?
☐ YES
☐ NOT REQUIRED

IS ESSENTIAL IMAGING DISPLAYED?
☐ YES
☐ NOT APPLICABLE

SIGN OUT

NURSE VERBALLY CONFIRMS WITH THE TEAM:

☐ **THE NAME OF THE PROCEDURE RECORDED**

☐ **THAT INSTRUMENT, SPONGE, NEEDLE AND OTHER COUNTS ARE CORRECT**

☐ **HOW THE SPECIMEN IS LABELLED** (INCLUDING PATIENT NAME)

☐ **WHETHER THERE ARE ANY EQUIPMENT PROBLEMS TO BE ADDRESSED**

☐ **SURGEON, ANAESTHESIA PROFESSIONAL AND NURSE REVIEW THE KEY CONCERNS FOR RECOVERY AND MANAGEMENT OF THIS PATIENT**

Figure 8.2 Surgical Safety Checklist adapted for Australia and New Zealand (Royal Australian College of Surgeons; adapted from World Health Organization, 2009b)[1]

environment. Lingard et al. (2004) found a communication failure rate of 30% in the operating room. Halverson et al. (2011) reported 56 communication failures in 76 hours occurring in the operating room before the conduct of a team training curriculum, whereas, following training, 20 communication failures over 74 hours were observed. Nagpal et al. (2010a) identified information transfer failure rates of 62% for pre-procedural teamwork and 53% for postoperative handover. Furthermore, in an Australian study, Gillespie, Chaboyer & Fairweather (2012) reported a communication failure rate of 57% in surgical procedures observed in the operating room. In another Australian study, Braaf et al. (2012) identified a failure rate of 28% across the perioperative pathway.

Research has also been undertaken into the types of communication failures identified. Knowledge of this information can help in developing strategies and policies aimed at addressing particular areas of concern. According to Lingard et al.'s (2004) work in the operating room, communication failure types comprised problems such as poor timing (45.7% of instances), problems with content where information was missing or inaccurate (35.7%), problems with purpose where disagreements were not resolved (24.0%) and problems with audience where key people were not included (20.9%). In the observational work across the perioperative pathway conducted by Braaf et al. (2012), the following communication types were found: purpose (41%), content (40.9%), occasion (9.9%) and audience (8.1%). While there appears to be marked variation in the proportions of failure types per operating room, it is clear that each type – purpose, content, occasion and audience – plays an important role in how communication occurs in practice.

Aside from considering the prevalence and types of communication failures, it is vital to explore outcomes associated with communication failures. Knowledge of these outcomes can be used in educating health professionals to develop understandings of how good communication influences safe surgical care. By identifying outcomes over time, it would be possible to track how changes in strategies and policies can lead to improved outcomes. In the observational work undertaken by Braaf et al. (2012), communication failure led to health professionals engaging in more frequent communication encounters, working with missing information, enduring an increased workload and experiencing confusion in clinical practice.

Other outcomes included tensions between health professionals of similar or different healthcare disciplines, inefficiencies in surgical and anaesthetic practices, delays in work processes, documentation errors, rushed clinical tasks, procedural errors, and wasted resources. Specific patient outcomes that were attributed to communication failures involved delays or cancellation of surgery, near miss events, adverse events, and longer operation times. Specific staff outcomes attributed to communication failures related to health professionals having to work overtime and increased harm to staff members, such as needle stick injuries and back injuries. Communication failures were also examined in terms of outcomes of care in Gillespie and colleagues' (2012) work. They found the number of communication failures contributed to increasing the expected length of the operation.

Practice example 8.1

Below is an observational excerpt relating to a patient who was scheduled to have elective surgery in a public hospital. The patient had an allergy to an intravenous contrast dye that was to be used during her surgical procedure. To prevent possible adverse reactions relating to the dye, she was required to receive a premedication regimen over a course of several hours. Unfortunately, her anaesthetist never prescribed the premedication regimen due to increased busyness of the perioperative environment and problems with communication.

The 69-year-old female patient was booked for an elective repair of a thoracic aortic aneurysm. She arrived in the surgical ward of the hospital a couple of days before her pending surgery. The patient was allergic to intravenous contrast dye. This allergy was noted by the anaesthetist during his preoperative visit on the day prior to surgery. The vascular registrar had documented in the medical history that the patient should have a series of intravenous hydrocortisone injections and an intravenous diphenhydramine dose as a part of her premedication regimen. The purpose of this premedication regimen was to counter any allergic effects from the contrast dye that would be used during surgery. Unfortunately, these orders were not written down by the anaesthetist. According to hospital protocol, the following orders should have been documented as 'premedication: 200 mg of hydrocortisone, to be administered intravenously 13 hours, 7 hours and 1 hour prior to the surgery, and 50 mg of diphenhydramine, to be administered intravenously 1 hour prior to the surgery'. The process of writing up the premedication orders was the responsibility of the anaesthetist. As the anaesthetist was speaking with the patient, however, he was interrupted by his pager. In answering his pager, the anaesthetist was called to the recovery room. Another patient was experiencing laboured breathing in the recovery room and the theatre staff needed assistance. Due to the interruption, the anaesthetist was trying to complete his session with the patient quickly, but he had forgotten to write up the hydrocortisone and diphenhydramine orders. The anaesthetist did, however, write up orders for diazepam and metoclopramide, which were routinely prescribed as premedication to patients.

The afternoon nurse noticed the comment made by the vascular registrar in the patient's medical record, but she did not relay this information at handover to the night-time nursing staff. Similarly, the vascular registrar did not verbally communicate with medical staff during the medical handover about the premedications. As a result, none of the afternoon or night-time staff realised that the patient required premedication orders for hydrocortisone and diphenhydramine.

The patient was transferred to the operating room at 7 a.m. on the day of surgery. On arrival to the operating room, the patient was welcomed by the nurse in the holding bay who noticed that the patient was allergic to intravenous contrast dye. However, she did not check if any premedication had been prescribed or administered to prevent allergic

continued ›

Practice example 8.1 continued ›

reactions from the contrast dye. The patient was wheeled on a trolley into the operating room. The anaesthetist induced the patient with general anaesthesia, and proceeded to monitor her vital signs and conscious state.

A **time out** procedure was then conducted. The surgeon asked everyone to hurry up with the time out because he just wanted to get on with the procedure. During the time out, the scout nurse raised a concern about the patient's allergy to intravenous contrast dye. The theatre team glanced at the anaesthetist for advice. The anaesthetist checked the premedication orders, and realised his mistake. No hydrocortisone and diphenhydramine had been administered prior to surgery. As it was important for the patient to have the hydrocortisone intravenous injections over several hours before surgery and to have the diphenhydramine one hour before surgery, the anaesthetist commented that the surgery could not continue and that it would need to be rescheduled. The surgeon sighed and, saying nothing, he walked out of the operating room with a look of disgust. After the anaesthetist administered the reversal agents for anaesthesia and removed the endotracheal tube, the patient was wheeled into the post-anaesthetic care unit. The anaesthetist was frustrated with himself for neglecting to document the premedication orders. As the patient began to wake up, the anaesthetist told her that there were some concerns with giving her the contrast dye, and the surgical team needed to wait till tomorrow where they could make the necessary adjustments to her medications and perform the surgery. He did not mention that two important medications were not prescribed and administered prior to her surgery. The patient returned to the surgical ward, feeling upset and confused.

> **time out**
>
> a process that occurs in the operating room following anaesthetic induction and before surgical incision. It involves health professionals pausing to communicate with each other about any concerns they may have about the upcoming surgery.

Analysis and reflection

In the observational excerpt, miscommunication occurred on a number of levels and involved different individuals. The anaesthetist was distracted during an interruption and as a result he forgot to document an important premedication regimen that led to rescheduling of surgery. The vascular registrar had documented in the medical record the importance of prescribing this premedication regimen, but neither the nursing nor the medical staff in the surgical ward conveyed this information during handover. On checking the patient's notes and allergy status in the holding bay, the holding bay nurse did not detect the omission.

There were concerns with how the time out was carried out. The intent of time out is never to direct blame on one person for a particular task not completed properly. Unfortunately, the surgeon displayed signs of impatience and he did not seem to take the time out process seriously. He considered the checklist as an impediment to the workflow of the operating room, and he wanted to get on with completing the surgical procedure.

No one told the patient the actual cause for the rescheduling of her surgery. Vague information was given to her during her recuperation in the post-anaesthetic care unit, where she was still quite drowsy from the anaesthetic. There was no further follow-up about the cause of the reschedule after the patient had returned to the surgical ward.

Reflective questions

1. Ask work colleagues, friends and family members if they have experienced any problems relating to surgery. If their response is affirmative, ask them how the problems were communicated to them by health professionals caring for them. Determine the adequacy of the explanations provided to them.
2. The process of taking stock to complete a time out requires health professionals to slow down in the operating room and to reflect on their practices. Ask yourself how difficult it would be to stop what you are doing in an operating room and to expect other health professionals to do the same. Think about what strategies can be used in the operating room to complete a time out properly, and to give it the time it deserves.

Implications for practice

Careful attention should be paid by health professionals when communicating with each other, particularly at strategic time points of surgery – before entry into the operating room, immediately before any surgical incision is made, and immediately before the patient leaves the operating room. These time points have been identified by the World Health Organization (2009a) as the most critical to achieving patients' safety in surgery. Unfortunately, it is commonly taken for granted that surgeons, anaesthetists, nurses and theatre technicians do not regularly collaborate with each other at key time points and about key aspects of the surgical procedure (Miller, Abrams, Earles, Phillips & McCleeary, 2011).

While health professionals may argue that work pressures inhibit such collaborations, ineffective collaboration paradoxically leads to communication failures that subsequently manifest as inefficiencies in surgical and anaesthetic practices, delays in work processes and longer operation times (Braaf et al., 2012; Gillespie, Chaboyer & Fairweather, 2012).

Structured communication tools should be strategically used at the key transition points of care in surgery. Such tools can promote clear and precise information, assist in decision-making and enable goal-directed care (Nagpal et al., 2010b). For instance, structured handover protocols can be developed for particular environments or points on the surgical pathway, such as the holding bay and the post-anaesthetic care unit, to ensure accurate and complete details are relayed between health professionals.

Hierarchical norms of behaviour appear to dominate in surgery, sometimes leading to communication failures. It is important that interdisciplinary training and education are undertaken by health professionals with the aim of fostering mutual understanding of the different roles and responsibilities of each discipline group. However, hierarchical norms of behaviour are often firmly entrenched and they are not going to change readily through training and education. The use of role models and change champions in the perioperative pathway can help to promote information sharing, active decision-making and shared communication (Mills, Neily & Dunn, 2007). By fostering patterns of good communication within teams, it is more likely that these patterns can filter through to other health professionals in the perioperative settings.

As patients move along the perioperative pathway, there needs to be increased accessibility of documentation in an electronic format. In order to maximise access to current and accurate data, it is imperative that patient documents (such as surgeons' reports, specialists' reports, anaesthetists' records of medications administered during surgery) and observation charts are readily available electronically. It is important that managerial documents relating to surgery are also available electronically, including operating room lists, surgeons' and anaesthetists' schedules, pathologists' and radiologists' availability for diagnostic and imaging services respectively, safety and sterilisation status of equipment and instruments, and location of key equipment and instruments.

Theoretical links

The above issues can be framed theoretically as follows. Clinicians' behaviours and ways of communicating in and around surgery are structured by decades of training and habituation. On the one hand, dominance is assumed by those who have surgical expertise: everyone is to conform with their wishes and commands. Surgical dominance is justified on the basis of two kinds of arguments or 'discourses'. The first is about hierarchy. Hierarchy is justified on the basis of surgeon's expertise and seniority. The other is about productivity. This is justified with reference to bureaucratic and organisational demands that compel the surgical team to complete their work activities efficiently and within a particular time frame. Communication that takes hierarchy and productivity as given and justified has often been associated with communication failures among health professionals, which subsequently result in adverse events (Braaf et al., 2013; Stevens & Rogers, 2009).

On the other hand, submissive behaviours and ways of communicating are also evident, but these tend to be displayed on the part of nurses and non-surgical medical staff (Riley & Manias, 2006). In affect, submissive and dominant behaviours and ways of communicating are two sides of the same coin. Both contribute to clinical incidents, albeit in their own ways. One example is truncated time outs and completion of checklists due to the refusal on the part of certain members of the surgical team to become involved and take the activity seriously. Another example is a hastened informed **consent** process to avoid delaying the surgical schedule, denying the patient the information they need about the surgical procedure to be performed or the anaesthetic medications to be administered.

> **consent**
> the process involved in a patient agreeing to the surgical procedure to be conducted. For a valid consent, the patient understands the information provided, freely and voluntarily agrees to the procedure, and is competent to provide consent.

Conclusion

Communication about surgery occurs through complex webs of care as patients move along the perioperative pathway. Clear links exist between communication failure and the occurrence of adverse patient outcomes, some of which result in catastrophic events. It is crucial that health professionals who provide surgical care are able to communicate effectively with each other and with patients and family members to ensure surgical safety. A variety of checklists and tools are available to assist health professionals in their communication encounters. These need to be adopted, regularly implemented, and routinely updated within the various environments associated with the perioperative pathway. It is also important for health professionals to identify and address dominance and submission within the surgical team, to consider their effect on communication during surgery, and to counter them as they create avoidable risks for patients.

Practice example 8.2

Read the following example and reflect on the patient's situation using the questions below.

A 72-year-old male patient was admitted for surgical removal of an infected aortic stent and graft repair of the abdominal aorta. The stent was placed in the aorta two years previously for treatment of an abdominal aortic aneurysm. During the current admission, the anaesthetist placed a small spinal drain in the lower region of the spinal cord to remove cerebrospinal fluid from the spinal area. Removal of cerebrospinal fluid would ultimately lower the pressure in the spinal cord and reduce the chance of postoperative paralysis.

The patient went to the operating room, and the infected stent and graft repair of the abdominal aorta was completed without any complications. The patient returned to the surgical ward, where the spinal drain remained in place for 48 hours after surgery. After 48 hours, the anaesthetist visited the patient in the ward, and tried to remove

continued ›

Practice example 8.2 continued ›

the drain. His efforts were unsuccessful, resulting in the drain becoming stretched. As the anaesthetist was worried about causing future problems with the spinal graft, he referred the matter to a neurosurgical colleague. The neurosurgeon suggested that the drain should be removed under general anaesthesia in the operating room to prevent patient injury. The patient was put on the operating room list for the next day by the operating room manager. The anaesthetist and the neurosurgeon carefully documented the patient's plan of care in the medical record.

The patient was scheduled to be operated around mid-afternoon. However, due to delays in previous surgical procedures, the case was moved to the end of the day. An anaesthetist who was covering for the latter part of the day had arrived and began to prepare for the case. She did not read through the plan of care in the medical record, and noticed that the **operating list** for this case was labelled as 'Removal of spinal drain'. The covering anaesthetist was very experienced with managing spinal drains, and she did not seek any further information about the surgical removal of the drain. There was also no handover between herself and the patient's original anaesthetist about the problems relating to this particular spinal drain. The covering anaesthetist also did not follow up with clarification from the patient, who was waiting in the holding bay area for his procedure.

> **operating list**
> the daily list developed by managerial staff of an operating room that details patients' names, surgical procedures, the names of surgeons and anaesthetists, the theatre room and the intended time of surgery.

Through lack of awareness about the plan for the patient to have a general anaesthetic, the covering anaesthetist attempted to pull out the drain. In her vain attempt to pull out the drain, the catheter snapped, and a small part of the drain remained in the spinal canal. At that point, emergency surgery had to be conducted to remove the drain. While the patient was at risk of developing spinal cord complications, such as paralysis, no major complications resulted from the covering anaesthetist's actions.

Reflective questions

1. In considering the covering anaesthetist's care, at which points did she not adequately communicate with other individuals to clarify the plan of care during surgery?
2. There does not appear to be much involvement by nurses in this situation. What role could have been played by nurses in the surgical ward and the operating room to prevent the communication problems that occurred?

Reflective questions

1. Imagine you are a patient, and your surgeon does not spend time with you to explain your impending surgical procedure and what will be involved. How would you feel about this process of gaining consent for surgery?

2. There is the potential for many communication failures to occur during the perioperative pathway. Map out some of the main areas for communication failures along a patient's journey. What practical strategies can you suggest to prevent these communication failures?

Further reading

McCarthy, K., Hacking, M., Al Mufti, R., & Hewitt, J., (2004). *Vivas and communication skills in surgery*. Edinburgh: Churchill Livingstone.

This book covers important components to consider in communicating with patients who require surgery. Information is provided on how health professionals working in surgery can interact effectively with their colleagues and the reader's knowledge and understanding are tested effectively using sample questions.

Salmon, P., (2000). *Psychology of medicine and surgery: A guide for psychologists, counsellors, nurses and doctors*. Somerset, NJ: Wiley.

This book demonstrates how beliefs, emotions and behaviours of health professionals, patients and family members can affect communication and coping in diagnosis and treatment. It provides a comprehensive account of why people feel and behave as they do in dealing with disease and surgery.

Stahel, P. F., & Mauffrey, C. (Eds.). (2014). *Patient safety in surgery*. New York: Springer.

This comprehensive book provides extensive information about all facets of safety affecting patients during surgery. The aim of the book is to improve safety and quality of care for patients undergoing many different types of surgical procedures.

Web resources

Association of Perioperative Registered Nurses comprehensive checklist:
http://www.aorn.org/Clinical_Practice/ToolKits/Correct_Site_Surgery_Tool_Kit/
    Comprehensive_checklist.aspx
WHO surgical safety checklist and implementation manual:
http://www.who.int/patientsafety/safesurgery/ss_checklist/en

References

Australian Commission on Safety and Quality in Health Care. (2012). *National safety and quality health service standards*. Sydney: Author.

Braaf, S., Manias, E., Finch, S., Riley, R., & Munro, F. (2012). Communication failure across the perioperative pathway. *International Journal of Person-Centered Medicine*, 2(4), 698–706.

—— (2013). Healthcare service provider perceptions of organisational communication across the perioperative pathway: A questionnaire survey. *Journal of Clinical Nursing, 22*(1–2), 180–191.

Department of Health. (2014). *Supporting patient safety. Sentinel event program. Annual report 2011–12 and 2012–13.* Melbourne: State of Victoria, Department of Health.

Elder, M. (2014). *Surgical procedure volumes: Global analysis.* Rockville, MD: Kalorama.

Gillespie, B. M., Chaboyer, W., & Fairweather, N. (2012). Factors that influence the expected length of operation: Results of a prospective study. *British Medical Journal Quality & Safety, 21*(1), 3–12. doi:10.1136/bmjqs-2011-000169

Halverson, A. L., Casey, J. T., Andersson, J., Anderson, K., Park, C., Rademaker, A. W., & Moorman, D. (2011). Communication failure in the operating room. *Surgery, 149*(3), 305–310. doi:10.1016/j.surg.2010.07.051

Lingard, L., Espin, S., Whyte, S., Regehr, G., Baker, G. R., Reznick, R. et al. (2004). Communication failures in the operating room: An observational classification of recurrent types and effects. *Quality & Safety in Health Care, 13*(5), 330–334. doi:10.1136/qhc.13.5.330

Miller, M. J., Abrams, M. A., Earles, B., Phillips, K., & McCleeary, E. M. (2011). Improving patient-provider communication for patients having surgery: Patient perceptions of a revised health literacy-based consent process. *Journal of Patient Safety, 7*(1), 30–38. doi:10.1097/PTS.0b013e31820cd632

Mills, P., Neily, J., & Dunn, E. (2007). Teamwork and communication in surgical teams: Implications for patient safety. *Journal of the American College of Surgeons, 206*(1), 107–112. doi:10.1016/j.jamcollsurg.2007.06.281

Nagpal, K., Vats, A., Ahmed, K., Vincent, C., & Moorthy, K. (2010a). An evaluation of information transfer through the continuum of surgical care: A feasibility study. *Annals of Surgery, 252*(2), 402–407. doi:10.1097/SLA.0b013e3181e986df

Nagpal, K., Vats, A., Lamb, B., Ashrafian, H., Sevdalis, N., Vincent, C., & Moorthy, K. (2010b). Information transfer and communication in surgery: A systematic review. *Annals of Surgery, 252*(2), 225–239. doi:10.1097/SLA.0b013e3181e495c2

Riley, R., & Manias, E. (2006). Governing time in operating rooms. *Journal of Clinical Nursing, 15*(5), 546–553.

Royal Australasian College of Surgeons, Australian and New Zealand College of Anaesthetists, Royal Australian and New Zealand College of Ophthalmologists, Royal Australian and New Zealand College of Obstetricians and Gynaecologists, Australian College of Operating Room Nurses, & Perioperative Nurses College of the New Zealand Nurses Organisation. (2009). Surgical safety checklist (Australia and New Zealand). Retrieved June 17, 2014 from http://www.surgeons.org/media/12661/LST_2009_Surgical_Safety_Check_List_%28Australia_and_New_Zealand%29.pdf

Stevens, J. P., & Rogers, S. O. (2009). Communication and culture: Opportunities for safer surgery. [Editorial]. *Quality & Safety in Health Care, 18*(2), 91–92. doi:10.1136/qshc.2009.032177

Weiser, T. G., Regenbogen, S. E., Thompson, K. D., Haynes, A. B., Lipsitz, S. R., Berry, W. R., & Gawande, A. A. (2008). An estimation of the global volume of surgery: A modelling strategy based on available data. *Lancet, 372*(9633), 139–144. doi:10.1016/s0140-6736(08)60878-8

World Health Organization. (2009a). *Implementation manual WHO surgical safety checklist.* Geneva: Author.

——. (2009b). *Who guidelines for safe surgery: Safe surgery saves lives.* Geneva: Author.

Acknowledgement

Some concepts presented in this chapter were derived from research supported by an Australian Research Council Linkage Project Grant (project number: LP0883265).

Note

1 This checklist has been adapted from the World Health Organization Surgical Safety Checklist by the Royal Australasian College of Surgeons in consultation with the Australian and New Zealand College of Anaesthetists, the Royal Australian and New Zealand College of Ophthalmologists, the Royal Australian and New Zealand College of Obstetricians and Gynaecologists, the Australian College of Operating Room Nurses and the Perioperative Nurses College of the New Zealand Nurses Organisation. It is not intended to be comprehensive, additions and modifications to fit local practice are encouraged.

9

Communicating with people with cognitive impairment

Sam Davis and Aileen Collier

Learning objectives

This chapter will enable you to:
- identify contributory factors that impact on the safety of people with cognitive impairment in healthcare settings;
- recognise the role of communication in providing a safe environment for people with cognitive impairment, particularly dementia;
- integrate person-centred principles into practice to minimise risk and maximise quality care for people with cognitive impairment.

Key terms

Cognitive impairment
Delirium
Dementia
Malignant social positioning
Person-centred care

Overview

cognitive impairment
communication, attention, memory, thinking and problem-solving difficulties usually associated with dementia and delirium.

Cognitive impairment manifests as dementia, or the gradual decrease in one's ability to think or remember things. Dementia is brought about by Alzheimer's or related neurological diseases. The number of Australians with dementia is expected to reach 900 000 million by 2050 (AIHW, 2012).

The number of people living with dementia is unlikely to alter in the near future even if there are advances in treatment.

At present, these large numbers mean that more than half of all people living in aged care in Australia have **dementia**. Further, one in every 100 people admitted to hospital have a diagnosis of dementia and 5% of attendances at the general practitioner (GP) involve the management of people with dementia (AIHW, 2012).

The challenges of caring for people with dementia cut right across the healthcare sector. People with dementia are vulnerable to healthcare environments because their declining cognitive abilities decrease their capacity to adapt to change, remain independent, and vocalise their needs. All clinicians, independent of their specialty and/or site of care, need to communicate effectively if the care needs of people with cognitive impairment and their families are to be addressed. In this chapter we will provide some resources to help clinicians communicate with and provide safe care for people who are cognitively impaired.

> **dementia**
> an umbrella term for a number of diseases characterised by progressive decline of brain functions causing changes in memory, perception, personality, language, and cognitive skills, and resulting in difficulties with activities of daily living. People with dementia are at high risk of developing delirium, or temporary confusion.

Introduction

Cognitive impairment is not associated with any one particular disease or with any one age group. Cognitive impairment is associated with stroke (Man et al., 2011), traumatic brain injury (Nash et al., 2014), developmental disabilities, chronic disease (Abete et al., 2014; Fan & Meek, 2014), chronic stress and mental illness (Marin et al., 2012).

While age is the primary risk factor for cognitive impairment, other risk factors include family history, education level, physical inactivity and elements such as exposure to pesticides or toxins as well as chronic conditions. Failure to understand and address the underlying causes of cognitive impairment can have a profound impact on the outcomes of care. People with cognitive impairment 'are at greater risk of adverse outcomes than people who do not have cognitive impairment' (Draper, Karmel, Gibson, Peut & Anderson, 2011), including **delirium**.

Delirium is a common condition, affecting up to 50% or more of older people in hospitals and residential care (Harding, 2006). Features of delirium include reduced clarity of awareness of the environment with reduced ability to focus, sustain or shift attention; memory impairment; disturbance of sleep–wake cycle; speech or language disturbance; disorientation to time and place; emotional disturbance; psychomotor behavioural disturbance such as agitation; and hallucination or other misinterpretations (Clinical Epidemiology and Health Service Evaluation Unit, 2006, p. 25).

> **delirium**
> a state of mind caused by an underlying physical condition, characterised by acute onset (usually hours to days) and tending to fluctuate over the course of the day (American Psychiatric Association, 2000).

Delirium remains underdiagnosed in most healthcare settings (Edlund et al., 2006). Undiagnosed delirium leads to negative outcomes for older people. They may have to be kept in hospital for longer, and this means they are at greater risk of experiencing complications (such as an infection or mismedication) and even dying (either in hospital or soon after discharge). Delirium may also lead to a loss of independence and it may exacerbate cognitive decline (van Munster & de Rooij, 2014). It can cause significant distress for people and their families (Morita et al., 2004). Delirium has been classified into three subtypes (Edlund et al., 2006):

1. the hyperactive–hyperalert (restlessness, agitation, aggression);
2. the hypoactive–hypoalert (latency in reaction and response to verbal stimuli, psychomotor slowing;
3. the mixed type.

Delirium is often distinguished from dementia by virtue of its acute course and reversibility but, as Meagher (2001) points out, the boundary between delirium and dementia can be blurry, particularly where a person has 'comorbidities, a prolonged delirious state, Lewy body dementia (with its fluctuating course and symptoms that frequently include psychosis), and delirium symptoms that persist beyond the acute treatment phase'. Nevertheless, it is important for us to remember that 'the presentation of delirium is the same regardless of whether dementia is present because symptoms of delirium will dominate when they co-occur' (Meagher, 2001).

Rather than relying on medications and/or constraints, clinicians should communicate effectively as this is critical to recognising and responding to someone with cognitive impairment. In particular clinicians need to be aware of and attuned to the possibility of the presence of hypoactive (latent) delirium.

Furthermore, we need to attend to what Hutchinson and Brawer (2011) describe as analogic communication. Analogic communication refers to all embodied communication, including non-verbal cues (Hutchinson & Brawer, 2011). Patients or residents may display through analogic communication that they are uncomfortable, such as by a worried expression or nervous movements. In particular, attention to environmental factors that could be exacerbating delirium is important. Examples are sensory deprivation (for example, a windowless room) or sensory overload (for example, too much noise and activity); isolation from family and friends; absence of familiar objects around the person; frequency of room changes; and, perhaps most frequently overlooked, whether the person has visual or hearing aids and whether they are in place (Meagher, 2001).

Communication with people experiencing cognitive impairment can be challenging. The very nature of cognitive impairment is that the deficit to mental functioning makes it difficult for the person to relate to others in terms of articulating meanings and interpreting what is being communicated. Yet communication is vital to ensuring safe, quality care that meets the individual needs of a person. You need to be acutely aware of what and how you are communicating and how the cognitively impaired person could receive your communication and, in turn, respond to you and others. We consider these issues later in the chapter. First, let's turn to a practice example to orient our subsequent discussion about communication approaches and strategies.

Practice example 9.1

Tom (79 years old) was diagnosed with Alzheimer's disease a couple of years ago. He lives at home with his wife, Betty. Following a visit to the GP, he was admitted to the local hospital. Tom, an extremely tall man, has been finding it difficult to get comfortable in the hospital bed. Since admission, four days ago, he has been pacing up and down the ward a lot, even though he is very tired. He has been causing the nursing staff some concern.

For example, Tom stares at people fiercely, which they find intimidating. He suddenly shouts at other people as they walk across his line of sight, pointing and giving them a 'look of disgust'. Yet, when the ward gets really busy, he just sits in the chair beside the nurses' station, turning the pages of the various magazines and newspapers from a table nearby.

Every once in a while he tears a piece of paper from what he is looking at and jumps up from the chair and tries to give it to staff passing by, insisting that they take it. When they refuse or say they will look later, he gets very upset.

On his second day in the hospital, Tom started rearranging things in the ward. He moved a television to face a different way and moved chairs from people's besides and lined them up along the corridor. Tom has been refusing to comply with requests specific to personal care routines and eating. Because he has been sitting near the nurses' station at meal times, one registered nurse had his breakfast put on a table in front of him there but when they came to take the tray, he had barely touched it. He did keep his cup of tea and finished it.

Yesterday, he hit out at nursing staff who were trying to get him to put clean pyjamas on. When his wife came to visit later in the day, she had no difficulties getting him to put clean pyjamas on, with some prompting on what to do and minor assistance with the buttons on the top. Although no assessment of his behaviour has been completed, ward staff have noted on his medical record that he is 'agitated and aggressive'.

Analysis and reflection

The hospital environment presents a daunting, unfamiliar world to the person with dementia and is generally over-stimulating, frustrating and confusing. For staff charged with delivering care in the acute setting, people with dementia present significant challenges which usual workplace routines are ill-equipped to accommodate. In the scenario in practice example 9.1, the experiences of Tom and the staff exemplify these problems.

Often, nursing staff are frustrated by having to manage patients who are aggressive, and believe that they could be doing more important tasks (Moyle et al., 2010). These are the very staff often displaying negative attitudes towards people with dementia. Just as worrying is that senior staff often express concern about how patient's cognitive challenges impede the delivery of technical aspects of care (Moyle, 2010).

To address patients' agitation and aggression, nursing staff often request pharmacological interventions; that is, they drug patients (Weitzel et al., 2010). However, people with dementia are at higher risk of potentially serious adverse effects from antipsychotic medication, making it a poor course of action, and one which can often promote further behavioural and clinical issues (Banerjee, 2009). When patients are aggressive, they are often restrained – this can further exacerbate the aggression. Even when staff have strong reservations about using restraints, the culture of work and organisational policies may lead them to initiate the use of restraints (Ludwick, O' Toole & Meehan, 2012).

Therefore, being formally identified as agitated and aggressive does not bode well for Tom. Consider for a moment the situation from Tom's perspective. As a person with dementia, he may be struggling to understand the ward environment or to verbally express his thoughts and feelings. He may be experiencing some of the effects of dementia, such as a decreased attention span, impaired judgment, decreased insight and diminishing visual and spatial abilities. The behaviours associated with dementia should be first considered as a form of communication – *communication of an unmet need.*

Unfortunately, patients' unmet needs are commonly overlooked as part of clinical assessment. The usual practice in any healthcare setting is to collect information and then make a judgment based on that information – this is clinical assessment. Using a commonsense label ('aggressive') to describe patients' behaviour in formal documentation is *not* assessment. On the contrary, such labelling is likely to promote adverse behaviours in colleagues and invite avoidable negative outcomes.

When a person is struggling to understand what is going on around them, they will feel vulnerable. When they express that vulnerability in ways that are not the norm, this is because they are ill and likely suffering from cognitive impairment. To classify patients on the basis of such behaviours and risk stigmatisation of the patient is unprofessional.

> ## Reflective questions
>
> 1. How might Tom's behaviour be viewed differently?
> 2. What should be explored and considered to appropriately assess his agitated state and resistance to personal care routines?
> 3. What information might help better understand Tom's experiences and reactions to being in the hospital ward?
> 4. What is it about the hospital ward environment that might be triggering Tom's responsive behaviour?

Implications for practice

Inappropriate staff communication frequently precipitates undesirable patient responses or 'responsive behaviour'. Responsive behaviour tends to be invited through the use of 'elderspeak' (infantalising communication) and 'resistiveness' to care (Williams et al., 2009). Examples of 'elderspeak' include 'using a singsong voice, changing pitch and tone, and exaggerating words, speaking very slowly, using limited vocabulary, using pet names (diminutives) such as 'honey' or 'dear', using collective pronouns such as 'we' – for instance, 'Would we like to take a bath now?' – and using statements that sound like questions' (Touhy & Jett, 2013). Elderspeak is a stark example of ageist communication, but a general lack of respect for the person with dementia is frequently conveyed through talking to others such as colleagues or family and friends about the person as if they were not present, or limiting or focusing interaction to care tasks only.

Likewise, messages conveying higher levels of control are associated with patients' resisting care – resistiveness (Williams & Herman, 2011). As Williams and colleagues (2012) point out, balancing the directive dimensions of care with a tone signalling respect and patience is an effective and efficient way to ensure the patient sees no reason to resist care.

A person-centred approach to communicating with people with dementia begins with acknowledging that the patient is trying to communicate something, and that it is important enough to that person for others to make the effort to understand. Consider that the person with dementia may not be able to change the way they communicate, but you can. Strategies for better communication here include the following:

- Involve the person in discussions in their presence – don't talk 'over' them.
- Use positive phrasing (avoid 'don't' and 'no') – make positive suggestions and directions.
- Avoid open-ended questions such as 'What would you like?' or 'What do you want?'

Communicating with people with dementia

The following advice is from the NHS (UK) document http://www.nhs.uk/Conditions/dementia-guide/Pages/dementia-and-communication.aspx:

- Keep your tone of voice positive and friendly.
- Don't stand too close to the person while talking as it can intimidate them – either be on the same level or lower than they are, which is less intimidating (keep in mind any cultural considerations of interaction).
- Touching or holding the person's hand while talking to them can help to reassure them and make you feel closer – watch their body language and listen to what they say to see whether they're comfortable with you doing this.
- Use eye contact to look at the person, and encourage them to look at you when either of you are talking.
- Try not to interrupt them, even if you think you know what they're saying.
- Try not to finish the person's sentences – instead, look for clues in their body language, expression and tone to suggest words, and check with them to see whether you've understood them correctly.

Above all, sharing information is the key to maintaining safety in the care of a person with dementia. Remember that the way in which information is communicated can have far-reaching consequences if the language itself is not person-centred. Staff behaviour and language must reflect respect and dignity for the personhood of all individuals.

It is easy for us to fall into the habits of using terms and phrases and not realise the messages that are actually conveyed. The language we use in verbal and written forms has a significant influence on those around us – whether the person with dementia, their family or other health professionals. Remember that using labels that identify a person with a task, a condition or a behaviour undermines personhood.

Guidelines for improving the language of dementia care

Eliminate negative, generalised labels for people with dementia from the vocabulary of staff, signage, and all documentation, including medical records and care plans. Examples of unacceptable descriptors include 'feeder', 'wanderer', 'toileter', 'screamer', 'agitated', 'difficult', 'behavioural', 'unmanageable' [and] 'redirect'.

Encourage the use of more positive and, more specifically, descriptive language to refer to the needs of people with dementia, e.g., 'Person who needs help eating,' rather than 'feeder'; 'energetic and exploratory,' rather than 'restless and wandering'; 'needs help in the toilet' rather than 'needs toileting'.

Instead of labelling a person with dementia as 'agitated' in notes and care plans, describe the situation and what was done, e.g., 'Person is talking loudly about his wife and pacing in his room – he calmed down when I asked him to tell me about his wife.' (Department of Health Services, 2014)

Finally, by asking the following questions, you will be able to remind yourself and your colleagues to practise **person-centred care**:

person-centred care
care that emphasises the personhood of those living with dementia and their relationships and values and shows respect, trust and recognition of the uniqueness of individuals in caring relationships.

- What do I know about this person and how will it help me build a relationship that I can use to achieve good outcomes in the therapeutic context?
- How can I show respect for this person so that I can gain their trust and make them feel safe in my care?
- What can I do to engage them so that communication can occur that will enhance the care outcomes?
- Does this person have needs that will affect how assessment and treatment will progress?
- What do I need to do to validate their perspective of themselves, those around them and their experiences in the course of providing care?

Theoretical links

The dominant theory of dementia care in the twenty-first century is that which has developed from the work of Tom Kitwood. His term 'person-centred' serves to highlight that the person treated is central in the patient–clinician partnership, and that this partnership is 'both respectful and reciprocal'. Kitwood's theory aims to retrieve the personhood of people living with dementia in order to '[open] up the way for a more personal and optimistic view of care giving' (Kitwood, 1990, p. 177).

Personhood is a dynamic that manifests in and as social interaction (Penrod et al., 2007). A patient's personhood can be respected, or negated, depending on how the patient is treated or *positioned* in interactions.

The concept of **malignant social positioning**, introduced by Kitwood (1997), refers to negative interactions between people with dementia and their carers. Malignant social positioning involves the carer disempowering and diminishing the patients' personhood. Kitwood contends that poor care involves malignant social positioning as a form of payback. Such care puts people with dementia under even more stress than they experience from the effects of the dementia alone.

> **malignant (social) positioning**
> positioning that occurs when a person with dementia is spoken about in derogatory or negative terms. For example, the person may be characterised as not interesting, or even as 'incomplete'.

Factors detrimental to the safety, clinical outcomes and well-being of people with dementia are well-documented. In the acute sector, one such factor is the 'harmful pathway' (George, Long & Vincent, 2013, p. 356). Once positioned as aggressive, patients with dementia are at high risk of adverse events. They may receive inadequate assessment and treatment and even inappropriate interventions (such as over-medication or restraint). A series of such adverse events is referred to as 'cascade iatrogenesis'. Here, 'iatrogenesis' means 'healthcare-caused harm or wrong', and a cascade is a *chain* of such harms and wrongs (George, Long & Vincent, 2013, p. 357). Other factors leading to unsafe care for people with dementia include 'ageism' and related negative organisational values. Ageism manifests in health professionals' negative stereotypes of older people (Wells et al., 2004).

These factors may produce the following substandard care effects. Healthcare workers often give low priority to the care needs of people with dementia. Hospitals and aged care facility environments are often focused more on risk management than on trying to improve the cognitive functioning and well-being of people with dementia (Moyle et al., 2010). People with dementia often have distressing acute hospital experiences (Cowdell, 2010). Healthcare institutions frequently deliver task-oriented care that does not recognise the uniqueness of the patient (Edvardsson, Winblad & Sandman, 2008). Health services often have poor physical environments that do not reflect 'enabling design' – building and interior design that recognises the needs of cognitively impaired patients (Calkins, 2009).

Conclusion

Our approach to people with cognitive impairment as persons and the environment we create for them underpin the issues with care delivery and outcomes in any healthcare setting. Being person-centred in our care and in the design of care environments is essential for optimal care delivery. It requires health professionals and designers to think about the effect of what they do on the person as a whole.

While there are many definitions of person-centred care and associated terms, common to all is the importance of relationships and partnerships underpinned by inclusive communication. Killick (2004) points out that if a health professional is not able to connect with the person or patient with dementia, they are likely to withdraw into themselves and reduce their efforts to communicate.

Practice example 9.2

As Tom progressed on his dementia journey, Betty found it increasingly difficult to care for him at home, even with community care support. She found the fact that Tom seldom spoke any more particularly difficult. Reluctantly Betty agreed that a move to a residential aged care facility was the only option. The only appropriate vacancy was a two-hour drive away. Betty didn't find this too worrying, however, as their oldest daughter and three grandchildren lived just 10 minutes away from the facility.

Tom enjoyed visits from his daughter and grandchildren who would come two or three times a week. Smiles, hugs and kisses were plentiful. However, the daughter was always in a hurry and seldom stayed for more than a half an hour. When they left, Tom would sit in his room staring out of the window for hours. Betty would drive up on a Tuesday evening and stay at her daughter's house. She would go to the aged care facility at 9 a.m. on Wednesday morning and stay all day, driving home just before dinner time. Tom looked forward to her visits and would be sitting in a chair at the door waiting for her on Wednesday mornings. The staff often saw them holding hands, or Betty would be stroking his arm while she was talking to him.

Betty has been amazed at the change in Tom since he has moved to the home. He is far more independent than before he moved in, and although he still doesn't say very much, he has taken charge of one of the raised garden beds to grow vegetables – something he hasn't done for years. In recent weeks he has developed a friendship with a woman in the home whom he introduces to everyone as 'his sister' Nancy. They sit together at mealtimes, she reads the newspaper to him, they walk the garden paths and watch the birds together. 'Nancy' is often making something in craft activities while Tom watches on. Many of these crafts end up as gifts for Betty when she visits. Betty has told staff that his sister Nancy died when he was just a teenager.

Betty and the staff see the value and enjoyment both Tom and 'Nancy' are getting out of the relationship. However, the staff indicated to Betty that although their daughter is still visiting two or three times a week, she seldom brings the grandchildren to visit as often and while Tom is always very pleased to see her, he often paces up and down, shouting for about a half an hour after she leaves. No one can make out what he is saying

continued ›

Practice example 9.2 continued ›

but it is distressing for Tom and other residents, especially 'Nancy', whom he has pushed away on a number of occasions and then ignored for the rest of the day. On those days, he usually eats alone in his room, if he can be tempted to eat at all. Betty is now very concerned as this is a side of Tom she has not seen and she doesn't feel able to talk to her daughter about it as she fears it will stop the visits altogether. Nancy's family have also raised concerns, having witnessed his change in behaviour when visiting one day. Some staff are now referring to Tom as 'agitated' and have begun to perceive the relationship between 'Nancy' and Tom as unhealthy.

Reflective questions

Tom's behaviour just described tells a story – he is trying to communicate something but those around him are unable or unwilling to understand. You have been asked to take the lead in determining the issues and working with Tom, his family and other staff to develop strategies to address the situation.

1. What are the risks to safety and care delivery if issues are not addressed?
2. What role will communication play in developing strategies to resolve matters?
3. How will person-centred practice guide you in developing these strategies?

Further reading

Brooker, D. (2007). *Person-centred dementia care: Making services better.* London: Jessica Kingsley Publishers.
This book provides clear guidelines on how to put key aspects of person-centred care into action. The author re-establishes the meaning of person-centred care in practice.

Clinical Epidemiology and Health Service Evaluation Unit. (2006). *Clinical practice guidelines for the management of delirium in older people.* Melbourne: Author.
This document is an initiative of the Australian Health Ministers' Advisory Council's (AHMAC) Health Care of Older Australians Standing Committee (HCOASC) and the Australian Department of Health and Ageing. It provides recommendations for the management of delirium and accompanying resources.

McCarthy, B. (2011). *Hearing the person with dementia: Person centred approaches for families and caregivers.* London: Jessica Kingsley Publishers.
This is a practical book outlining the effects of dementia on communication and providing communication guidance for person-centred care.

Web resources

Come into my world: http://nursing.flinders.edu.au/comeintomyworld

Commonwealth of Australia, *Delirium in older people*: http://www.health.gov.au/internet/main/publishing.nsf/Content/delerium-guidelines.htm

References

Abete, P., Della-Morte, D., Gargiulo, G., Basile, C., Langellott, A., Galizia, G. et al. (2014). Cognitive impairment and cardiovascular diseases in the elderly. A heart-brain continuum hypothesis. *Ageing Research Reviews, 18*, 41–52.

AIHW. (2012). *Dementia in Australia*. Canberra: Author.

American Psychiatric Association. (2000). *Diagnostic and statistical manual of mental disorders* (4th ed.). Washington, DC: Author.

Banerjee, S. (2009). *The use of antipsychotic medication for people with dementia: Time for action*. London: Department of Health.

Calkins, M. (2009). Evidence-based long term design. *Neurorehabilitation, 25*(3), 145–154.

Clinical Epidemiology and Health Service Evaluation Unit. (2006). *Clinical practice guidelines for the management of delirium in older people*. Melbourne: Author.

Cowdell, F. (2010). The care of older people with dementia in acute hospitals. *International Journal of Older People Nursing, 5*(2), 83–92.

Department of Health Services. (2014). *Person-directed dementia care assessment tool*. Bureau of Aging and Disability Resources. Wisconson: Author. Retrieved March 12, 2015 from https://www.dhs.wisconsin.gov/publications/p2/p20084.pdf

Draper, B., Karmel, R., Gibson, D., Peut, A., & Anderson, P. (2011). The hospital dementia service project: Age difference in hospital stays for older people with and without dmentia. *International Psychogeriatrics, 23*(10), 1649–1658.

Edlund, A., Lundstrom, M., Karlsson, S., Brännström, B., Bucht, G., & Gustafson, Y. (2006). Delirium in older patients admitted to general internal medicine. *Journal of Geriatric Psychiatry and Neurology, 19*(2), 83–90.

Edvardsson, D., Winblad, B., & Sandman, P. O. (2008). Person-centred care of people with severe Alzheimer's disease: Current status and ways forward. *The Lancet Neurology, 7*, 362–367.

Fan, V. S., & Meek, P. M. (2014). Anxiety, depression and cognitive impairment in patients with chronic respiratory disease. *Clinics in Chest Medicine, 35*(2), 399–409.

George, J., Long, S., & Vincent, C. (2013). How can we keep patients with dementia safe in our acute hospitals? A review of challenges and solutions. *Journal of the Royal Society of Medicine, 106*, 355–361.

Harding, S. (2006). Delirium in older people. Canberra: Commonwealth of Australia.

Hutchinson, T. A., & Brawer, J. R. (2011). The challenge of medical dichotomies and the congruent physican–patient relationship in medicine. In T. A. Hutchinson (Ed.), *Whole person care: A new paradigm for the 21st century* (pp. 31–43). New York: Springer.

Killick, J. (2004). Dementia, identity and spirituality. *Journal of Religious Gerontology, 16*, 59–74.

Kitwood, T. (1990). The dialectics of dementia: With particular reference to Alzheimer's disease. *Ageing and Society*, *10*(02), 177–196.

——. (1997). *Dementia reconsidered: The person comes first*. Buckingham: Open University Press.

Ludwick, R., O' Toole, R., & Meehan, A. (2012). Restraints or alternatives: Safety work in care of older persons. *International Journal of Older People Nursing*, *7*(1), 11–19.

Man, B. L., Wong, A., Chan, Y., Lam, W. A., Hui, C., Leung, W. et al. (2011). Cognitive and functional impairments in ischaemic stroke patient with concurrent small vessell and large artery disease. *Clinical Neurology and Neurosurgery*, *113*(8), 612–616.

Marin, M. F., Lord, C., Andrews, J., Juster, R., Sindi, S., Arsenault-Lapierre, G. et al. (2012). Chronic stress, cognitive functioning and mental health. *Neurobiology of Learning and Memory*, *96*(4), 583–595.

Meagher, D. J. (2001). Delirium: Optimising management. *British Medical Journal*, *322*(7279), 144–149.

Morita, T., Hirai, K., Sakaguchi, Y., Tsuneto, S., & Shima, Y. (2004). Family-perceived distress from delirium-related symptoms of terminally ill cancer patients. *Psychosomatics*, *45*, 107–113.

Moyle, W., Borbasi, S., Wallis, M., Olorenshaw, R., & Gracia, N. (2010). Acute care management of older people with dementia: A qualitative perspective. *Journal of Clinical Nursing*, *20*, 420–428.

Nash, S., Luaute, J., Bar, J., Sancho, P., Hourse, M., Chossegros, L. et al. (2014). Cognitive and behavioural post-tramuatic impairments: What is the specificity of a brain injury? A study with the ESPARR cohort. *Annals of Physical Rehabilitation and Medicine*, *57*(9-10), 600-617.

Penrod, J., Kolanowski, A., Fick, D., Loeb, S., & Hupcey, J. (2007). Reframing person centred nursing care for persons with dementia. *Research Theory Nursing Practice*, *21*(1), 57–72.

Touhy, T. A., & Jett, K. F. (2013). *Elbersole and Hess' towards healthy ageing: Human needs and nursing response*. Philadelphia: Elsevier Health Sciences.

van Munster, B., & de Rooij, S. (2014). Delirium: A synthesis of current knowledge. *Clinical Medicine*, *14*(2), 192–195.

Weitzel, T., Robinson, S., Barnes, M. R., Berry, T. A., Holmes, J. M., Mercer, S. et al. (2010). The special needs of the hospitalised patient with dementia. *Medsurg Nursing: Official Journal of the Academy of Medical-Surgical Nurses*, *20*(1), 13–18.

Wells, Y., Foreman, P., Gething, L., & Petralia, W. (2004). Nurses' attitudes toward aging and older adults-examining attitudes and practices among health service providers in Australia. *Journal of Gerontological Nursing*, *30*(9), 5–13.

Williams, K. N., Boyle, D. K., Herman, R. E., Coleman, C. K., & Hummert, M. L. (2012). Psychometric analysis of the emotional tone rating scale: A measure of person-centred communication. *Clinical Gerontologist*, *35*(5), 376–389.

Williams, K. N., Herman, R., Gajewski, B., & Wilson, K. (2009). Elderspeak communication: Impact on dementia care. *American Journal of Alzheimer's Disease and Other Dementias*, *24*(1), 11–20.

Williams, K. N., & Herman, R. E. (2011). Linking resident behaviour to dementia care communication: Effects of emotional tone. *Behavior Therapy*, *42*(1), 42–46.

10

Therapeutic communication with people experiencing mental illness

Jennifer Plumb

Learning objectives

This chapter will enable you to:
- express why it is important that every health and welfare service professional knows how to communicate therapeutically with a person in mental distress;
- identify the basic principles of therapeutic communication with a person in mental distress, including building rapport and trust, seeing the whole person, and adopting an attitude of 'unconditional positive regard';
- identify basic techniques for communicating with a person who is experiencing a crisis which puts their own safety, or the safety of others, at risk.

Key terms

Empathy
Mental health
Psychiatry
Respect
Therapeutic communication
Verbal de-escalation

Overview

It is estimated that almost half of the population will experience a mental illness at some time in their lives (Australian Bureau of Statistics, 2009). It is therefore almost certain that whatever health profession you enter, you will encounter people experiencing acute symptoms of mental illness at the time they come to you for help.

Your ability to communicate and connect with someone in such a situation can be the difference between them getting timely and appropriate support or deteriorating further. So, if you are tempted to skip over this section because you do not intend to work in the field of mental health, we encourage you to think again.

Even though research shows that the attitudes and actions of healthcare staff can have profound effects on the clinical and life outcomes of people living with **mental health** difficulties, communication with **respect** by professionals is unfortunately often the exception rather than the rule (Clarke, Dusome & Hughes, 2007; Rose et al., 2013).

This chapter focuses on increasing your confidence in interacting with people experiencing acute emotional distress in the context of mental illness. You will learn basic principles underpinning high-quality **therapeutic communication**, which can be applied more widely to any professional encounter where a person is emotionally distressed.

> **mental health**
> psychological well-being.
>
> **respect**
> positive attitude towards another. It involves granting another person the right to be who they want to be, and say and think what they want to say and think.
>
> **therapeutic communication**
> a technique of healing through interaction. It is the establishment of a connection which incorporates choice of words, body language and tone of voice which together demonstrate to a distressed person an attitude of respect, compassion and hope.

Introduction

When the other person is hurting, confused, troubled, anxious, alienated, terrified, or when he or she is doubtful of self-worth, uncertain as to identity, then understanding is called for. The gentle and sensitive companionship of an empathic person ... provides illumination and healing. In such situations deep understanding is, I believe, the most precious gift one can give to another. (Rogers, 1995, p. 161)

Many sectors of health care have become increasingly dominated by technologies that extend the skills of health professionals, allowing them to see inside the body, to pinpoint pathology, and to monitor vital signs. The practice of mental health care is, in contrast, a largely technology-free zone. With the exception of pharmaceutical interventions, and despite advances in genomics, the clinical practice of mental health care happens principally through interaction.

The difference between good and poor quality mental health care very often lies in the quality of the relationship between the patient and the professional (for example, Green et al., 2008; Priebe et al., 2011). Here, communication is not separate from the 'real work' of treatment and healing. Communication is the 'real work' – the main tool of treatment – for professionals working with people experiencing mental illness.

The use of principles of therapeutic communication by health and welfare professionals, whether or not they work in mental health care, can have a significant impact on people experiencing mental illness.

> Preventing psychological harm means protecting the art and humanity of medicine as much as the science. It requires recognition that professional words and behaviour are potentially as toxic as therapeutic. (Rees, 2012, p. 446)

We have two strong sources of evidence confirming the importance of appropriate communication with patients experiencing mental illness. First, interactions characterised by judgmental or stigmatising attitudes can exacerbate a person's mental illness, erode their self-respect, and make it less likely that they will try to seek help in the future (Hansson et al., 2013; Reavley et al., 2014; Thornicroft, Rose & Kassam, 2007).

Second, people with severe mental illness have a life expectancy of between 10 and 20 years less than their peers. This excess mortality mostly stems from preventable physical illnesses that have nothing directly to do with mental illness (Lawrence, Hancock & Kisely, 2013; Nordentoft et al., 2013). This is a poor reflection on the quality of primary care and general hospital care provided to this group of people.

A further sign of failure to engage therapeutically with patients experiencing a mental illness is the fact that people who die by suicide are more likely to have had recent contact with health services (through a hospital admission for a physical health complaint or through a visit to their GP) than they are to have been in contact with specialist mental health services (Ahmedani et al., 2014; Luoma, Martin & Pearson, 2002; O'Neill, Corry, Murphy & Bunting, 2014). This research confirms the importance of communicating with such patients in ways that appropriately acknowledge their needs.

Clearly, the safety and quality of health care for people experiencing mental illness is far from optimal. Given the importance of responding to patients experiencing mental illness with appropriate communication, the way the interaction unfolds between the person and the professional plays a crucial role in determining whether health service encounters help or hinder their recovery and whether recommended treatment (whether for mental or physical health) is effective (Burgess et al., 2008; Clement et al., 2012; Sirey et al., 2001).

We now examine the principles of therapeutic communication through two clinical practice scenarios.

Practice example 10.1

This example presents the perspective of a person attending a health service and experiencing distress.

I sit opposite the doctor with tears running down my face, my hands uselessly shredding tissues into little balls that fall to the floor as I try to tell her how this feels. I have never known such a complete inability to control or soothe or describe the absolute blackness inside. Three days ago, she changed my medications, and my body and mind are no longer mine. I shake, my clothes are soaked in sweat. I cannot use words. She sits impassively behind her clipboard, carefully writing notes. 'I can't get through this day.' I

continued ›

throw this at her, again and again. She shifts in her chair, hands over a new prescription, a slightly different dose. My desperate phone messages from yesterday, never acknowledged. The too-sudden change of drugs, never discussed. I go back out onto the street, clutching the prescription. This city, my home, feels foreign. I am lost.

A different, new doctor. My friend takes me to her that same day. We sit in the waiting room for a long time. In between the procession of patients, the doctor comes over to explain – 'I am so sorry – it's such a busy afternoon'. At last, it's my turn. She comes back to the waiting room, says my first name, smiles, shakes my hand, introduces herself. She smiles at my friend, asks her name. Walking to her room, she points me to a chair close to hers, asks if I like peppermint tea. She returns with two cups of steaming minty comfort, places them together on the table between us. She types notes as we talk. Between her halting two finger efforts at the keyboard, she leans towards me, her eyes meet mine: 'You're having a tough time of it, aren't you. What's happened?'

She is interested, I think. The words start to come. She takes it seriously. She nods, she frowns, her eyes radiate kindness and concern. She explains to me why I am feeling this way – what is happening in my brain and what the drugs have done. Fear and panic recede. This will fade. She seems to get how hard it is to think about the next step. She writes down what I need to do, just tonight and tomorrow morning. A list, with times and tasks. Stay with your friend. Eat something. Take this drug, this much, this time. Tomorrow, see my nurse, this time, this address. 'I will call you first thing,' she says. And she does.

Analysis and reflection

The differences between the two interactions in practice example 10.1 and the impacts they had on the writer of this extract illustrate important aspects of helpful, as against harmful, communication.

Note that the healing quality of the communication is, from the writer's perspective, separate to the formal, technical tasks of **psychiatry** such as the mental state examination, risk assessment, and decisions about medication. Even though the first doctor may have been fulfilling these requirements, we can see that for the writer in the midst of her distress, something key to her recovery was missing. While the first doctor leaves her feeling disoriented, the second doctor makes it seem possible to 'keep going'.

While the first doctor remains impassive behind a clipboard as she busily writes clinical notes, the second intersperses her note-writing with time dedicated solely to talking. In doing so – making eye contact, expressing **empathy**, and communicating

> **psychiatry**
> a branch of medicine that specialises in the treatment of disorders such as schizophrenia and psychosis.
>
> **empathy**
> a mental state whereby a person, experiencing compassion, shows they are affected by another person's suffering, and takes steps to alleviate that person's suffering.

recognition of distress – she makes the writer feel like she is being taken seriously. Empathy asks the question, 'How have this person's experiences led them to see/feel/think and act in the way they do?' (Elliott et al., 2011, p. 134).

The first doctor appears to do little to validate this person's experience or acknowledge her pain. During the interaction, she keeps an emotional distance and the writer finds it hard to bridge the gap to express how she is feeling.

The second doctor's initial encounters with the writer in the waiting room were important in establishing rapport. Her acknowledgement of the long wait established a frame of respectful communication, and also reduced the writer's uncertainty about what was happening. Calling the writer by her first name only, shaking her hand and smiling, and acknowledging the presence of her friend were all acts that reduced the power differential between doctor and patient and made it clear that the doctor saw the writer as a person rather than simply a 'case'.

The simple gesture of offering a cup of tea established a sense of comfort and security within which the interaction could proceed. While this may seem unusual in a run-of-the-mill healthcare setting, and may not be appropriate with people who are highly agitated or aggressive, in this case it was a very effective way to share a normalising experience and create a caring connection.

Reflective questions

Imagine that you have already qualified in your chosen profession and that you encounter the person who wrote practice example 10.1. She may have come to you about some other health problem but breaks down in front of you. Or she may have come to you directly for help with her distress (for example, if you work in an emergency department).

1. How might you feel if she were crying in front of you, unable to say what is wrong?
2. What might you instinctively want to do or say, and what effect might that have on her?
3. What manner, tone of voice, body language could you adopt to help her feel less distressed?
4. What could you do practically to help her feel less distressed?
5. How would you decide the next steps to take?

Implications for practice

Research by and with people experiencing mental illness reveals a common set of professional attitudes and interactions that help them or harm them during times of acute distress (see for example Gunasekara et al., 2014; Noble & Douglas, 2004). Many of them will be familiar from the scenario above. Let's spell out a few important communication principles.

Be aware of your impact on the other person: even brief negative encounters with health and welfare services can have lasting impacts on a person's self-regard, compounding the distress caused by the illness itself (Corrigan, 2004; Hansson, Stjernswärd & Svensson, 2014; Markowitz, 1998; Rüsch, Angermeyer & Corrigan, 2005). An intelligent and articulate man living with schizophrenia told the author that he was hurt when he had called a government helpline with a question about his benefits. The person on the other end started talking loudly and slowly to him as soon as he mentioned his illness. The patient's hurt did not register for the person on the helpline.

See the whole person: when you encounter a person experiencing distress, remember that illness is not their defining feature. They have a past, they have unique experiences, and even if they do not feel them at that moment, they have hopes, preferences and strengths. Attempting to connect with these other aspects of a person can be valuable both in creating a sense of hope and in connecting them to the 'here and now', particularly if they are responding to internal stimuli such as hallucinations (Bowers et al., 2009).

Think about how you can tailor your interaction so that it is appropriate to the individual. This means finding out about and considering the different needs associated with (for example) diverse cultural, religious and linguistic backgrounds and people who have experienced abuse or trauma.

Build rapport and trust: simple kindnesses are incredibly important to someone who is distressed or who has disclosed mental illness to you (Borg & Kristiansen, 2004). You can show your care by the expression on your face and the tone of your voice, just as you would with any person you care about. Depending on the circumstances, this care might involve attending to physical comfort or avoiding compromising the person's dignity (for example, by leaving them alone and distressed in a public waiting room).

Empower the other: when someone is very distressed, they can feel as though things are getting out of their control (Goddard, 2011). It is important to offer options for next steps, and ask about preferences. This is central to a recovery-oriented model of mental health support, in which people are empowered by professionals to make their own choices and to build on their strengths and preferences to live a meaningful life with or without symptoms. It is also vital to recognise that family members and other supporters can in many cases be a resource for the person's ongoing well-being. Loved ones can often feel excluded and ill-informed about what is happening. Only involve them if the person consents, however.

Create continuity and consistency: consistency of care is an important aspect of therapeutic interactions between services and people experiencing mental illness (Burns et al., 2009). If possible, if you have started to build trust and rapport with a person and if they will continue to access your service, try to ensure that they can speak to or be treated by the same person each visit.

Theoretical links

During recent years, the ideal of 'person-centred care' has become popular in health policy circles (Freeth, 2007; Stewart, 2001). The importance accorded to the individual patient's experience is partly related to the increased role of choice in the healthcare industry, and partly to a recognition that a positive experience of treatment and care can have a significant impact on clinical outcomes. In mental health care, this principle is integral to the conduct of recovery-oriented models of care (for more information about the recovery approach, see the *National Framework for Recovery Oriented Mental Health Services* in the 'Further reading' list at the end of this chapter).

The idea is nothing new. A theory of a 'person-centred approach' to therapeutic interaction with people experiencing mental distress was developed by a psychologist, Carl Rogers, as early as the 1950s. Together, the principles introduced in previous sections encompass an attitude which Rogers called 'unconditional positive regard' (Rogers, 2007).

Unconditional positive regard is part of a theory of psychotherapy that is more complex than we can do justice to here (see Freeth (2007) to learn more about Rogerian theory). The essence of the concept is for the caregiver to hold a hopeful, calm, and respectful attitude towards the distressed person, unconditionally. It does not mean that you have to agree with what they are saying, or that you cannot set limits on acceptable behaviour. However, for the time you are interacting with them, you try to put your own judgments aside and aim for an empathic understanding of a person's actions or words as coming from a place of fear, anxiety or unbearable pain. For many people, the feeling of being accepted *despite* their distress can be novel and healing (Hunter et al., 2013; Rogers, 1995).

Conclusion

To conclude, we have seen that calmly 'being with' someone who is very distressed, and being able to tolerate that distress for long enough to establish a connection, presents a unique communication challenge to health professionals. This is especially the case if the distress is induced by hallucinations or delusions. However, from the perspective of the person experiencing mental illness, what is often all that is needed is simply being treated and talked to as a valued human being:

> For decades I waited, waited for the people who were allocated to help me, to listen. To listen with their hearts and minds, without preconceptions or judgements … Madness does not strip you of the basic human needs to be valued, treated with respect and regard, and 'loved'. It is through thoughtful relationships with family, friends and health professionals that we seek understanding and solace. (Debra Lampshire in Geekie et al., 2012, p. xvii).

Practice example 10.2

We now move on to a second scenario, in which an attempt is made to show unconditional positive regard when a person expresses their distress in a more aggressive way. Below, you will find an edited transcript of nurses performing a role-play. This was part of a training session on how to deal with a communication dilemma that commonly arises when people who are involuntarily detained in hospital angrily demand to leave.

The training focused on **verbal de-escalation** techniques, which aim to prevent aggressive distress escalating to a point where physical restraint is needed. This scenario illustrates the fact that even though this person is expressing their distress in a very different way to the person who told their story in the practice example 10.1, the same principles of therapeutic communication can still be used.

> **verbal de-escalation**
> interaction with a person who is expressing distress which threatens their own safety or that of others. It involves using empathic and verbal techniques to exert a calming effect on the person's behaviour and avert the need for physical or chemical restraint (see Richmond et al., 2012).

Note that in this dialogue the nurse (N) does not always adhere to the principles of therapeutic communication and attitude. See if you can spot where the nurse deviates from some of the principles outlined in the section 'Implications for practice' above.

Role-play

Brian is very agitated. He is in his room in the mental health ward and wants to go home.

Nurse: Brian, look, I understand that you've been having a bit of a rough day ... I wanted to come and see if you were up to speaking about it.

Brian: [Angrily] Why am I here? I've been here for weeks. Why can't I go home?

N: As I think you understand, the team came to see you earlier in the week and they felt you weren't at your usual level.

B: [Angrily] Do you know me? Do you know me?

N: [Using a calm tone] At the moment, you are showing symptoms of being unwell from how we understand your mental illness.

B: I'm not unwell. I'm not throwing up.

N: I think at the moment you will need us to get through this rough time.

B: Why? I wanna go home.

N: It is in your best interests that you stay with us at this stage, OK ... We just want to monitor you at the moment.

B: [Sadly, more calmly] I want my own bed.

N: I know you do. I think it's a good idea to stay here and we'll bring some of your things in from home to make you feel a bit more ... at home. ... We're organising for you to have a few friends and family come and visit and hopefully they will assist us in making you feel more comfortable.

continued ›

Practice example 10.2 continued ›

B: [Hopeful] Can they come today?

N: They certainly can come today … are there any belongings that you'd like
            them to bring?

B: I want my pillow. The pillows here make creaky noises when I roll over and
            it wakes me up … they're plastic, I think. You might want to change them.
            Can I have my own pillow?

N: Do they? That's a great idea. You can absolutely. I will organise that myself.

[Role-play ends; other nurses begin discussing how the interaction went.]

Trainer: Great. What you want to do in de-escalation is open up a dialogue … rather
            than throwing things at you, you actually want to connect with them.

Colleague: Some of your language you used was really good. Like when he said about
            the pillow, you really acknowledged his experience and that empowers
            [Brian] to be able to inform you of something.

Reflective questions

1. Explain how you think Brian might have been feeling before, during and after this
    incident. Why might he have been agitated?
2. What are the key differences between the situations described in the first practice
    example and in the second one?
3. How might these differences affect how you might communicate with the
    person experiencing distress if faced with the second situation compared to
    the first?
4. How could the therapeutic communication principles introduced to you in practice
    example 10.1 be used in a situation such as this one where distress is expressed more
    aggressively?
5. How did the nurse in practice example 10.2 succeed in using some of these principles?
    What could they improve?
6. Think about and plan how you might use Rogerian principles in your next interaction
    with an emotionally distressed person – whether this person is experiencing mental
    illness or not.

Further reading

Australian Government. (2013). A national framework for recovery oriented mental health
    services. Retrieved September 14, 2014 from http://www.health.gov.au/internet/
    publications/publishing.nsf/Content/mental-pubs-n-recovgde-toc

Therapeutic communication forms a central part of the recovery philosophy of mental health care. The appendix to this document illustrates in detail the practical skills and capabilities health professionals need to engage therapeutically with people experiencing mental illness, including 'promoting a culture and language of hope and optimism'.

Blofeld, J., Sallah, D., Sashidharan, S., Stone, R., & Struthers, J. (2003). *Independent inquiry into the death of David Bennett.* Cambridge: Norfolk, Suffolk and Cambridgeshire Strategic Health Authority.

Although some of the issues addressed in this UK inquiry report go beyond the scope of this chapter, the document is a compelling illustration of the importance of therapeutic interaction to the safety of care.

Freeth, R. (2007). *Humanising psychiatry and mental health care: The challenge of the person-centred approach.* Abingdon: Radcliffe Medical Press.

This is a comprehensive guide to the theory and practice of Rogerian person-centred care, and a discussion of the challenges the approach still presents to the accepted relationship between health services and people with mental health difficulties.

Goddard, M. (2011). On being possibly sane in possibly insane places. *Psychiatric Services, 62*(8), 831–832.

This is a short and vivid first-hand account of a doctor's experiences of becoming acutely mentally ill and his subsequent treatment by the health system in the US. He describes being treated in a way that made him feel frightened, disempowered and no longer in control of what happened to him.

National Institute for Health and Clinical Excellence. (2011). Service user experience in adult mental health: Improving the experience of care for people using adult NHS mental health services. Retrieved September 14, 2014 from http://www.nice.org.uk/guidance/CG136

This is a detailed description of what people experiencing mental illness should be able to expect from their service providers, and the site provides links to a wealth of other resources about optimising experiences of care.

Rees, C. (2012). Iatrogenic psychological harm. *Archives of Disease in Childhood, 97*(5), 440–446.

Written by a paediatrician, this paper examines the concept of how psychological harm can be caused by the experience of general health care, and how non-mental health clinicians can avoid this.

··

Web resources

Australian Commission on Safety and Quality in Health Care: http://www.safetyandquality.gov.au/our-work/mental-health
Mental Health First Aid: http://www.mhfa.com.au
National Mental Health Consumer and Carer Forum: http://www.nmhccf.org.au
National Voices: http://www.nationalvoices.org.uk

··

References

Ahmedani, B. K., Simon, G. E., Stewart, C., Beck, A., Waitzfelder, B. E., Rossom, R. et al. (2014). Health care contacts in the year before suicide death. *Journal of General Internal Medicine, 29*(6), 870–877.

Australian Bureau of Statistics. (2009). National survey of mental health and wellbeing: Summary of results. Cat no.: 4326.0, 2007. Canberra: Author.

Borg, M., & Kristiansen, K. (2004). Recovery-oriented professionals: Helping relationships in mental health services. *Journal of Mental Health, 13*(5), 493–505.

Bowers, L., Brennan, G., Winship, G., & Theodoridou, C. (2009). *Talking with acutely psychotic people: Communication skills for nurses and others spending time with people who are very mentally ill*. London: City University.

Burgess, D. J., Ding, Y., Hargreaves, M., van Ryn, M., & Phelan, S. (2008). The association between perceived discrimination and underutilization of needed medical and mental health care in a multi-ethnic community sample. *Journal of Health Care for the Poor and Underserved, 19*(3), 894–911.

Burns, T., Catty, J., White, S., Clement, S., Ellis, G., Rees-Jones, I. et al. (2009). Continuity of care in mental health: Understanding and measuring a complex phenomenon. *Psychological Medicine, 39*(2), 313–323.

Clarke, D. E., Dusome, D., & Hughes, L. (2007). Emergency department from the mental health client's perspective. *International Journal of Mental Health Nursing, 16*(2), 126–131.

Clement, S., Brohan, E., Jeffery, D., Henderson, C., Hatch, St. L., & Thornicroft, G. (2012). Development and psychometric properties the barriers to access to care evaluation scale (bace) related to people with mental ill health. *BMC Psychiatry, 12*(1), 36.

Corrigan, P. (2004). How stigma interferes with mental health care. *American Psychologist, 59*(7), 614–625.

Elliott, R., Bohart, A., Watson, J., & Greenberg, L. (2011). Empathy. In J. C. Norcross (Ed.), *Psychotherapy relationships that work: Evidence-based responsiveness*. New York: Oxford University Press.

Freeth, R. (2007). *Humanising psychiatry and mental health care: The challenge of the person-centred approach*. Abingdon: Radcliffe Medical Press.

Geekie, J., Randal, P., Lampshire, D., & Read, J. (2012). *Experiencing psychosis: Personal and professional perspectives*. Hove: Routledge.

Goddard, M. (2011). On being possibly sane in possibly insane places. *Psychiatric Services, 62*(8), 831–832.

Green, C., Polen, M. R., Janoff, S. L., Castleton, D. K., Wisdom, J. P., Vuckovic, N. et al. (2008). Understanding how clinician-patient relationships and relational continuity of care affect recovery from serious mental illness: Stars study results. *Psychiatric Rehabilitation Journal, 32*(1), 9–22.

Gunasekara, I., Pentland, T., Rodgers, T., & Patterson, S. (2014). What makes an excellent mental health nurse? A pragmatic inquiry initiated and conducted by people with lived experience of service use. *International Journal of Mental Health Nursing, 23*(2), 101–109.

Hansson, L., Jormfeldt, H., Svedberg, P., & Svensson, B. (2013). Mental health professionals' attitudes towards people with mental illness: Do they differ from attitudes held by people with mental illness? *International Journal of Social Psychiatry, 59*(1), 48–54.

Hansson, L., Stjernswärd, S., & Svensson, B. (2014). Perceived and anticipated discrimination in people with mental illness: An interview study. *Nordic Journal of Psychiatry, 68*(2), 100–106.

Hunter, C., Chantler, K., Kapur, N., & Cooper, J. (2013). Service user perspectives on psychosocial assessment following self-harm and its impact on further help-seeking: A qualitative study. *Journal of Affective Disorders, 145*(3), 315–323.

Lawrence, D., Hancock, K., & Kisely, S. (2013). The gap in life expectancy from preventable physical illness in psychiatric patients in Western Australia: Retrospective analysis of population based registers. *British Medical Journal, 346*(f2539), 1–14.

Luoma, J. B., Martin, C. E., & Pearson, J. L. (2002). Contact with mental health and primary care providers before suicide: A review of the evidence. *American Journal of Psychiatry, 159*(6), 909–916.

Markowitz, F. E. (1998). The effects of stigma on the psychological well-being and life satisfaction of persons with mental illness. *Journal of Health and Social Behavior, 39*(4), 335–347.

Noble, L. M., & Douglas, B. C. (2004). What users and relatives want from mental health services. *Current Opinion in Psychiatry, 17*(4), 289–296.

Nordentoft, M., Wahlbeck, K., Hällgren, J., Westman, J., Ösby, U., Alinaghizadeh, H. et al. (2013). Excess mortality, causes of death and life expectancy in 270,770 patients with recent onset of mental disorders in Denmark, Finland and Sweden. *PLoS One, 8*(1), e55176: 1–11.

O'Neill, S., Corry, C. V., Murphy, S., & Bunting, B. P. (2014). Characteristics of deaths by suicide in Northern Ireland from 2005 to 2011 and use of health services prior to death. *Journal of Affective Disorders, 168*, 466–471.

Priebe, S., Dimic, S., Wildgrube, C., Jankovic, J., Cushing, A., & McCabe, R. (2011). Good communication in psychiatry–a conceptual review. *European Psychiatry, 26*(7), 403–407.

Reavley, N., Mackinnon, A., Morgan, A., & Jorm, A. (2014). Stigmatising attitudes towards people with mental disorders: A comparison of Australian health professionals with the general community. *Australian and New Zealand Journal of Psychiatry, 48*(5), 433–441.

Rees, C. (2012). Iatrogenic psychological harm. *Archives of Disease in Childhood, 97*(5), 440–446.

Richmond, J. S., Berlin, J. S., Fishkind, A. B., Holloman, G. H., Zeller, S. L., Wilson, M. P. et al. (2012). Verbal de-escalation of the agitated patient: Consensus statement of the American Association for Emergency Psychiatry Project Beta De-escalation Workgroup. *Western Journal of Emergency Medicine, 13*(1), 17–25.

Rogers, C. (1995). *A way of being.* Boston, MA: Houghton Mifflin Company.

——. (2007). The necessary and sufficient conditions of therapeutic personality change. *Psychotherapy: Theory, Research, Practice, Training, 44*(3), 240–248.

Rose, D., Evans, J., Laker, C., & Wykes, T. (2013). Life in acute mental health settings: Experiences and perceptions of service users and nurses. *Epidemiology and Psychiatric Sciences, 16*, 1–7.

Rüsch, N., Angermeyer, M. C., & Corrigan, P. W. (2005). Mental illness stigma: Concepts, consequences, and initiatives to reduce stigma. *European Psychiatry, 20*(8), 529–539.

Sirey, J. A., Bruce, M. L., Alexopoulos, G. S., Perlick, D. A., Friedman, S. J., & Meyers, B. S. (2001). Stigma as a barrier to recovery: Perceived stigma and patient-rated severity of illness as predictors of antidepressant drug adherence. *Psychiatric Services, 52*(12), 1615–1620.

Stewart, M. (2001). Towards a global definition of patient centred care. *British Medical Journal, 322*(7284), 444–445.

Thornicroft, G., Rose, D., & Kassam, A. (2007). Discrimination in health care against people with mental illness. *International Review of Psychiatry, 19*(2), 113–122.

Acknowledgement

The author acknowledges the kind contribution of clinical expertise to this chapter by Dr Tony Florio.

Communicating in partnership with service users: what can we learn from child and family health?

Nick Hopwood

Learning objectives

This chapter will enable you to:

- understand some of the key features of partnership approaches, and how they differ from expert-centred models of care;
- understand the role of verbal and non-verbal communication in partnership-based work;
- understand the complementary links between partnership approaches and ecological approaches, which take wider influences into consideration;
- understand how conceiving partnership in terms of a 'strengths-based approach' can help provide a way to use your valuable professional expertise while remaining faithful to principles of partnership.

Key terms

Ecological approach
Learning
Partnerships
Pedagogy
Service users
Strengths-based approach

Overview

This chapter explores communication as a crucial basis for establishing effective **partnerships** between child and family health professionals and health service users. It focuses

partnerships
reciprocal and respectful ways of working characterised by openness, mutual expertise, trust, negotiation and shared decision-making. Partnership contrasts with approaches in which professionals set the agenda, make decisions, and occupy the role of 'expert' while others' knowledge is regarded as secondary. In this chapter reference is made to the family partnership model (FPM; Davis & Day, 2010) as a specific partnership framework that has been widely implemented in Europe and Australasia.

learning
processes that enable people to know more or different things, to be different, and to act differently.

pedagogy
the theory about the processes that are understood to bring about learning. While it is similar to 'teaching', the latter often implies a formal educational setting (like a school) and a 'teacher'. In contrast, pedagogy points to the idea that many non-teaching health professionals are in fact engaged in helping and obliging colleagues and novices to learn.

service users
patients, clients, and consumers.

on health services that support families with young children, but the key concepts and lessons learned are applicable more widely. An example in which a number of features of partnership are on display is provided, and this is then used to show how thinking about partnership in terms of **learning** and **pedagogy** can be useful, particularly in showing how to use professional expertise effectively.

Introduction

Relationships between healthcare professionals and the people they help are changing. One important reason for this is that **service users** are increasingly encouraged and expected to play a role in their own care. They may be involved in the design and planning of their care, and consulted about the appropriate standards of care. Professionals are not seen as the only 'experts' in the equation, but as bringing important expertise to a situation in which others have valuable knowledge to contribute, too. This involvement can be referred to as *co-production* or *partnership* (Dunston et al., 2009).

The emphasis on co-production and partnership no doubt results from rising pressures on health services due to an increasing need to manage chronic conditions. There remain many features of health care where a strong expert-led approach is still needed, but when professionals are helping others cope with long-term health challenges and risks, a more consultative and joint process is called for.

Partnership approaches have caught on widely in child and family health services, where there are now several models of care that have been trialled and implemented (Davis & Day, 2010). These approaches play a prominent role in services that specifically aim to enhance health and well-being for families with young children. Child and family health professionals may work in homes, neighbourhood centres, children's centres, schools, community health or primary care settings, day stay or residential units, hospitals, and via telephone support services. They include nurses, health visitors, social workers, speech and language specialists, occupational therapists, psychologists, and practitioners from a range of medical disciplines such as psychiatry and paediatrics.

Child and family health services can provide support for parents prior to and after the birth of new children, screen for and address mood disorders among parents and children, help families cope with challenges associated with chronic health conditions, and build resilience in families by fostering relationships between families and their communities. Because the family unit is so important in shaping the health and wellbeing of all its members (Bronfenbrenner, 1979, 2005) services engage not with individuals but with *families*.

When working with parents and children, it is important to make sure they feel listened to and respected, and that they are not disappointed when inappropriate expectations are not met. Research has showed that family members were much less likely to follow through on advice from professionals when they did not feel involved in decisions relating to their care, or when they could not express their views, concerns and desires without being judged (Davis & Fallowfield, 1991).

Communication in partnership with family members requires skills of 'active listening' (allowing others to speak and finishing speaking only when they are done). Active listening demonstrates that you are listening attentively, and with empathy. This strategy also means questioning vulnerable people without fuelling anxiety, and showing an unconditional positive regard for the people you are trying to help. This happens verbally and through non-verbal cues, including body posture, gaze, facial expressions and gestures. Parents and children should feel that they can express their feelings and describe their experiences without being judged, and that they have a say in setting the agenda and deciding what happens.

The family partnership model (FPM) suggests there are a number of stages involved in the helping process. All the stages build on a relationship between the professional and the family. The stages also help to maintain and develop this relationship. The process begins with exploration, or listening to parents without judging. Then professionals explore how parents understand their situation, and might work to explore alternative understandings before setting goals. Goals are negotiated and reflect parents' priorities and values. Strategies to work on those goals are planned jointly, with family members actively involved in their implementation. Outcomes are reviewed, and it may be that further work is then done together, perhaps working on different goals.

Partnership approaches mean that professionals do not solve problems for others. Instead they help to build problem-solving abilities, confidence, and self-esteem by helping family members learn about parent–child interaction and themselves developing strategies to anticipate and cope with challenging circumstances.

Practice example 11.1

In this example Ruth, a nurse, is working with Kirsty who has been struggling to get her 18-month-old son Harry to fall asleep (settle) in the evening, and to self-settle when he wakes up during the night. The setting is a residential service where professionals are on hand to support families around the clock for a period of five days. Kirsty is becoming exhausted; the situation is placing strain on her relationship with her husband, and affecting Kirsty's ability to join in her local mothers' group and other community activities with Harry.

continued >

Practice example 11.1 continued ›

Kirsty has told Ruth that getting Harry to 'self-settle' is an important priority for her and her family, and Ruth has suggested that they try a different approach to settling. They will give Harry a chance to learn to settle by waiting until his cries indicate distress before going in to comfort him. Ruth has explained that she knows this will be hard for Kirsty, and that if Kirsty feels it is too much at any point they can try something else. They negotiate a goal, which is to challenge the family themselves to try a new settling approach and see how it goes.

Kirsty gives Harry a cuddle, tells him it is time for sleep, puts him down, gives him a kiss, and then turns to leave the room. As she does so, Harry begins to cry gently. Ruth touches Kirsty on the shoulder and nods, indicating they should go and stand outside together. Ruth reassures Kirsty: his immediate cries were expected. Ruth stands in a calm, relaxed posture and makes frequent eye contact with Kirsty, whose body is more tense.

Ruth asks Kirsty what she thinks Harry's cries mean. Kirsty isn't sure. Ruth says, 'Well, he's not screaming, and there are some silences there, so I think he's just protesting.' Kirsty nods, and Ruth explains that although it can be distressing for parents when their children cry, protest cries are very normal – children are just like adults and find change hard, and crying is a way to communicate this.

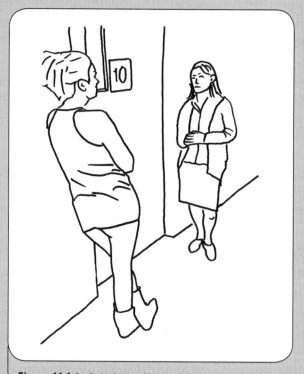

Figure 11.1 Ruth (right) and Kirsty (left) outside the nursery

continued ›

Practice example 11.1 continued ›

Over the next 15 minutes, they listen to Harry's cries, and go into the nursery each time they become more distressed. Ruth reminds Kirsty of the strategy they had chosen: Kirsty will pat the mattress next to Harry and offer gentle 'Sush-sush-shusssshh', 'Time for sleep', 'It's OK mummy's here', and to leave again when Harry calms down. Throughout the process Ruth reassures and praises Kirsty, asks her how she is feeling, and closely monitors her body language for signs of anxiety; she reminds Kirsty that at any time she can go in and cuddle Harry if she feels that is what she wants to do.

After coming out of the nursery for the fourth time (see Figure 11.1), Ruth asks Kirsty how she feels it is going, and Kirsty responds, 'OK but it's hard because he's still crying when I leave.' Ruth says, 'I noticed that time that Harry didn't lift his hands up when you went in.' Kirsty hadn't noticed this, being more occupied with Harry's cries. Ruth explains that this means Harry isn't wanting or expecting to be picked up for a cuddle any more, and that this learning has been prompted by Kirsty's consistent actions of going in and patting the mattress whenever Harry indicates distress. Harry is learning that Kirsty isn't far away and is there when he needs her, but also is becoming more at ease in his cot as he settles for sleep.

Analysis and reflection

Looking at practice example 11.1, we can see different features of partnership-based communication in action. It enables us to reflect on how these features compensate and counteract situations where experts set the agenda for families, tell them what to do, or assume there is a need to solve problems for them.

Right from the start this episode is strongly shaped by Kirsty's particular needs and challenges. Indeed, *she* herself sets the priority to be Harry's learning to self-settle. Within the **ecological approach**, respecting Kirsty's own understanding of the problem – Harry's difficulty settling – is critical for her to begin moving towards restoring the whole family's well-being and connectedness, including restoring connections with other families in their community. If Harry can self-settle, then he and his parents will be better rested, Kirsty will have more energy to play with Harry in the daytime, she will feel more able to be the mother and wife she wants to be, and she will be more confident in joining in her mothers' group and other activities.

> **ecological approach**
> an approach that takes account of contexts within which events take place. Ecology pays attention to a variety of contexts, including social, cultural, historical, political and environmental contexts.

Helping Kirsty to realise her priorities, Ruth contributed her expertise drawing on a repertoire of settling strategies and offering several alternatives. While Ruth was there to support Kirsty throughout the process, Ruth was not the one settling Harry. While Kirsty might have learned something by watching Ruth settle Harry, the experience is much more meaningful because she is acting it out herself. This is a significantly more effective preparation for when Kirsty and her family return home.

Significantly, too, Ruth asked Kirsty how she interpreted Harry's initial cries. Even though Kirsty wasn't sure, this simple question showed that Ruth was interested in Kirsty's understanding of the situation. Ruth then didn't simply say, 'He's protesting', but instead pointed to features of the crying, features they both could hear. This enabled Kirsty to 'read' Harry's cries such that she knew that he did not need her immediate physical presence. This way of directing others' attention is important, not just because it brings part of Ruth's expertise out into the open, but also because it helps Kirsty learn what to listen for in future.

Likewise, when Ruth mentions Harry not lifting his hands, she is again drawing on her professional expertise, showing she knows what to look for and why it is important. Importantly, this is used to help shift the situation as Kirsty perceives it (Harry is still crying, so progress isn't being made) to one in which signs of positive change may become apparent.

Then when Ruth adds how normal this is and likens Harry and other young children to adults in finding change hard, she recognises that Kirsty finds the crying hard to cope with, and provides multiple forms of reassurance. Here Ruth is communicating her empathy for Kirsty; she does not dismiss Kirsty as overly sensitive or a bad mother, but rather shows an unconditional regard that acknowledges that Kirsty's tension comes from her strong maternal instinct. Rather than saying her anxiety around crying was 'wrong', Ruth helps Kirsty 'read' the cries at multiple levels. This helps to move Kirsty's anxiety to the background to some extent.

In all, Ruth questions and monitors Kirsty for physical cues indicating anxiety. In doing so, Ruth exploits several communication channels: language, emotion and touch. These multiple channels ensure that Kirsty is not confronted with language alone, and help her connect what is going on to her own bodily responses. Although Ruth has offered support, and reassurance that Harry's cries do not all indicate distress, Ruth does not assume that Kirsty's experience is the same as hers: she makes use of all available signs to assess the need to stop or try a different approach.

> **strengths-based approach**
> a strength-based approach focuses on those aspects of people's own behaviour that show promise and use these to scaffold (support) changes in knowledge and behaviour, rather than work from idealised models and predetermined behaviour goals.

Most importantly, Ruth creates a *transformative event* for Kirsty: she is able to expand Kirsty's impact on the world by assisting Kirsty in recognising and acting on real-world cues. In effect, Ruth enacts a **strengths-based approach**, using Kirsty's way of being in the world as her starting point, and not doubting that Kirsty is capable of using her own resources to enhance how she relates to and manages Harry.

Implications for practice

The limitations of approaches where experts dominate and problem-solve for families are well documented (Davis & Day, 2010). Even when professionals have the best intentions of working in partnership with families, it can be easy to slip back into expert-led models, or to get stuck in 'being nice' to parents and avoid presenting the challenge that is needed to help bring about the change that families would benefit from (Fowler et al., 2012). The example above points to a number of questions that can be used to check and improve the quality of the partnership:

1. Has the process begun by listening to the family (or client, or patient) without judging? Yes, Ruth listened to Kirsty's challenges relating to Harry's settling and why it was so important to address them.

2. In what ways are family members being given control over any course of action, and active involvement in trying new strategies? Ruth suggested a new approach, sought Kirsty's approval, and then guided and supported Kirsty in actually doing the settling.

3. Is professional expertise being used and communicated in effective ways? It appears so: Ruth did not spell the approach out in principle and in full, but deduced what to say and how to guide Kirsty from the situation. For Ruth, partnership does not mean abandoning her expert knowledge base. On the contrary. But Ruth used aspects of Harry's cries to draw Kirsty's attention to what Harry might be experiencing. For Ruth, the situation and Harry's crying came first, and her expertise second.

4. Are all available communicative means being used to provide support and reassurance, demonstrating that you are listening to and empathising with family members? Yes. Ruth used touch, posture, eye contact, questioning and verbal commentary.

5. Are all available communicative means being used to monitor and assess how a situation is being experienced by others? Ruth neither assumed Kirsty was 'OK' with Harry's crying, nor that Kirsty's response was somehow 'wrong'. Ruth listened to Kirsty and looked for physical signs of anxiety that could prompt her to change her approach.

6. Is challenge being presented with appropriate support? Without challenge, there can be little change, and there is little change that is not challenging for those involved. The trick is to pitch challenge so that it is not overwhelming, given the support that is available. It is important to bear in mind what will happen when you aren't available for support yourself. Ruth negotiated a goal with Kirsty that was not fixed on Harry self-settling, but on Kirsty trying something new and taking on a challenge. This acknowledged that addressing the situation may not be easy for Kirsty. At the same time, it set Kirsty up for success. Tackling her own responses rather than stipulating some ideal end-point meant that if Harry did need a cuddle in the end, it would not be a failure. Ruth's guidance and sharing of expertise made the new approach do-able for Kirsty, while the constant monitoring ensured it did not push too far.

Theoretical links

We can think of partnership work as meaning that as a professional you have a *pedagogic* role; this means that you help others learn, rather than telling them what to do or solving problems for them. Three concepts can help understand how this works, and why your professional knowledge base and expertise are still important (Hopwood, 2013).

The first concept – 'zone of proximal development' – relates to the importance of creating situations where service users can benefit from your and your colleagues' expertise. As mentioned above, the literature refers to this as creating a zone of proximal development (ZPD), a 'pedagogic' or learning situation where others that are less skilled are able to spend time with, observe, learn from, and replicate the behaviour of those that are (somewhat) more skilled, given appropriate guidance and support (Vygotsky, 1978).

The second concept is partnership. Partnership is about helping others, such as parents, move from their current situation into a ZPD in which their understandings and actions can change. The idea is that when the support (often referred to as 'scaffolding') is withdrawn, people can now do these new things independently. As a professional, your expertise has an important role in determining where a particular person's ZPD is, what scaffolding might be appropriate, and when to withdraw it. In the example, Ruth judged that Kirsty's ZPD lay in areas relating to understanding Harry's cries as communicating different things (protest or distress), and in knowing how to demonstrate her presence without picking Harry up (patting the mattress, shushing).

In the last part of the excerpt we saw an example of a transformative event – our third concept (Hopwood & Clerke, 2012). This concept builds on the idea of the ZPD and links it to particular moments where people like Kirsty become able to act beyond their original capacity. Transformative events have three ingredients or steps. First, you can help someone notice something new about a situation. Ruth noticed Harry not lifting his arms up. Second, you can help someone understand why this is significant. Ruth explained that this meant Harry was not wanting or expecting to be picked up any more. Finally, you can help to attribute the change to others, so that their actions are seen to be having a tangible effect, however small. Ruth said that the change in Harry was due to Kirsty always going in when he was distressed, but patting the mattress rather than picking him up. In this way an event that might be deemed a failure is changed into something where a small but important change is noticed and the person you are helping is the person bringing it about. Your professional expertise is crucial at every step, but the transformation happens for family members.

Conclusion

The idea of partnership is integral and central to the values and professional ethics of many health professionals. In the context of child and family health, professionals are strongly committed to helping those who are struggling, and to ensuring that all children get the best possible start in life. Most professionals seek to help parents and would *not* describe their role as about judging parents as good or bad, or providing parents with a standard recipe for effective parenting. However, without an explicit framework, it can be difficult to turn the desire to help people in a respectful, collaborative, strengths-based, and capacity-building way.

The FPM is one example of a number of frameworks that describe the skills required and processes involved in developing partnership. In this chapter we have seen how partnership links to ecological approaches that focus not on individuals, but on relationships including the whole family within a community setting. These approaches acknowledge ways in which seemingly small and isolated issues can in fact have much wider implications.

To be effective in partnership you have to go beyond being 'nice' to the people you are helping. You may often have to support them in taking on challenges, and risk drawing their attention to things they had not noticed before. Seeing the process as one of learning, focusing on people's strengths, and seeing your pedagogic role as fostering those strengths can help with this. Framed in that way, the partnership model provides a framework in which your expertise is important, but does not take over, and in which you can present challenges and help others see progress being made as a result of what *they* are noticing, changing and doing. Getting this right involves a specialised kind of communication, including but not limited to being able to listen and encourage others to talk openly, demonstrate your empathy and positive regard negotiate and reach joint decisions, and share your expertise in a way that others can understand.

Practice example 11.2

Tania, mother of Katrina (three years old) and Miro (nine months old), has come for her first appointment at a toddler clinic for help managing Katrina's temper tantrums. She arrives 15 minutes late for her appointment, with Miro in a push-chair, and Katrina holding her hand. Tania looks exasperated. Sarah, a toddler specialist, leads them to a room and immediately Katrina begins playing with the toys, and Tania puts Miro down near some other toys. Unprompted, Tania tells Sarah that Katrina often goes into tantrums that 'come from nowhere', and more and more often, Katrina is vomiting in the peak of each tantrum. She says, 'I've tried everything and the only thing that works is giving her sweets, so now I give her sweets to try to avoid her kicking off.' Meanwhile, Katrina has been playing quietly with one set of toys, and Miro has crawled over to his sister, and grabbed a ball that Katrina was rolling down a spiral track. Katrina finds another ball, and they play together for a while. Then Katrina goes over to a dolls' house, and shortly afterwards starts hitting a doll against the wall and then throws the doll across the room towards Tania. Tania remarks, 'See, she just doesn't play nicely, and if I tell her off, she'll scream, so I give her sweets.'

Reflective questions

Depending how the toddler specialist responds, this episode could mark the beginning of a relationship and process founded on principles of partnership, or it could quickly become an experience in which Tania's feelings of inadequacy as a mother are reinforced, and her wariness of attending services like the toddler clinic is accentuated. The following questions will help you reflect on how this could unfold in a productive and respectful partnership.

1. When Tania first mentions giving sweets to Katrina, what might you say in response? Would you:
    a. raise the issue of sugary foods and their links to tooth decay and obesity?
    b. explain that tantrums are attention-seeking behaviours and that by giving sweets Tania is reinforcing this behaviour in Katrina, so that to stop the tantrums she should ignore them?
    c. say that there are lots of other strategies that Tania might use in avoiding and responding to tantrums, and that you'd like to explain them to her so she can consider which she would prefer to try?
    d. ask her to say more about the sweets she is giving and what happens when she gives them? Something else?

2. Partnership is a 'strengths-based approach', but many parents find it hard to see strengths in themselves when things appear to be going so wrong. What opportunities can you see in the example to provide positive and concrete reinforcement of Tania as a parent, and to demonstrate your unconditional positive regard for her?

3. Tania believes that vomiting is an extreme (pathological) behaviour that means she is failing as a parent. How would you communicate a different point of view based on your expertise?

4. Tania wants Katrina to stop flaring into temper tantrums. Do you think this is the best goal to work on together? If not, how would you go about negotiating a different goal?

5. Clearly, Katrina's tantrums are affecting Tania. Do they have any wider implications or connections? How could you understand these tantrums in terms of an ecological approach? What other information would you need?

6. How would you go about assessing Tania's understanding of what causes tantrums, and how she might anticipate and respond to them? How will you determine an appropriate level of challenge for her, and what scaffolding (support and guidance) she will need? How will you manage the withdrawal of these supports?

7. Can you imagine how a transformative event might unfold in this setting? What could you be looking out for (noticing), why would it be important, and how could you link this to Tania's actions and strengths?

8. What checks will you use to ensure the partnership remains effective?
    a. How will you make sure you go beyond being nice?
    b. How will you check the level of challenge being presented is appropriate?

Reflective questions

While partnership practices have become widespread in child and family health settings, partnership and key concepts presented in this chapter apply more widely. Some of the questions below are general in nature. Others refer to the practice examples above. This should help you think through how the ideas from this chapter are relevant to your own work.

1. Think about the patients, clients or service users you work with.
   a. What forms of knowledge do they bring with them?
   b. How do you know this?
   c. What could you do differently to better understand their expertise and make use of it in the care you provide?
2. In what ways are patients, clients or service users in your context actively involved in their care? Do you think they might think that care is being done to them, or for them? Would it make sense for them to be more involved? If so in, what ways?
3. Could a strengths-based approach help improve outcomes in the kind of work you are familiar with? In other words, if you shifted from a focus on behaviours you would like to see, to a focus on what individuals and their families are currently doing and might be capable of together, would you do things differently? Might you need to refer to colleagues from other services? If so, whom?
4. While much work is still involved in treating patients, there are many instances where part of your job as a health professional is to help others learn.
   a. Could this be the case in aspects of your work now or in the future? Think about learning to live with chronic conditions, understand risk, make complex decisions about care options, and other situations.
   b. Can you think of ways in which concepts such as the ZPD, or transformative events, might be relevant to you?
5. Imagine you came across a mother like Kirsty (practice example 11.1), who seems exhausted and potentially experiencing a mood disorder or mental illness. How would you approach the issue, if at all? What might make Kirsty feel vulnerable or judged? How could you avoid this, without brushing it all under the carpet?
6. Imagine you came across a mother and daughter like Tania and Katrina (practice example 11.2), what might you do? For example, if Tania visited you as her general practitioner and you saw her giving sweets to calm her daughter down, would you say something? Again, how could you show empathy rather than judgment?

Further reading

Day, C., & Davis, H., (1999). Community child mental-health services: A framework for the development of parenting initiatives. *Clinical Child Psychology and Psychiatry*, 4(4), 475–482. doi:10.1177/1359104599004004004

This short paper explains more about linkages between services and service integration in a tiered model, including interprofessional work. It also discusses partnership in contexts relating to mental health (which have not been covered in this chapter).

Feeley, N., & Gottlieb, L. N., (2000). Nursing approaches for working with family strengths and resources. *Journal of Family Nursing, 6*(1), 9–24. doi:10.1177/107484070000600102
This paper describes a different approach to partnership (not specifically the FPM) within a nursing context.

Harrison, I., (2007). Working in partnership with parents using an attachment model: Some tips for clinicians working with parents and infants. *The Journal of the Child and Family Health Nurses Association (NSW) Inc., 18*(2), 2–5.
This is written by a psychiatrist and offers a very clear explanation of how the theory of attachment complements the idea of partnership.

Onyett, S., (2009). Working appreciatively to improve services for children and families. *Clinical Child Psychology and Psychiatry, 14*(4), 495–507. doi:10.1177/1359104509338878
This emphasises strengths-based approaches that are common to many partnership models.

Wright, L. M., & Leahey, M., (2009). *Nurses and families: A guide to family assessment and intervention* (5th ed.). Philadelphia: F A Davis.
This is a well-known practical guide to working in collaborative, strengths-based ways with whole families, linked to the family systems nursing model.

Web resources

Centre for Parent and Child Support (UK): http://www.cpcs.org.uk/index.php?page=about-family-partnership-model
Governance International: http://www.govint.org/good-practice/case-studies/the-family-partnership-model-in-practice-in-new-south-wales

References

Bronfenbrenner, U. (1979). *The ecology of human development.* Cambridge, MA: Harvard University Press.

——. (2005). *Making human beings human: Bioecological perspectives on human development.* Thousand Oaks, CA: Sage.

Davis, H., & Day, C. (2010). *Working in partnership: The family partnership model.* London: Pearson.

Davis, H., & Fallowfield, L. (1991). *Counselling and communication in health care.* London: Wiley.

Dunston, R., Lee, A., Boud, D., Brodie, P. & Chiarella, M. (2009). Co-production and health system reform – from re-imagining to re-making. *Australian Journal of Public Administration, 68*(1), 1–14. doi:10.1111/j.1467–8500.2008.00608.x

Fowler, C., Rossiter, C., Bigsby, M., Hopwood, N., Lee, A., & Dunston, R. (2012). Working in partnership with parents: The experience and challenge of practice innovation in child and family health nursing. *Journal of Clinical Nursing, 21*(21–22), 3306–3314. doi:10.1111/j.1365–2702.2012.04270.x

Hopwood, N., (2013). Understanding partnership practice in primary health as pedagogic work: What can Vygotsky's theory of learning offer? *Australian Journal of Primary Health.* doi:10.1071/PY12141

Hopwood, N., & Clerke, T., (2012). *Partnership and pedagogy in child and family health practice: A resource for professionals, educators and students.* Hertsellung: Lambert Academic Publishing.

Vygotsky, L. S. (1978). *Mind in society: The development of higher psychological processes.* Cambridge, MA: Harvard University Press.

Note on ethics approval

This chapter draws on a study of partnership practices in child and family health settings. The research was approved by South Western Sydney Local Health Network Human Research Ethics Committee, reference HREC/10/LPOOL/186, and ratified by the University of Technology, Sydney Human Research Ethics Committee, reference 2011–095R.

Part 3

General health communication strategies

12

Improving care by listening: care communication and shared decision-making

Natalya Godbold and Kirsten McCaffery

Learning objectives

This chapter will enable you to:

- understand key experiences of patients which influence their expectations and willingness to communicate during care;
- develop strategies to encourage patients to communicate with you;
- understand the importance of listening to patients;
- develop strategies to actively involve patients in making decisions about their own care, and in taking charge of the care itself.

Key terms

Patient-centred care
Patient experiences
Patient perspectives
Person-centred care
Shared decision-making
Unpopular patient

Overview

This chapter explores communication priorities for patients, the issues they find important, and the implications of these preferences for how clinicians communicate with one another and with their patients. Central in this chapter are strategies for working with patients and/or their family members, to involve them in decision-making about and in monitoring of their own treatments and safety. The diverse cultural and linguistic expectations and demands posed by services catering for patients of different cultural backgrounds are also acknowledged.

Introduction

Patients go into health care looking for answers to their health-related problems. But a good proportion of patients find their experiences in care distressing and disempowering. In this chapter, we explore why patients have such negative experiences, and propose strategies to reduce their distress. These strategies include processes referred to as **shared decision-making** or SDM. SDM aims to involve patients in the decision-making processes affecting them. SDM thereby acknowledges **patient perspectives** during healthcare provision.

However, all attempts to empower patients, including SDM, can only ever partly succeed. We discuss the implications of this challenge for health practitioners and patients. We also examine how patients' negative experiences of health care can be a problem not just for patients but also for nurses, allied health staff, managers and doctors, as such experiences compromise patient safety and **person-centred care**.

We begin to exemplify these issues using the story of a real patient we will call Sean, though Sean is not his real name. Sean is a well-educated, well-presented and polite person. He writes professionally, and has edited many reports about the Australian healthcare system describing the ideal of **patient-centred care**. In 2013, Sean attended a major Sydney hospital for a simple procedure. The operation was successful, but due to postoperative bleeding, Sean stayed two nights for observation. Afterwards he blogged about his experiences.

> **shared decision-making**
> the interaction process between the healthcare practitioner and the patient who come together to devise treatment plans. Shared decision-making becomes possible when there is mutual listening and shared dialogue.
>
> **patient perspectives**
> the patient's views, needs and wants as defined and understood by the patient him- or herself.
>
> **person-centred care**
> care that acknowledges that both patients and professionals are people. Person-centred care is used to emphasise the importance of recognising that care is a human-to-human dynamic that may have different participants at its centre at different times, allowing for their different and potentially changing roles and contributions.
>
> **patient-centred care**
> care that is structured to benefit the patient. Patient-centred care is opposed to profession-centred and service-centred care. The latter are structured to benefit those working in the health system, potentially at the expense of the patient.

> [W]hen I'm finally released, [...] I call my partner to find he is already driving up and will pull up in front of the hospital to let me hop in. [...] 'Take me home,' I say and break down sobbing, full upper body up and down, my hand smashed into my face, in a way I haven't cried since Dad died.

Sean's health care was medically exemplary. His procedure was successful; his subsequent care was careful, and no medical errors occurred. He did not have to endure difficult pain or physical distress. Yet Sean's experience of health care was deeply distressing. He wrote on his blog:

> I was shocked at the chasm between what is hoped for and what I experienced. At no time did I feel central to my care, a true subject rather than an object. I'm shocked at my level of unhappiness and complaint. ... I found it so traumatic.

So why was the experience in hospital so difficult for him? Sean's blog post reveals a range of experiences common to patients like himself, including:

- lack of information about what has happened, is happening and will happen next;
- loss of control, including not being heard by hospital staff;
- the need to remain friendly with healthcare professionals so as not to jeopardise their goodwill and care.

Reflecting on his traumatic experience with a simple procedure, Sean wrote in his blog:

> As a well-educated, articulate and relatively confident individual, I would have imagined that I'd fare well in the health system, that I could use whatever skills, charm and education built up over my years to create some level of positive human interaction and be satisfied with the care I received. That was not the case. ... So many people I know ... have undergone major operations requiring much bigger procedures and longer stays in the hospital. How are they managing?

And, we can ask, what about the patients who are not as articulate or confident as Sean?

In this chapter, we explore what is common about the experiences of patients, and address strategies that may help them. We also examine how these experiences can be a problem for nurses and doctors as well as patients, by compromising patient safety and person-centred care.

Practice example 12.1

Consider the following story, again of a well-educated, articulate patient: Joe. Now in his forties, Joe has had kidney failure since his youth, necessitating in-hospital haemodialysis (cleaning of the blood). So, unlike Sean who had never been to hospital before, Joe is very experienced with hospitals, and is very knowledgeable about his condition. To receive haemodialysis as a treatment for kidney failure, patients need a fistula, created by joining a vein and an artery to form an enlarged blood vessel able to sustain ongoing access to the blood. Patients have a limited number of locations where a fistula can be created, so a functioning fistula must be carefully protected.

Joe was told by his vascular surgeon that, if he had trouble with his fistula, he should go to emergency and tell the triage nurses to call the vascular surgeon on duty. Joe's vascular surgeon assured him that the nurses would understand the urgent care required. So when Joe noticed a problem with his fistula, that is what he did. But instead of calling a vascular surgeon, the triage nurses told Joe to sit down to wait to be seen by one of the emergency doctors. 'This fistula needs to be seen by a vascular surgeon within about two hours,' he told the nurses. 'Go and sit down,' he was told. Joe lost the fistula, compromising his ability to receive life-sustaining dialysis. He required the expensive and painful construction of a new fistula. Even though Joe had information about what was happening, he couldn't make the nurses listen.

Reflective questions

1. What could Joe have done differently to get the information he wanted?
2. What might the clinicians have said to Joe to reassure him that he had been heard?
3. If the vascular surgeon was unable to come and an emergency doctor had to attend to Joe, how might the clinicians have discussed this with him?

Analysis and reflection

Let's now examine what happened to Joe in somewhat more detail. There are four main problems affecting his care: a lack of information, a loss of control, not being heard, and a greater need for patients to be friendly and cooperative. We discuss each of these in turn.

Lack of information

Joe clearly wanted information about what was happening, and he was given little. Though in the past patients may have been more passive in conversations about their care, these days more patients want to know what is happening to them and, especially, most patients want to know when and how their illness or condition will be fixed. Patients may even expect that healthcare professionals will be able to tell patients 'the answers' quite quickly. Often this can't be done. Diagnosis may not be the straightforward affair that patients might imagine, and it can require tests and involve different specialists. Moreover, care often involves waiting and responding to the body as it responds to treatments, and the speed and content of such responses cannot be determined or predicted accurately. So while it is reasonable for patients to want to understand their situation, it is not always possible to give them clear 'answers'.

Instead, it is important for health professionals to be clear about the processes involved in their care: to explain how things work. If patients ask for information, provide it, even if that means saying, 'I don't know yet', or 'I am not able to talk to you about that. You need to ask the doctor when they come.' Such answers demonstrate that there are processes for information provision in your workplace, allowing the patient to understand them and work within them. Even if you are unable to provide solid or clear answers, explanations about how things work enable you to connect with the patient and respect their need for information. Explanations further allow patients to think through their situation (Purtilo & Haddad, 2007). Importantly, too, encourage patients to take their questions further and alert them to opportunities to do so as they arise. We will return to this last point later.

Loss of control

Joe experienced a loss of control due to his illness. Patients such as Joe can no longer do everything they want to due to their condition. Any good health professional textbook explains how difficult such a change can be: changing one's abilities, ruining one's plans, maybe even changing one's life course. This includes a potential loss of physical and social function, stigmatisation, changed roles and identity, financial loss and loss of opportunities, some of which may be traumatic, even if others may represent a welcome reduction in duties and demands (Anderson & Bury, 1988; Purtilo & Haddad, 2007).

When a patient enters a hospital or goes to see a doctor, however, there is another level at which they lose control, involving a whole new set of lost choices. First and foremost, they lose control over time; they can't decide when their care will commence or finish – that is at the discretion of doctors. They may notice others being seen before them, adding to the frustration of waiting. Then, if they are admitted into hospital, they must remove their clothing; they cannot choose what or when to eat or drink, and they may not be able to move freely due to catheters and cannulas. And they cannot decide what their treatments will be – even in the context of excellent patient-centred care. That is, a patient cannot get a particular treatment without a doctor agreeing to it and prescribing it. If they are given choices in their care, they often don't know what the different options mean, and therefore can't really compare outcomes. Moreover, all choices of treatment may appear equally unsavoury to the recipient, making their choice into one that feels forced because they cannot choose to escape the situation painlessly.

There is little that any individual healthcare professional can do to restore all these levels of a patient's lost control in the short term. Beyond helping to ameliorate the patient's illness or condition, the best strategies to use in everyday interactions with patients who are dealing with loss of control are acknowledgement and connection, and giving them things they can control (Purtilo & Haddad, 2007). For these reasons, as a health professional you should agree and acknowledge the patient's frustration or loss when they complain about their lost choices. You might sometimes even be responsible yourself and could acknowledge that, for instance, long waiting times are a problem, and you could apologise for them.

But empathy may not enable the professional to achieve everything for the patient. Therefore, you should also help a patient regain some control by showing them how to assist with or manage their own care. This can be very simple at times. Explain, for instance, how to care for their cannula, by not moving the hand their cannula is in. Explain what is required for them to be discharged, so that they can work towards that goal – for instance, by providing usable samples, by walking, by passing tests, and so forth. All this can contribute to a patient's sense of knowing what is happening to them, and having a degree of control over their care.

Not being heard

When Joe showed the triage nurses his failing fistula, they apparently did not recognise the urgency of the situation, nor did they appear to listen to his requests for urgent help. Perhaps they did call for a vascular surgeon, but the surgeon did not come. What matters, ultimately, is that Joe felt that he was not heard. And, significantly, the fistula failed. When a patient knows that they lack control, and feels that they are not being heard, it is natural for them to feel frightened, angry and depressed. Moreover, patients sometimes know that they will have to return to this healthcare facility again, so the experience of not being heard creates fear not only for a present single situation, but potentially a long-term fear of similar, future situations. Patients begin to feel unsafe in the long term.

All this means we need to listen to patients, and 'hear' the cues and information they may be able to provide. We need to take patients' concerns and wishes seriously. If Joe's triage nurses did call a vascular surgeon, they should have told Joe about it. We also need to *show* that we are listening (see Chapter 3). If the nurses had explicitly acknowledged Joe's request for a vascular surgeon, he might not have been so upset about having been treated by an emergency doctor. Then he might still feel safe to go to emergency with other problems, because he might feel that at least frontline staff there would respond respectfully and knowledgeably.

The need for patients to be friendly and cooperative

We have discussed how patients lack control over their situation and the processes which might help them. For the reasons described earlier, healthcare professionals are *partly* in control. And research shows that healthcare professionals provide different standards of care to patients they like, compared to patients they don't like: unpopular patients wait longer, receive less information, and experience interactions with fewer friendly elements such as jokes, smiles or chats (Stockwell, 1984). Patients know that unpopular patients receive different, substandard care (Werner & Malterud, 2003). This knowledge may affect how all patients interact with healthcare staff in two ways (Braun Curtin & Mapes, 2001; Godbold, 2013):

1. They may complain less. Your patient may not tell you when something is going wrong. They might not tell you when they are scared or upset. If you ask how they are, they may say 'Good!' even when they are experiencing pain and symptoms, or when they are feeling unsafe.
2. They may ask fewer questions. This means that your patient may not ask for information, even when they need it.

An outcome of these two strategies is that patients may feel even *less* in control, have *less* information, and feel even *less* able to make themselves heard. So for patients who attempt to be cooperative, the other experiences described here can be even harder to bear, and you as a professional may never hear a thing about it. In fact, you may even think they like you, when in fact they don't! 'Feigned niceness' is hard work for patients, and it may distract healthcare providers.

Implications for practice

Despite the system you may work in, there are strategies you can use to aim for good experiences for your patients. First, remember that even the briefest interaction you have with a patient can serve to create therapeutic relationships. Crawford and Brown (2011) argue that warmth and human engagement can be communicated even in the short snatches of time you may have with patients, without slowing your work down.

Second, recognise that patients are already involved in their own care, even if they don't want to be. This is because the patient describes their illness and because they move in and with the ill body in ways that slow or assist the healing process; because they self-care; and because they decide when to bring changes to the attention of a medical professional. So even if a patient doesn't want to know anything about their care, if you, for example, tell them that they need to keep their cannula hand still to avoid damaging the vein and having to get a new one put in, most people will carefully keep their hand still. And if you tell them that it should last three days and then needs to come out, some people will even remind the new shift three days later that they need a new cannula.

Third, think of the patient as part of the healthcare team – like an apprentice in their own care. Of course, patients are different from apprentices in that they usually don't want to be patients. Even so, many people are keen to be active in their care, for their own safety. Patients may be inexpert and quite untrained, or they may already be quite skilled and adept with their own care, depending on their previous experiences and their interest in self-care. Many patients are interested in remaining as well as possible, and as safe as possible – two big incentives to involving them in knowing about their care. Treat patients as apprentices by asking what they know about their situation, by talking them through your thoughts and decisions, and by teaching them about the equipment around them like their cannula or their blood pressure equipment. By treating patients as apprentices, you encourage them to think about their own safety. You also create connections for talking about care, which might encourage patients to ask questions and talk to you. Many patients need active, repeated encouragement to ask questions, and they will notice how their questions are received. If you set up the situation properly, the patient may think they will be more popular by talking and asking. This is a healthy outcome.

Here is a summary of the suggestions made so far:

- Tell patients about the processes of the service or system they are in; the processes of their care, including how to care for themselves; and how to work towards their discharge. Watch your patients to see how much they want to be involved in their own care and how much they already know. Take notice of what they tell you (and how).
- Move beyond exchanges like, 'How are you feeling this morning?' 'Great!' Ask about specific, likely symptoms or sources of pain, and when and how often they last felt them.
- Watch patients moving: do their words match their capacities?
- If patients speak up about problems, encourage that and respond constructively. Make it clear that hearing about their experiences is an important and useful part of their care.
- Use shared decision-making processes to include patients in decisions about care.
- Keep patients informed about the processes and systems they are involved in or are experiencing and, if they are interested, explain the equipment you are using, too.

Theoretical links

We suggest there are three important theoretical concepts that have relevance for thinking about how to involve patients in their care. The first is SDM. SDM helps people make informed decisions consistent with their personal preferences and values. It supports patients and providers to communicate more effectively about health and exchange relevant information. SDM is now an explicit health policy goal in many industrialised nations (Australian Commission on Safety and Quality in Health Care, 2009; NHS RightCare, 2012).

The SDM approach can provide a framework for communicating with patients about healthcare choices to help improve conversation quality. It can be viewed as a continuum (Guadagnoli & Ward, 1998) where the extent to which the patient or the clinician takes responsibility for the decision-making processes varies. At each extreme are clinician-led decisions and patient-led decisions, with many other possible positions in between (Guadagnoli & Ward, 1998; Levinson, Kao, Kuby, & Thisted, 2005). The level of patient involvement will vary according to various factors, such as the patient's own preference to be involved, the social context in which the decision is occurring, and the disease that is at issue.

Regardless of whether the patient or clinician takes the lead in the decision-making process, joint discussion about the health issues under consideration should at least occur. Shared decision-making aims to create communicative, respectful environments in which patients should feel that they understand the processes of their care. Systematic research reviews show that patient outcomes such as knowledge about options, accuracy of risk perception, decisional uncertainty and the match between patient values and choice are significantly improved through the use of shared decision-making interventions such as decision aids (Stacey et al., 2013).

Patient 'empowerment' is a second important theoretical concept. Since the early 1970s clinicians have been encouraged to view patients as 'empowered' and capable of involvement in their own care. Empowerment may improve clinical outcomes and increase patients' sense of ownership of their care and treatment (Department of Health, 2001). But not all patients want to be 'in control' of their care (Aujoulat, d'Hoore & Deccache, 2007). Moreover, patients' options for control are limited by factors such as the healthcare system, urgency, finances and mobility (Lupton, 1997). It is partly their loss of control to illness that brought them to clinicians for help. Power to diagnose, recommend treatments and perform procedures remains with clinicians (Roberts, 1999).

The **'unpopular' patient** is our third theoretical concept. Some patients are 'unpopular' with health professionals (Highley & Norris, 1957; Koekkoek et al., 2011; Stockwell, 1984). 'Good' patients follow instructions and don't ask too many questions (Stacey et al., 2009). Some

> **unpopular patient**
> a patient who is made to wait longer, receives less information, and experiences fewer friendly gestures such as jokes, smiles or chats, this happens when healthcare professionals provide different standards of care to patients they like compared to patients they don't like (Stockwell, 1984; Werner & Malterud, 2003).

practitioners dislike patients who research their condition on the internet or try to 'know too much' about their illness (Broom, 2005).Treatment of 'unpopular' patients is different from that received by 'good' patients – for example, they may wait longer for care and their questions may be ignored (Stockwell, 1984; Werner & Malterud, 2003). Patients must balance the tensions between being 'empowered' and being 'good', while also being ill. How can they be both in control and cooperative? And how are they to understand what is happening to them, without asking too many questions?

Conclusion

You could argue that Sean's distress was a reaction to the trauma of undergoing a procedure and staying several days in an unfamiliar environment. Any patient may experience this. Perhaps medical care can't help but be distressing. But some of the experiences which Sean found traumatic could be easily addressed. Why not aim to improve our interactions so that patient's experiences are more positive – and so that they are more inclined to return when they need more care? Meanwhile there can be no argument that Joe's experiences of not being heard had serious consequences leading to costly interventions and the loss of one of his few potential sites for dialysis.

It is important to recognise that problems faced by patients cannot be addressed by any single 'fix' nor resolved 'once and for all'. For patients as for clinicians, health care is an evolving process of understanding and responding to the need for care. However, moment by moment, healthcare practitioners do have opportunities to support patients' experiences. This chapter has explored key problems in communicating with patients, as seen from their perspective. It has put forward a range of practical strategies which you might use: give patients useful information; hear what they have to say and show what you have done about it; get patients actively involved in their care, thereby obtaining elements of control; and encourage patients and their families to continue to talk with you about their symptoms and worries. These skills will enable you to provide truly person-centred (rather than patient's-body-centred) care.

Practice example 12.2

Mary has come to hospital for an exploratory laparoscopy to find a cause for her urine retention. During that procedure, the surgeon found lots of endometriosis, which was removed on the spot. Now Mary is fretful and demanding. She rings for the nurses every half an hour, complaining of pain, wanting the doctor to come, and asking when she can go home. She is snappy and discourteous and implies nurses are withholding information from her about what happened during the procedure.

Reflective questions

1. Do you think Mary could be labelled as an unpopular patient? If yes, why?
2. Which of the common patient experiences (lack of information, loss of control, not being heard, the need to remain friendly) could be relevant to Mary? When and why?
3. How might you respond to Mary's fretful and demanding behaviour? Identify a pool of potential tactics for your dealings with Mary that might address each of the potential issues highlighted in question 2. For example, what questions might you ask? What could you do differently?
4. How and when might shared decision-making processes be useful to involve Mary in discussions of her treatment options? (Hint: Was she expecting to have endometriosis removed? Does she know what endometriosis is?)

Reflective questions

1. Do all patients want to be involved in shared decision-making?
2. How might you 'read' whether a patient would prefer more or less involvement in their own care? How kind of question might you ask to determine if and how much a patient might like to be involved in decision-making processes or self-care?

Further reading

Porritt, L. (1990). *Interaction strategies: An introduction for health professionals.* Melbourne: Churchill Livingstone.

This book presents skills and strategies with which healthcare workers can help patients make decisions about their treatment. The author explores the interactional nature of communication and the importance of being able to recognise verbal and non-verbal communication processes; she also points out a range of common blocks which may occur.

Purtilo, R. B., & Haddad, A. (2007). *Health professional and patient interaction* (7th ed.). St. Louis, MO: Saunders.

Strategies for respectfully communicating with patients are illustrated through useful examples and scenarios. The authors explore the role and importance of respect in healthcare interactions in a range of settings, and present patient's perspectives on common situations in health care.

Web resources

Ask Share Know: http://www.askshareknow.com.au
Cancer Institute NSW: http://www.cancerinstitute.org.au/patient-support/what-i-need-to-ask
Option grid: http://www.optiongrid.org

Ottawa Hospital Research Insititute, *Patient decision aids*: http://decisionaid.ohri.ca/decguide. html

Ottawa Hospital Research Institute Inventory of Decision Aids: http://decisionaid.ohri.ca/ azinvent.php

References

Anderson, R., & Bury, M. (Eds.). (1988). *Living with chronic illness: The experience of patients and their families*. London and Boston: Unwin Hyman.

Aujoulat, I., d'Hoore, W., & Deccache, A. (2007). Patient empowerment in theory and practice: Polysemy or cacophony? *Patient Education and Counseling, 66*(1), 13–20.

Australian Commission on Safety and Quality in Health Care. (2009). *National Safety and Quality Framework: A national framework for improving the safety and quality of health care*. Sydney: Author. Retrieved January 21, 2011 from http://www.safetyandquality.gov.au

Braun Curtin, R., & Mapes, D. L. (2001). Health care management strategies of long-term dialysis survivors. *Nephrology Nursing Journal, 28*(4), 385–392.

Broom, A. (2005). Virtually Healthy: The impact of internet use on disease experience and the doctor-patient relationship. *Qualitative Health Research, 15*(3), 325.

Cass, A., Lowell, A., Christie, M., Snelling, P. L., Flack, M., Marrnganyin, B., & Brown, I. (2002). Sharing the true stories: Improving communication between Aboriginal patients and healthcare workers. *Medical Journal of Australia, 176*(10), 466–470.

Crawford, P., & Brown, B. (2011). Fast healthcare: Brief communication, traps and opportunities. *Patient Education and Counseling, 82*(1), 3–10. doi:10.1016/j. pec.2010.02.016

Department of Health. (2001). The expert patient: A new approach to chronic disease management for the 21st century. Retrieved October 15, 2011 from http://www. dh.gov.uk/en/Publicationsandstatistics/Publications/PublicationsPolicyAndGuidance/ DH_4006801

Godbold, N. (2013). Tensions in compliance for renal patients – how renal discussion groups conceive knowledge and safe care. *Health Sociology Review, 22*(1), 52–64.

Guadagnoli, E., & Ward, P. (1998). Patient participation in decision-making. *Social Science & Medicine, 47*(3), 329–339.

Highley, B. L., & Norris, C. M. (1957). When a Student Dislikes a Patient. *American Journal of Nursing, 57*(9), 1163–1166.

Koekkoek, B., Hutschemaekers, G., van Meijel, B., & Schene, A. (2011). How do patients come to be seen as 'difficult'? *Social Science & Medicine, 72*(4), 504–512. doi:http://ezproxy. uws.edu.au:/login?url=http://dx.doi.org/10.1016/j.socscimed.2010.11.036

Levinson, W., Kao, A., Kuby, A., & Thisted, R. (2005). Not all patients want to participate in decision making. *Journal of General Internal Medicine, 20*(6), 531–535.

Lupton, D. (1997). Consumerism, reflexivity and the medical encounter. *Social Science & Medicine, 45*(3), 373–381. doi:10.1016/s0277–9536(96)00353-x

NHS RightCare. (2012). Shared decision making. Retrieved from http://www.rightcare.nhs.uk/ index.php/shared-decision-making

Purtilo, R. B., & Haddad, A. (2007). *Health professional and patient interaction* (7th ed.). St. Louis, MO: Saunders.

Roberts, K. J. (1999). Patient empowerment in the United States: A critical commentary. *Health Expectations, 2*(2), 82–92.

Stacey, C. L., Henderson, S., MacArthur, K. R., & Dohan, D. (2009). Demanding patient or demanding encounter? *Social Science & Medicine, 69*(5), 729–737.

Stockwell, F. (1984). *The unpopular patient.* London: Croom Helm.

Werner, A., & Malterud, K. (2003). It is hard work behaving as a credible patient: Encounters between women with chronic pain and their doctors. *Social Science & Medicine, 57*(8), 1409–1419. doi:10.1016/S0277–9536(02)00520–8

13

Intra- and interprofessional communication

Jill Thistlethwaite, Marie Manidis and Cindy Gallois

Learning objectives

This chapter will enable you to:
- define teamwork;
- define collaborative practice;
- define values-based practice;
- understand the nature of intra- and interprofessional work and communication;
- reflect on your own professional identity and how this may affect working with others;
- consider the effects of professional tribalism on collaboration and communication.

Key terms

Collaborative practice
Multidisciplinary team
Professional identity
Teamwork
Values-based practice

Overview

Contemporary health care is predominantly delivered to patients and clients by a range of health professions working in either defined and co-located teams or looser collaborations. Each health profession has a defined set of roles and responsibilities, values and identities, and its own jargon and hierarchy. Good communication is important among health professionals to avoid misunderstandings and to provide optimum patient care and outcomes. Effective **teamwork** is necessary in the complex environments where health care is provided. Well-performing teams have regular meetings to set goals and review performance. Dysfunctional teams have problems including conflict and lack of trust between members. Health professionals who work collaboratively need to share their values and scope of practice to avoid poor communication.

> **teamwork**
> a way of working that involves 'listening and constructively responding to points of view expressed by others, giving others the benefit of the doubt, providing support to those who need it, and recognizing the interests and achievements of others' (Katzenbach & Smith, 1993, p. 15).

The practice examples in this chapter illustrate intra- and interprofessional communication issues, one involving spoken and the other written communication. One central issue is continuity of care, as this relies on adequate handover of the care of patients (orally and accompanied by patient records) among health professionals when they change shifts or when patients are referred from one team or location to another.

Introduction

Health care is complex, frequently highly specialised and delivered by a growing number of health professional groups. Each health profession defines its own roles, and within each profession there are different subdisciplines, each with their own demarcations of responsibilities. For example, medical doctors may be surgeons, cardiologists, pathologists, and so forth. Nurses may be advanced practice nurses, nurse practitioners, remote area nurses, enrolled nurses, and the like. For their part, allied health professions have their own role and status demarcations.

Each professional group and subgroup has its own values and priorities, jargon and hierarchy. This creates the potential for miscommunication and adverse patient or client events. (Note that the health professions may refer to the consumer of care in different ways: patient, client, or service user.) Most patients will interact with several types of health professional during an acute or chronic illness. Such professionals may be collaborating quite intensely in a co-located team (in the operating room, or on a ward), or they may be in looser collaborations and have quite infrequent interactions (in community settings).

Effective teamwork means providing quality health care in whatever environment, whatever its complexity (Romanow, 2002). Effective teamwork also presupposes that clinicians cope with technological advances in diagnosis and patient management (Institute of Medicine, 2001). Both these kinds of team effectiveness are crucially dependent on effective communication: are team members able to talk about problems that arise, are they able to exchange important knowledge, and are they able to help each other come to terms with new technologies and information?

It has been clear for some time that effective communication is a marker of good teamwork and it leads to fewer errors (JCAHO, 2005). By the same token, suboptimal communication is a marker of ineffective teamwork, and is a prime cause of patient safety problems and poor patient outcomes. Ineffective teamwork was found to be at the heart of problems affecting acute hospital services in New South Wales. The Garling report, reporting on a state-wide investigation into New South Wales emergency health services in 2008, recommended that 'clinical education and training should be undertaken in a multidisciplinary environment which emphasises **multidisciplinary team** based patient-centred care' to help prevent further problems (Garling, 2008, p. 11).

> **multidisciplinary team**
> a team comprised of professionals from different backgrounds

Note that there are several words that are frequently used synonymously: interprofessional; multi- and interdisciplinary; and multiprofessional. However, we feel that 'interprofessional' teamwork best describes what is at issue here: how to achieve 'two or more professions working together as a team with a common purpose, commitment and mutual respect' (Freeth et al., 2005). We define multiprofessional teamwork as carried out by professionals working in parallel with little interaction and infrequent communication.

For us, optimal team functioning requires professionals to be able to do two things. First, they need to be able to negotiate a common purpose and shared goals. Second, they need to have regular meetings where they reflect on their performance (Dawson, Yan & West, 2007). Health professionals who identify themselves as working in teams but who do not meet frequently to set goals and reflect on performance report less job satisfaction and more burnout, and have a greater likelihood of being involved in adverse events (Dawson, Yan & West, 2007). Important skills to learn for teamwork include communication in general but also more specific competencies:

- interprofessional communication;
- patient-/client-/family-/community-centred care;
- role clarification;
- team functioning;
- collaborative leadership;
- interprofessional conflict resolution (CIHC, 2010).

Dysfunctional teamwork leading to poor intra- and interprofessional communication has five common features. The first is a lack of trust. Trust is defined as the willingness to rely on others' skills and judgment. A lack of trust may be due to not knowing the scope of practice and role and skills of other health professionals: what they are responsible for and capable of doing. In the healthcare environment you need to be able to ask each other what your responsibilities are and to discuss the limits of your practice.

The second, fear of conflict, means that one professional may avoid questioning another's behaviour. Avoiding questioning colleagues for fear of conflict is a prime cause of adverse events. Fear of conflict may also result in a lack of commitment to establishing common goals. A team member may not agree with the stated goals but is afraid to let this be known. Remember that conflict can be productive if there are agreed ground rules for all communication, and all communication involves mutual respect so that each team member feels able to speak and is listened to.

It may be though that there is undue pressure to share each other's personal and professional values within the team. Values here mean 'standards by which our actions are selected' (Mason et al., 2010, p. 71). Such pressure to agree on values may explain why at times team members fear conflict will arise when questioning team values. Such questioning is particularly problematic when team values are out of alignment with patients' values. This may create difficult situations for clinicians who feel torn between conforming with their team and providing patient-centred care.

Being able to question and renegotiate values to ensure they remain patient-centred means that practice is 'values-based'. **Values-based practice** is 'a blending of the values of both the service user and the health and social care professional, thus creating a true, as opposed to a tokenistic partnership' (Thomas, Burt & Parkes, 2010, p. 15).

> **values-based practice**
> care that adheres to moral values such as empathy and person-centredness. Values-based practice can be distinguished from task-based practice. Where values-based practice unfolds in response to patients' needs, task-based practice is driven by pre-determined (and often clinician-defined) structures and activities.

Five characteristics of dysfunctional teams are as follows:

1. absence of trust;
2. fear of conflict;
3. lack of commitment;
4. avoidance of accountability;
5. inattention to results (Lencioni, 2002).

Practice example 13.1

An example of intra-professional conflict is between hospital doctors in different specialties. This conflict was expressed through clinicians' contributions to the patient's written medical record (chart). In this case (taken from Hewett, Watson & Gallois, 2013), a patient's chart across a single afternoon revealed escalating conflict between an emergency medicine specialist and a gastroenterology registrar (a junior doctor receiving training as a specialist) in a large hospital. The conflict concerned the treatment for a patient with an upper gastro-intestinal bleed. This serious and potentially life-threatening condition requires immediate treatment. Best practice guidelines indicate that an upper endoscopy (examination via inserted camera of the upper gastro-intestinal tract) should be performed to diagnose (and in some cases treat) the cause of the bleed as soon as possible, and certainly within 24 hours of admission.

A department of emergency medicine (DEM) resident medical officer (RMO, a recent medical graduate receiving general hospital training) initially reviewed the patient on presentation to the DEM. Summarising his colleagues' discussion and decision, this RMO wrote in the chart that the patient should go for admission and endoscopy ('scope'). The first entry in the medical record appears at 2:30 p.m. (1430 hours); pseudonyms are used for all doctors.

continued ›

Practice example 13.1 continued ›

[Extract 1:] 1430h Discussed w DEM reg (Dr [Allan]): to be admitted medically. Spoke with Med Reg 4B Dr [Baker] – she will kindly r/v but suggests discussing with endoscopy reg re ?urgent scope. D/W Dr [Young, registrar in gastroenterology] – will try and arrange scope for today. Pt fasting since 7am. [signature]

More than two hours later, at 4:50 p.m., the emergency department (ED) consultant (Dr Wilson, the emergency medicine specialist), who had not previously been involved in the patient's care, wrote the following:

[Extract 2:] 21/4/05 DR [Wilson] ED 1650: Phone call from Dr [Young]: wanting bed in DEM post-procedure advised none available no endoscopy will be performed as no bed available post-procedure (as per Gastro consultant decision).

An hour and a half later (at 6:00 p.m.), the gastroenterology registrar (Dr Young) recorded a one-and-a-half page entry of narrative text, which began:

[Extract 3:] 21/4/05 Dr Young, GE reg. I was paged about this man at 1330h. I saw him in DEM immediately after I completed the urgent procedure I was doing (about 1430h). I consented him and booked a bed + explained the priority for a bed to the ED nurses at this time. I also spoke to the involved Med Reg. I arranged to do the case [procedure] in the endoscopy unit at the end of our pm list with an anaesthetist.

Later in the entry, the gastroenterology registrar continued:

[Extract 4:] No bed was available for the patient at 1630. I discussed the need for him to return to DEM after the case with Dr [Young]. Dr [Young] declined to accept the patient back to DEM. I called the bed manager ... and was again told there was no possibility of a bed. I again spoke with Dr [Young] who advised me that the case could not be done.

The gastroenterology registrar then described referring the problem to the hospital's Chief Executive Officer (CEO), a significant escalation of the conflict. The CEO was able to broker a solution. The final statement from the gastroenterology registrar (before the endoscopy report) concluded:

[Extract 5:] The case therefore was done in [the operating theatre], after hours, when it could have occurred in the endoscopy unit during hours.

Analysis and reflection

The record starts in a fairly straightforward way (extract 1), and illustrates the cryptic style in which doctors are trained to write in charts. The medical and nursing records are often kept separately, particularly if in paper format. Note that nurses are trained to use a more narrative style in the patient record, which places more emphasis on patients' behaviour and progress. This style difference can lead to inter-group conflict, mainly exemplified by nurses and doctors claiming not to understand each other's chart entries (or in the case of doctors, not always reading them carefully). In extract 1, there is an expression of thanks to the registrar in general medicine (Med Reg 4B: 'she will kindly review'), and trust that she can arrange things with the gastroenterology department. There was also a note about the urgency of the situation and the need for an endoscopy that day.

Things did not proceed smoothly, however. A conflict about the patient appeared in the chart soon after presentation at the ED, as extract 2 shows. Two hours later, the emergency medicine specialist, Dr Wilson, had intervened and was laying responsibility for any adverse consequences at the door of Dr Young, the gastroenterology registrar, as well as indicating a lack of trust of Dr Young and Dr Young's senior consultant. In contrast to the cryptic style used in extract 1 which had concentrated on the patient's condition and intended treatment, extract 2 presents a longish narrative description of the conversation about bed availability. This departure from standard cryptic medical notation often appears when there is intra-professional conflict among doctors.

In the final entries (extracts 3, 4 and 5), which are all part of a longer narrative, no discussion of the patient or his condition or treatment appears. Rather, the discussions between doctors in gastroenterology and emergency are detailed by Dr Young, the gastroenterology registrar. Dr Young appears to be concerned to set down the gastroenterology department's side, which is that an endoscopy cannot be performed unless the patient has a bed to go back to. Dr Young blames the other departments, particularly emergency, which is specifically named four times in the extracts. Dr Young describes the consequences of the conflict (that the procedure was performed late and out of hours in surgery, when it should not have been). Again, however, no mention is made in this long narrative of the patient, his condition or progress, or his treatment, other than that the endoscopy was eventually performed. Dr Young seems to be mainly concerned to detail the conflict. The patient has been forgotten, at least temporarily.

These extracts show escalating distrust and conflict between, in this case, the emergency and gastroenterology doctors. The context and history are relevant: a significant history of interdepartmental conflict relating to contested responsibilities for patient care. As the RMO in the ED was probably not aware of this context, the initial entry was polite and accommodating. A clear and deliberate statement was made about the patient's fasting status, critical information for the gastroenterology team in planning the timing of the procedure.

By contrast, the entry by the ED consultant (Dr Wilson) was unheralded. It signalled distrust of the motivations of the gastroenterology doctors (to claim an ED bed), reflecting inter-group conflict and escalating hostility between the groups. The entry prompted a detailed defence by the gastroenterology registrar. He concluded with a statement about the perceived inefficiency and waste stemming from the ED's refusal to continue the care of the patient after the endoscopy.

Reflective questions

1. What are the inter-specialty, intra-professional and interprofessional communication lessons for doctors and other health professionals, both junior and senior, that arise from practice example 13.1?
2. Why is practice example 13.1 best explained in terms of professional identity and inter-group conflict, rather than in terms of individual communication skills?
3. How could the conflict in this example be defused? How could the doctors have resolved it without going to the hospital CEO?
4. What could the hospital do, in terms of policy and practice, to minimise conflicts of this kind?

Implications for practice

Practice example 13.1 illustrates the impact on communication between professionals when their **professional identity** is challenged or questioned. Professional identity can arise and become salient within a single profession (for example, surgeons and physicians, or nurses and nurse practitioners), as well as between or among professions (for example, doctors, nurses and physiotherapists). Tribal conflicts can be very serious, and can be detrimental to patient care.

professional identity
the values and practices that are commonly associated with a professional role and become integral to a person's sense of self to form their professional identity.

Indeed, the case in practice example 13.1 is a stark example of the ways in which inter-group conflict and lack of trust can have serious consequences – sometimes even lethal ones – for patients. In this case, the patient's treatment was delayed because doctors from two departments could not resolve their conflict. This problem did not stem from lack of clarity or comprehensiveness in communication, although that was one of the results of the conflict. Instead, the problem came from a conflict over bed allocation, one that took priority over the patient's welfare and good treatment. The conflict could have been resolved by one department or the other agreeing to accept the patient, but both departments felt justified in holding their ground. Such conflicts could be resolved in the longer term by hospital-level policy that clarifies the process of admission from the ED, so that patients always have a path to admission when this is necessary.

As is very frequently the case, the cause of the problem was ambiguity in the hospital's procedures, and this ambiguity is exploited by different groups to their advantage. Thus, it was not clear who was responsible for finding a bed, or who was responsible for the patient's care. Instead of locating the cause of the problem in the hospital, its policies or the system, however, the doctors blamed each other, allowing their group identity to supersede what should be their common goal: best patient care.

The implications for practice of this are that health professionals should be very aware of the consequences of rigid professional identification. Rigid professional identification here means that a professional from one group is incapable of enacting their unique expertise without engaging in rivalry with another professional group.

It is further important to remember that identity, inter-group tensions and conflict can be communicated in writing as well as in speech, even in something as stylised and formal as a medical record. Additionally, identity, tension and conflict can be signalled through embodied conduct; that is, through people using their bodies to include or exclude others.

Finally, professional identity is very helpful in building confidence, creating networks, and imparting values to health professionals. But if identity becomes so important that it causes lack of trust and conflict, patients and health professionals will suffer as a consequence. Thus, it is essential in practice to communicate with people from different professions as fellow health professionals to create common ground. Professionals need to remind themselves to put the patient first, as all health professionals share the goal of best patient care. It is helpful to seek out members of other professions in informal contexts to build understanding and trust, and it is worth seeking every opportunity to train or work together. This is particularly so when health professionals are at the same level (for example, all junior doctors in different specialties, or all senior practitioners), because it is easy to build a shared identity around levels of experience and seniority.

Theoretical links

As students you will develop your own professional identity, which will affect your working with other professionals. Identity is how one defines oneself to oneself and to others (Lasky, 2005). Professional identity is an ongoing process of formation and transformation because of one's shifting experiences and fortunes over time (Giddens, 1991).

Social identity theory (SIT) takes these ideas somewhat further. SIT hypothesises that we may define ourselves in terms of the group (tribe) to which we belong (Tajfel & Turner, 1979). Turner (1982) later suggested that this identification with our own social group (or in-group) may lead to suspicion of and bias against other groups (out-groups). We then stereotype out-group members, and we make unfavourable comparisons between their attributes and those of our own in-group. This is a process that Turner referred to as 'inter-group differentiation'. One example of this is that nurses may regard occupational therapists (OTs) as interested in intellectual problems and quite innovative, but also as snobbish, more likely to have wealthier families, but less well organised, kind and nurturing. OTs may regard nurses as less resistant to change, while gossiping more. Both groups may rate their own profession as being more interested in people than the other (Westbrook, 2010).

'Cognitive dissonance' may occur for individuals when their values conflict with those of their own group (Festinger, 1962). Indeed, 'health professionals' success or failure in their professions is explained by the degree of alignment between their embodied or unconscious self-identity and the views, values, attitudes and behaviours espoused

collaborative practice
ways of working that involve team members enacting tasks together to accomplish practice goals.

by their chosen profession role' (Thistlethwaite, 2012, pp. 25–26). The alignment between self-identity, professional identity and interprofessional identity is thus fundamental to **collaborative practice**.

Conclusion

When professionals privilege their status and interests over the needs of the patient, or over the needs of their fellow professionals, they are in breach of the principles of patient-centredness and patient safety. Patients (and families) are often aware of inter-group conflicts, and will feel unsafe as a result of those conflicts (Iedema et al., 2011). Conflicts arise when professionals use their particular expertise as a basis for engaging in rivalry with members of another professional group. But such conflicts and the behaviours that produce them go against the interests of the patient, and they should not be allowed to undermine patients' care. Nor should such conflicts be condoned by anyone working in health care and claiming to be a healthcare professional.

Because patients are presenting with increasingly complex health problems requiring attention from different services and specialties, healthcare professionals need to work together to ensure that patients receive appropriate, coherent and continuous care. This means healthcare professionals need to communicate not just more frequently, but also more effectively than they have to date. In this context, inter-group conflicts are unprofessional and potentially dangerous.

Practice example 13.2

Below is another example examining interprofessional communication between health professionals interacting in the ED of a semi-rural hospital (Manidis et al., 2010). It highlights complications in the chain of communication that takes place between several clinicians. The clinicians look after Denton, a 79-year-old man who has been smoking 18–20 cigarettes a day for 60 years and is now suffering from chronic obstructive pulmonary dysfunction (COPD). He arrives at the ED with increasing shortness of breath and a raised temperature. He spends over five hours in the ED and is finally admitted to the ward at 17:45 p.m.

At various times staff try to establish whether Denton is a CO_2 retainer. Carbon dioxide (CO_2) retention occurs in some patients with COPD, and this retention may increase if they are given a high dose of oxygen to relieve their shortage of breath, but this may cause further problems with their breathing. Therefore, it is important to know the status of COPD patients if considering oxygen therapy.

continued >

Practice example 13.2 continued ›

Table 13.1 Denton and interprofessional communication in the emergency department (ED)

Clinician	Time	Knowing about Denton's CO_2 status	Tells	Outcome
N2 asks Z1 on Denton's arrival in the ED about his CO_2 retainer status	12:45 p.m.	Unclear whether N2 learns Denton is a CO_2 retainer	No evidence that N2 hands over this evidence to N5, the new nurse; more likely he doesn't as she questions D1 later about this	Subsequent clinicians don't know whether Denton is a CO_2 retainer
IC1 hands over to IC2	14:00 p.m.	Says she doesn't know anything about Denton	We know IC1 speaks to N2 but don't know if they share any case knowledge	None recorded
N5 stops to ask D1 if Denton is a 'collapse'	14:25 p.m.	N5 asks D1 if Denton is a 'collapse'; D1 explains that Denton is not a 'collapse'; he is suffering from pulmonary fibrosis and shortness of breath	No evidence of N5 telling anyone	N5 does not know if Denton is a CO_2 retainer; clarifies that he is not a collapse
N5 asks D1 if Denton is a CO_2 retainer	14:30 p.m.	Is told patient is a CO_2 retainer	No evidence of N5 telling anyone	Reduces oxygen a bit as D1 advises; D1 says Denton is a CO_2 retainer
D1 talks to D3, registrar, by 'phone to admit Denton to hospital	16:08 p.m.	Believes patient is a CO_2 retainer	Tells registrar he thinks Denton is a CO_2 retainer	Registrar now thinks Denton is a CO_2 retainer
D2 talks to D1 regarding Denton's CO_2 retainer status	16:15 p.m.	D2 using Denton's previous notes tells D1 Denton is not a CO_2 retainer [via the reference to Denton's blood bicarbonate level]	D2 tells D1	D1 finds out Denton is not a CO_2 retainer only after Denton has been in the ED for four hours

Note: N2, N5 = staff nurse; IC1/IC2 = in charge nurses; D1 = junior doctor; D2 = senior doctor; D3 = medical registrar; Z1 = paramedic

Critical information about Denton is 'lost' or 'distorted' in the complex chain of staff changes, absences, poor handovers, and attempts to reconstruct what is known about the patient. As noted, a key question in Denton's case (and for the clinicians who care

continued ›

Practice example 13.2 continued ›

for him) pertains to his 'CO_2 retainer status'. When Denton arrives by ambulance just after midday, N2, following hospital protocols for a patient presenting with COPD, asks the paramedic whether he (Z1) knows if Denton is a CO_2 retainer or not. The paramedic replies 'no' but it is not clear from the audio recording whether the 'no' means, 'No, he is not a CO_2 retainer', or 'No, we don't know if he is a CO_2 retainer'. The nurse does not ask for clarification, and the paramedic does not check what she has understood during this ambiguous exchange. There is no evidence that N2 talks to D1 about Denton's CO_2 status at this time or later.

Several hours later, at 14:00 p.m., the nurse in charge of the ED (IC1) hands over to IC2 at the end of her shift, though there is little to report and she states she does not know very much about Denton. At 14:25 p.m. N5, who is standing in for a colleague, asks the junior doctor D1 at the bedside about Denton, saying she (too) doesn't know much about him, but asks D1 if Denton was a 'collapse'. D1 says Denton was not a collapse.

N5 leaves and when she returns a short while later at 14:30 p.m. to care for Denton, she questions the junior doctor (D1) about Denton's CO_2 status. D1 has not volunteered this information to N5 previously. At the time of her question it would appear that N5 has not had time to read Denton's notes; nor has she found out from N2, N3 or the IC nurses if Denton is a CO_2 retainer. Therefore, she seeks to clarify Denton's status. D1 tells her Denton is a retainer, but it is not obvious why he thinks this.

Finally, after four hours of treatment in the ED, at 16:08 p.m. over the phone D1 tells the registrar (D3) admitting Denton to the medical ward that he thinks Denton *is* a CO_2 retainer. As he talks to the registrar, D1 is yet to learn at 16:15 p.m. from D2 that Denton is after all *not* a CO_2 retainer. D2 checked Denton's levels of 'bicarb' from his medical records relating to a previous admission and explains to D1 why Denton is not a CO_2 retainer.

Working alone at Denton's bedside, the difficulties of 'knowing about' Denton for each nurse and the junior doctor are evident. Each works and questions repetitively but in isolation from colleagues; each is disconnected from other members of the care team; as a group they are challenged by not all being in the same place at the same time, at times not being able to find or understand records, inaccurate information sharing, and frequently poor collegiate relationships in constructing what they know about a patient.

Reflective questions

1. What are the intra- and interprofessional communication lessons that arise from practice example 13.2 for (a) ED managers, (b) nurses, (c) junior doctors, and (d) senior doctors?

2. No one asks Denton what his CO_2 status is: should he be aware of this? Do you think the health professionals would or should trust his knowledge of his own status?

3. How should knowledge and information about patients such as CO_2 status be handed over and shared between health professionals?
4. Does each health profession require different or the same information about the patient? What is the role of the patient record for sharing information?

Further reading

Hammick, M., Freeth, D., Copperman, J., & Goodsman, D. (2009). *Being interprofessional*. Cambridge: Polity Press.

This is an easy-to-follow guide on interprofessional approaches to healthcare work. The book emphasises the urgent and increasing need for health practitioners across all disciplines to collaborate better with each other.

Web resources

Canadian Interprofessional Health Collaborative (CIHC) (2009): http://www.cihc.ca/files/CIHC_Factsheets_CP_Feb09.pdf

World Health Organization (WHO). *Framework for Action on Interprofessional Education and Collaborative Practice*: http://www.who.int/hrh/resources/framework_action/en

References

Canadian Interprofessional Health Collaborative (CIHC). (2010). Retrieved from http://www.cihc.ca/files/CIHC_IPCompetencies_Feb1210r.pdf

Dawson, J. F., Yan, X., & West, M. A. (2007). *Positive and negative effects of team working in healthcare: Real and pseudo-teams and their impact on safety*. Birmingham: Aston University.

Festinger, L. (1962). *A theory of cognitive dissonance*. London: Tavistock.

Freeth, D., Hammick, M., Reeves, S., Koppel, I., & Barr, H. (2005). *Effective interprofessional education: Development, delivery and evaluation*. Oxford: Blackwell Publishing.

Garling, P. (2008). Final report of the Special Commission of Inquiry: Acute care services in NSW public hospitals. NSW: State of NSW through the Special Commission of Inquiry.

Giddens, A. (1991). *Modernity and self-identity*. Cambridge: Polity.

Hewett, D., Watson, B., & Gallois, C. (2013). Trust, distrust, and communication accommodation among hospital doctors. In J. Crighton, & C. Candlin (Eds.), *Discourses of trust* (pp. 36–51). Basingstoke: Palgrave Macmillan.

Iedema, R., Allen, S., Britton, K., & Gallagher, T. (2011). What do patients and relatives know about problems and failures in care? *BMJ Qual Saf, 12*(21), 198–205.

Institute of Medicine. (2001). *Crossing the quality chasm: A new health system for the 21st century*, Washington, DC: National Academy Press.

Joint Commission on the Accreditation of Healthcare Organizations (JCAHO). (2005). *Sentinel event statistics: December 17, 2003*. Oak Terrace, IL: Author.

Katzenbach, J. R., & Smith, D. K. (1993). *The wisdom of teams: Areating the high-performance organization*. Boston: Harvard Business School Press.

Lasky, S. (2005). A sociocultural approach to understanding teacher identity, agency and professional vulnerability in a context of secondary school reform. *Teaching and Teacher Education, 21*(8), 899–916.

Lencioni, P. (2002). *The five dysfunctions of a team*. Lafayette: The Table Group.

Manidis, M., McGregor, J., Slade, D., Scheeres, H., Dunston, R., Stanton, N. et al. (2010). *Communicating in the emergency department: Report for Gosford Hospital*. Sydney: University of Technology.

Mason, T., Hinman, P., Sadik, R., Collyer, D., Hosker, N., & Keen, A. (2010). Values of reductionism and values of holism. In J. McCarthy & P. Rose (Eds.), *Values-based health and social care. Beyond evidence-based practice* (pp. 70–96). London: Sage.

Romanow, R. J. (2002). Building on values: The future of health care in Canada. Final report (pp. 1–356). Ottawa: Commission on the Future of Health Care in Canada.

Tajfel, H., & Turner, J. (1979). An integrative theory of inter-group conflict. In W. G. Austin & S. Worchel (Eds.), *The social psychology of intergroup relations* (pp. 33–47). Monterey: Brooks/Cole Publishing Company.

Thistlethwaite, J. E. (2012). *Values-based interprofessional collaborative practice*. Cambridge: Cambridge University Press.

Thomas, M., Burt, M., & Parkes, J. (2010). The emergence of evidence-based practice. In J. McCarthy & P. Rose (Eds.), *Values-based health and social care. Beyond evidence-based practice* (pp. 3–24). London: Sage.

Turner, J. C. (1982). Towards a cognitive redefinition of the social group. In H. Tajfel (Ed.), *Social identity and intergroup relations* (pp. 15–40). Cambridge: Cambridge University Press.

Westbrook, M. T. (2010). Professional stereotypes: How occupational therapists and nurses perceive themselves and each other. *Australian Occupational Therapy Journal, 25*, 12–17.

Communicating care: informed consent

Katherine Carroll and Rick Iedema

Learning objectives

This chapter will enable you to:
- describe key characteristics of a good informed consent procedure;
- explain how consent processes may differ when working with Indigenous Australians;
- discuss how the concepts of relational autonomy, embodied knowledge, experiential knowledge, and emotion can assist in understanding patients' decision-making;
- reflect upon how you might structure verbal informed consent encounters;
- consider how different information and styles of communication may be practiced in verbal and written informed consent material.

Key terms

Embodied knowledge
Experiential knowledge
Informed consent
Relational autonomy
Socio-economic contexts

Overview

Informed consent involves giving patients information about treatment options and possible risks. This information is provided to facilitate patients' decision-making. Informed consent

> **informed consent**
> the process of ensuring that the patient consents to being subjected to medical treatments.

aims to enable a patient to weigh up their own values, goals and concerns together with scientific evidence.

Patients are asked to engage in informed consent prior to treatments or interventions, and when those treatments or interventions are part of a scientific study. Informed consent may involve verbal communication, and it may include written information that the patient is asked to review and carefully consider (Jordens, Montgomery & Forsyth, 2013). The patient is required to sign the consent form as evidence of having read about and agreed to the treatment.

To facilitate this process, informed consent documents contain accessibly written, scientifically determined, detailed information. This information covers the relevant treatment or intervention, its potential side effects, the various risks that may be involved, and a relatively linear account of the treatment trajectory (Franklin & Kaufman, 2009; Rid & Dinhofer, 2009).

This chapter discusses the principles of informed consent as it occurs in everyday communication in clinics, acute hospital wards and general practice. It considers how the decision-making of patients, their families, and their care providers is shaped not just by individuals' personal preferences, but also by their **socio-economic contexts**, cultural backgrounds and expectations, personal experiences and emotions. Decisions are further likely to be shaped by the broader cultural climate created by health, legal and educational institutions which create policies, regulations, and professional cultures and subcultures in the healthcare system.

> **socio-economic contexts**
> the social and economic circumstances that surround us. These circumstances may include 'multi-cultural immigration', 'student strikes', 'the mining boom' and the 'global financial crisis'.

Introduction

Advances in medicine and technology produce many new treatment options for patients (Brown & Webster, 2004). In addition to this, the increased prevalence of chronic disease and co-morbidities in the population gives rise to new ethical and treatment challenges for patients, as well as for their families, and for healthcare providers. To come to terms with the implications of the various treatment options and with their own diseases, patients and their loved ones, in conjunction with their treating health professionals, need to deliberate about which treatments, interventions and kinds of research participation are preferable.

Informed consent is posited as the solution to some of these complex medical choices and related ethical problems. Informed consent is particularly important when it comes to making choices associated with as yet untested treatments when these are made available to patients in research clinical trials (Corrigan, 2003). Overall, informed consent has been shown to lead to greater patient satisfaction, improved patient outcomes, fewer medical errors, and lower rates of malpractice claims (Cordasco, 2013).

Informed consent: main principles

Informed consent is undergirded by the four bioethical principles: autonomy, beneficence, non-maleficence and justice (Beauchamp & Childress, 1994; Little, 2009). These principles guide how health professionals should treat patients, how doctors should undertake procedures in new fields such as regenerative, preventative and personalised medicine, and how the researcher should conduct innovative scientific and clinical trials.

In particular, scientific and clinical progress requires consent from patients, and this can be achieved only through effective communication between patients and their health professionals. For example, it is possible now to genetically screen embryos and foetuses for disease and disability (Boardman, 2013). But the information such screening produces about embryos and foetuses may have important implications for a woman's current and future pregnancies (Hundt et al., 2006; Kerr & Franklin, 2006). It is important then for parents to engage in 'genetic counselling' where this information and its health implications are discussed, and where they can make informed decisions about their future.

Another example is the field of regenerative medicine and research, where there is a growth in demand for fresh eggs (oocytes) to be donated by young, fertile women. However, young women must give informed consent before they undergo invasive treatment with unknown effects on their future fertility (Carroll & Waldby, 2012).

It is important to recognise that consent may rest not just with the individual. Families and guardians may also need to be drawn into the consent process. Consider people in advanced industrialised nations: they are suffering more chronic conditions and co-morbidities, and they are living longer. They are more likely to live a long life and then die in a hospital where medical technologies and highly skilled medical, nursing and allied health professions will keep them alive for longer than in the past. It is in intensive care units where families are often faced with an uncertain prognosis of their unconscious or incapacitated loved one, and where they will need to make complex decisions about the withdrawal or continuation of treatment (Guyer, 2006; Mesman, 2008; Murray, 2000).

One bioethical concept that has special importance in informed consent is the principle of autonomy. Autonomy is the 'respect for personal self-government' (Naffine & Richards, 2012, p. 49). That is, autonomy harbours recognition of the role that a patient plays in decisions about their body and personhood (McGrath & Phillips, 2008). One of the ways in which autonomy is respected in medical practice is through seeking voluntary consent for medical treatments or procedures from a person who is mentally competent to understand and give consent (Jordens, Montgomery & Forsyth, 2013). Factors to consider include positive factors, such as the absence of coercion in the decision-making process, and negative factors, such as incentives (payment or discounted treatment in return for research participation).

While the notion of individual autonomy is basic to Western bioethics, Indigenous cultures of Australia place the family unit and community group at the core of decisions made about their care, treatment or interventions (McGrath & Phillips, 2008). This means that, rather than consulting just with the individual about an intervention, health professionals also need to include the family, and they may be required to include certain people in tribal positions (McGrath & Phillips, 2008). For this to succeed, it is important to have knowledge of the 'right people' in the family and community network to approach for informed consent (McGrath & Phillips, 2008).

The achievement of a 'fully' informed consent may not be possible. However, informed consent is said to be one given freely by the patient or research participant when there is full understanding of what is involved, with full knowledge of any risks and their likelihood, and without any coercion (Corrigan, 2003; Little, 2009). Informed consent also involves the care provider or researcher providing complete, accurate and understandable information (Little, 2009). This means that the information needs to be comprehended, weighed up and decided upon by the patient or research participant (Little, 2009; Little et al., 2008; Rid & Dinhofer, 2009).

Clearly, the person or people making the decisions will require certain linguistic and cognitive competencies. Ascertaining patient understanding of information presented during informed consent is not always possible or easy (Jordens, Montgomery & Forsyth, 2013). Therefore health professionals need to consider carefully how best to deliver information to patients and research participants to facilitate the decision-making (Mouce, 2013). Nurses, doctors and allied health staff are required to engage in different techniques and interventions to communicate more effectively, and plan how that information should be presented (Jordens, Montgomery & Forsyth, 2013; Mouce, 2013). This is all the more important because consent forms contain increasingly detailed information of risks and they are increasingly lengthy (Jordens, Montgomery & Forsyth, 2013). This means that health professionals need to consider how much information to deliver, how quickly and in what language, and how to ascertain the patient's comprehension. Part of this process is that health professionals need to consider the likely effect of stress and anxiety on patients' understanding and recall of the treatment information (Mouce, 2013).

Practice example 14.1

It is just 48 hours after 'Nancy', a 25-year-old married woman, has given birth to premature twins (a boy and a girl).[1] The twins were born 10 weeks before their due date and were severely growth restricted *in utero*. The twins have a very low birth weight (VLBW), particularly the baby girl. Both babies have been admitted to the neonatal intensive care unit (NICU). The twins are expected to survive; however, due to their

continued ›

Practice example 14.1 continued ›

prematurity and VLBW the neonatologist is particularly concerned about preventing necrotising enterocolitis (NEC). NEC is a severe and sometimes fatal disease of the gastrointestinal system which often occurs in premature and VLBW infants (Neu, 2011). Breastmilk is very important for premature babies because it has been found to prevent NEC (Sullivan et al., 2010). Donor breastmilk – breastmilk donated by lactating women – is recommended ahead of infant formula when a mother's own milk is unavailable (American Academy of Pediatrics, 2012; World Health Organization UNICEF, 2003).

Nancy also has a five-year-old child, and while visiting the twins last night she told the NICU nurse that she had a lot of trouble producing sufficient breastmilk for her first child. The nurse identified Nancy's anxiety, and provided her with information about donated breastmilk (DBM) from the human milk bank. The nurse also discussed Nancy's lactation history with the neonatologist the following day during the morning ward round. They agreed that if Nancy could not produce sufficient volumes of breastmilk for both of the twins, it would be best to feed them with DBM from the hospital's human milk bank.

During the morning ward round the neonatologist decided that the baby girl was medically stable but hungry. The baby was therefore ready to begin milk feedings later that day. In the afternoon the neonatologist approached Nancy and her husband Michael to begin informed consent for the use of DBM. Informed consent in this case centred not only on the written material provided to patients, but also involved a discussion with the neonatologist (Figure 14.1).

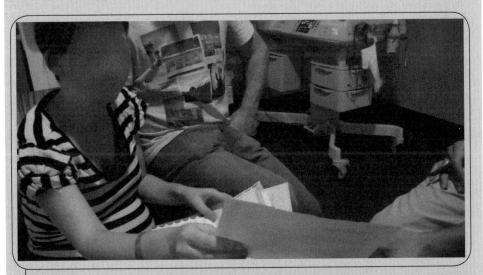

Figure 14.1 Neonatologist (right) discussing informed consent documents with parents (left) in a neonatal intensive care unit. Informed consent is supported by both written material and opportunities to engage in discussions with health professionals.

continued ›

Neonatalogist:	Now that she is breathing well without any tube in her nose or lungs, and she is a bit more than 48 hours old, it's time for us to start thinking about giving her some milk. You already know that what we would like to do is give her breastmilk. The reason we particularly want to give her breastmilk is because for a long time she has been stressed while growing inside, and she hasn't been growing well since about 26 weeks' gestation. We know that babies who have been pretty stressed for a long time before they are born often take a long time for their bowel to start working properly again. So we like to give those babies human breastmilk. So any breastmilk that you are able to express and bring down, it will go to her first.
Mother:	Fine.
Neonatologist:	The nurse said you had difficulties with your first baby supplying enough breastmilk?
Mother:	Yes.
Neonatologist:	Because we really want to give her breastmilk I want to have a conversation with you about donor breastmilk.
Mother:	Fine.
Neonatologist:	I understand that yesterday you received an information pamphlet from the nurse?
Mother:	Yes.
Neonatalogist:	Had you heard that we had a breastmilk bank here at the hospital before?
Mother:	No! [Laughs]
Neonataologist:	Have you had time to read the breastmilk pamphlet?
Mother:	I did today.
Neonatologist:	Did that make sense?
Mother:	Yeah, yes.
Neonatologist:	So if there wasn't enough breastmilk from your own expressing, what we would like to do is that rather than give her formula, and rather than keep the drip running unnecessarily, we would like to use breast milk from people who are donors.
Mother:	Yes.
Neonatologist:	So there are about 6–12 people who currently donate breastmilk to the breastmilk bank here at the hospital. There are very strict criteria: if you smoke you cannot donate, if you smoke marijuana you can't donate, if you have more than two standard drinks of alcohol a day you get ruled out as well. If you have hepatitis B or C, HIV or a whole series of medical conditions, then you cannot donate. If you want to be a donor you have to undergo regular blood testing as well. If the blood tests are all good and you are in tip-top physical condition, the breastmilk that

continued ›

you donate is pasteurised. So if there are any bacteria or viruses in it, then they get removed prior to the milk being given to the baby. So, as a consequence of the blood tests and the pasteurisation, we believe the risk of babies getting any virus or bacteria are negligible. If you are unable to supply enough milk for your little girl then it would be really good to give her the rest of the milk as donor breastmilk.

Mother: Yep.

Neonatologist: Can you fill me in on your own expressing? Are you seeing a lactation consultant?

Mother: Yes. I saw them yesterday and I hand express every three hours. It is only day two since they were born, so I am getting a little bit stressed that nothing is coming out. In the meantime I am more than happy to do the donor milk.

Neonatologist: Your baby girl seems to be very feisty and strong which is really good. You have been given a consent form already!

Mother: Yes. I haven't signed it yet.

Neonatologist: That is ok. Have you read it?

Mother: Yep.

Neonatologist: It reiterates what the information pamphlet says. It starts out by saying that human breastmilk is the best thing for the baby. Then it states that if there is not enough from mum we have available resources in our breastmilk bank. It outlines some of the risks associated with donor breast milk, and the steps we go through to reduce risks to negligible levels. My name is Dr Chris, and that is my signature, and so what I would like you to do is to write your name there and there and then sign.

Mother: [Signs the consent form] So when can she get the donor breastmilk?

Neonatologist: If she is hungry tonight, what we can do is start thawing some milk and give her some tonight. She is sucking furiously on her dummy and she is being very patient!

Mother: [Laughs] Ahhh she is a good girl!

After the informed consent the researcher briefly interviewed the parents about their informed consent experience with the neonatologist.

Researcher: So when you first read about donor milk in the information pamphlet was there anything you were concerned about?

Parents: Infections. Yeah … infections.

Researcher: Why did you not ask the doctor about these?

Parents: He told us it was negligible … and so he reassured us.

continued ›

Practice example 14.1 continued ›

Researcher:	What is your expectation with donor milk and your own milk?
Mother:	I am hoping that by giving her the donor milk now … I am hoping in the long run to have my milk and the donor milk together, if I don't have enough. But we will see what happens.
Researcher:	Are there any extra bits of information about donor milk that you would have liked to have known but wasn't covered in the consent form or the conversation?
Parents:	No. It was all really covered. I think it will go well, and if I can't express enough milk then I need to give her something. Donor milk is the next best thing to my own breastmilk.

Analysis and reflection

Practice example 14.1 provides an example of an appropriately negotiated and optimally informed consent. How do we know this? Let us weigh up what happened in the case study against the seven principles collated by Cordasco (2013) from a review of the informed consent scientific literature. These seven principles are useful for practitioners when needing to work toward a more complete informed consent process (Cordasco, 2013, p. 462):

1. discussing the patient's role in the decision-making process;
2. describing the clinical issue and suggested treatment;
3. discussing alternatives to the suggested treatment (including the option of no treatment);
4. discussing risks and benefits of the suggested treatment (and comparing them to the risks and benefits of alternatives);
5. discussing related uncertainties;
6. assessing the patient's understanding of the information provided;
7. eliciting the patient's preference (and thereby consent).

Cordasco also identifies that supplemental written material, the use of decision aides, repeat-back methods, and video educational tools may also assist in patient comprehension, recall and shared decision-making.

The informed consent session between the neonatologist and the parents of the hospitalised premature twins covered many of the principles of 'good' informed consent. To increase the chances that the parents adequately understood the feeding options for their premature twins, information was comprehensively presented in both a written and verbal form. Decision-making time was provided to parents by giving them the written information statement 24 hours ahead of meeting with the neonatologist. A comprehensive explanation of the safety of DBM by the neonatologist is extremely influential over parental decision-making as through the consent process neonatologists can reposition DBM as something that was largely unknown by parents and perceived as potentially risky into a life-saving food with therapeutic properties (Carroll, 2014).

One of the key ethical principles of informed consent is disclosure and understanding of treatment alternatives, which suggests that health professionals should provide information on the outcomes associated with DBM and alternate feeding options (Miracle et al., 2011). The written material and conversation with the neonatologist adequately communicated the risks of not giving DBM to the baby girl and included the unnecessary use of an intravenous drip (parenteral nutrition) and unnecessary use of a lesser food source (formula). The magnitude of infection risk through the use of DBM was also identified and characterised by the neonatologist as 'negligible'.

During the informed consent process, the neonatologist also ascertained the parents' prior knowledge by asking whether the parents had ever heard of a human milk bank, and whether they had the opportunity to read the information statement and consent form. He also ascertained the mother's prior experience with lactation. The neonatologist was respectful of the mother's contribution of her own breastmilk by reiterating that Nancy's own breastmilk would always be used first – that is, ahead of donor milk – to feed her babies. This reassurance is critical for mothers who may worry about lactation, breastfeeding and relying on DBM. Reassuring the mother that DBM is used only when her own milk proves insufficient is therefore an important component of the clinical encounter and the informed consent process (Carroll, 2014; Swanson et al., 2012). The reassurance recognises that both emotion and medical recommendations are influential when it comes to decision-making about DBM (Carroll, forthcoming).

Reflective questions

1. How could the informed consent process between the neonatologist and parents be improved?
2. Which health professional provided informed consent in this case study? Could another NICU health professional (such as a nurse or lactation consultant) obtain the informed consent for DBM? If so, what would be some care quality and patient satisfaction implications?
3. In this hospital DBM is required to have informed consent, but the administration of artificial infant formula is not subject to informed consent. Is this ethical in light of the alternative treatment disclosure principle inherent in a good informed consent process?

Implications for practice

Informed consent is more than a bureaucratic procedure. In fact, informed consent has much in common with shared decision-making (see Chapter 12). Shared decision-making is the process of the health professional and the patient reaching a decision together. Whereas informed consent may be regarded as an outcome that follows the decision about which treatment to pursue, the way it manifests (or should manifest) in communication is through shared decision-making. Put more succinctly, informed consent is the outcome of a shared decision-making communication process.

In a recent paper, Hoffmann and colleagues provide the following practical example of how shared decision-making may underpin informed consent. As shown in Table 14.1, the first question is: 'Should we wait, do nothing, and see what happens?' The second is: 'What are your test or treatment options?' Then we ask, 'What are benefits and harms of these options?', and 'How do these benefits and harms weigh up for you?' Finally, we ask, 'Do you have enough information to make a choice?' Table 14.1 offers example phrases, as well as further comments about what each question entails (Hoffmann et al., 2014):

It is important to acknowledge not just the scientific evidence, as is Hoffmann and colleagues' principal concern, but also patients' socio-cultural and relational circumstances. Here, what is critical is 'active listening' (see Chapter 19). Active listening involves giving the patient an opportunity to express thoughts and feelings that ordinary conversation might not allow them to express (Egan, 2006). An example of 'active listening' is provided in Chapter 19.

· ·

Theoretical links

Both practice examples 1 and 2 highlight that patients and research participants do not make informed-consent decisions in isolation from their social, economic and cultural contexts. There are three key sociological concepts that health professionals utilise to think about informed consent in a way that goes beyond merely telling the mother (or patient) about the relevant scientific evidence. The first is **relational autonomy**. This concept is important, because the way we achieve informed consent needs to engage not just with scientific evidence, but also with the mother's (or patient's) identity, and their sense of what is an appropriate action and decision. Generally, what is considered appropriate tends to reflect the person's relationships with their family members and peers, and relationships again reflect broader community and social expectations.

> **relational autonomy**
> a term that emphasises that, as individuals, we, our thoughts, decisions and intentions, have emerged and grown out of our social relations. Accordingly, a person's autonomy is always only possible thanks to being entwined in social relations, and it can never stand in opposition to social relations.

The concept of 'relational autonomy' is used to emphasise the importance of these 'relational' issues, and of the need to respect the mother's (patient's) right (that is, their autonomy) to refer to these issues when consenting to care decisions (Ehrich et al., 2007; Friedman, 2000).

The definition of relational autonomy makes clear that relational autonomy contrasts with 'individualist autonomy' – a term that presumes people can make decisions entirely independently from their social relationships and contexts. Relational autonomy can be

Table 14.1 An example of one approach to shared decision-making (Hoffman et al., 2014)

Five questions that clinicians can use to guide shared decision-making	Example phrases (for the opening clinical scenario of a child with acute otitis media)	Comments
1. What will happen if we wait and watch?	'In children, most middle ear infections get better by themselves, usually within a week. The best options to control pain and fever are paracetamol or ibuprofen.'	Quantitative information can be provided where possible, either at this step or in step 3 where each option is described. When this is not possible, descriptive information can be provided (e.g., 'most people find that the symptoms go away by …'). Eliciting patient's expectations about management of the condition (e.g., 'What have you heard or do know about … ?'), including previously tested approaches and experiences, along with fears and concerns, is important and may occur here or later in the process.
2. What are your test or treatment options?	'Waiting for it to get better by itself is one option. Another option is to take antibiotics. Do you want to discuss that option?'	For some decisions (such as in this example), the options may be familiar to patients and need little elaboration at this step. In others, a more detailed explanation of each option and its practicalities, including options which are time-urgent, will be required.
3. What are the benefits and harms of these options?	'We know from good research that of 100 children with middle ear infection who *do not* take antibiotics, 82 will feel better and have no pain after 2–3 days. Out of 100 children who *do* take antibiotics, 87 will feel better after about three days of taking them. So, about five more will get better a little faster. We can't know whether your child will be one of the five children who benefit or not.' (A graphic representation of these numbers can also be shown at this point, and again after the harms information is discussed.) 'There are some downsides to antibiotics though. Out of 100 children who *do* take antibiotics, 20 will experience vomiting, diarrhoea or rash, compared with 15 who *do not* take them. That means about five children out of 100 will have side effects from antibiotics. But again, we can't know whether your child will have any of these problems. The other possible downside is antibiotic resistance – would you like to hear more about it?' (The option of delayed prescribing could also be discussed here. …)	In addition to descriptively discussing the benefits and harms of each option, the probability of each occurring, where this is known, should be provided. For dichotomous outcomes (e.g., having a myocardial infarction), this should be in the form of natural frequencies (i.e., the number out of 100 or 1000 people who experience the event) rather than relative risk. For continuous outcomes (e.g., number of days of pain, and level of anxiety as reported on an anxiety measure), this may be expressed by the estimated size of the effect (e.g., the average reduction in 20 points on anxiety on a tool that measured it as a score from 0 to 10). Decision support tools, if available, can be useful at this stage. Simple visual graphics can be particularly useful in helping to communicate the numbers. Principles of effectively communicating statistical information to patients should be followed, such as using natural frequencies (i.e., x out of 100), being aware of framing effects, and using multiple formats. The discussions of harms should extend beyond the risk of side effects and include other impacts that the option could have on the patient, such as cost, inconvenience and interference with daily roles, and reduced quality of life.

Table 14.1 (*cont.*)

4. How do the benefits and harms weigh up for you?	'With all I've said, which option do you feel most comfortable with?'	This step includes eliciting patients' preferences and working with them to clarify how each option may fit with their values, preferences, beliefs and goals. Some decision aids include formal value clarification exercises that may be used to supplement the conversation and/or enable the patient to reflect further following the consultation. Clarifying the patient's understanding of what has been discussed so far, using the teach-back method, can help to identify if any information needs to be repeated or explained in another way.
5 Do you have enough information to make a choice?	'Is there any more you want to know? Do you feel you have enough information to make a choice?'	This provides another opportunity to ask if the patient has additional questions. Patients may feel ready to make a decision at this stage or it may be jointly decided to defer the decision and plan when it should be revisited. The patient may wish to seek further information before deciding, discuss with family, or take time to process and reflect on the information received.

exemplified as follows. When faced with the decision about whether or not to terminate a pregnancy due to carrying a baby with Down syndrome, parents are unlikely to consult only formal evidence and clinical information about Down syndrome – both so central to the health professional's expertise. When faced with such important decisions, parents are also likely to obtain information from their social networks, the internet, religious and cultural figures, and they will rely on the first hand experiences told to them by family and friends (Hundt et al., 2006).

Second are two related concepts: 'embodied' and 'experiential' knowledge. **Embodied knowledge** is gained from one's own direct experience of living in the world. For example, you may have personal experience of a particular disease or treatment (Boardman, 2013). For its part, **experiential knowledge** can be gained from having a close association with someone who has had a particular illness, or with someone who has close experience of an illness (such as a parent of a sick child).

It is important that the health professional acknowledges embodied knowledge and experiential knowledge (Belenky et al., 1986; Held, 1993; Jaggar, 1993). For example, rather

> **embodied knowledge**
> knowledge that operates through parts of the body other than the conscious mind. Examples are that your feet 'know' where to place themselves on the footpath, and your shoulder 'knows' how to avoid an oncoming tree branch.
>
> **experiential knowledge**
> knowledge that arises from having experienced situations, relationships and events 'first-hand'. This knowledge is not like abstract, general scientific knowledge, but is gained through personally participating in situations, relationships and events.

than viewing a specific condition through a medical lens that may emphasise complications associated with a particular disability or disorder, experiential knowledge may give voice to positive aspects of life with a certain condition, or enable people to imagine living with a condition into the future (Boardman, 2013).

An example of how embodied knowledge can be applied to informed consent is in egg donation to stem cell research (Carroll & Waldby, 2012). Often women undergoing fertility treatment or *in vitro* fertilisation (IVF) are targeted to provide eggs to stem cell research as they are already undergoing 'egg harvesting' to assist their own treatment. Yet most IVF patients recognise only after having had the IVF treatment how precious their eggs are. This is because the treatment reveals that their egg supply is limited and the number of eggs is constantly dwindling due to the process of ageing. As these issues tend to arise for patients only as their IVF treatment progresses, patients gradually develop a sense of their eggs as a limited resource. They therefore have a greater capacity to give informed consent to donate 'spare' eggs to research towards the end of their IVF treatment, and not at the beginning (Carroll & Waldby, 2012).

The third concept is emotion. As the foregoing clarifies, attending to emotion is critically important in making decisions about treatment. One emotion is regret, a negative emotion that may be experienced as a consequence of a past choice. For example, after experiencing the ordeal of the highly risky and painful bone marrow transplant and chemotherapy for cancer treatment, some patients say that they would not consent to it again: they regret consenting to the chemotherapy (Little, 2009). Patients also have the capacity to experience 'prospective regret'. This refers to feeling regret for an adverse outcome that *might* occur as a result of a decision made in the present. It is common in everyday life to say, for example, 'I'm going to regret this …' (Little, 2009). Therefore it is possible to learn from the feeling of regret and acknowledge how regret and other emotions play important roles in people's decision-making (Little, 2009).

Conclusion

Informed consent is typically understood by health professionals as a 'rational choice' that refers to formal evidence and decontextualised information (Held, 1993). It is important, however, that we recognise the individual people, their backgrounds and relational ways of making decisions when asking them to consent to treatments. Sociological concepts such as 'relational autonomy', 'embodied/experiential knowledge' and 'emotion' broaden consent processes that may otherwise remain constrained by 'rationalist' thinking: thinking that relies on science and formal information, but not on personal experience, or socio-cultural insights and priorities.

A broader approach to informed consent attends to the important role that is played by emotions, previous experiences, embodied knowledge, and past decisions on the decision-making process (Carroll & Waldby, 2012; Little, 2009). By referring to biomedical principles in addition to sociological notions, health professionals have access to tools that should broaden how they engage in communication during informed consent. These concepts emphasise that patients' decision-making should not ignore their unique inter-personal, social, economic, and cultural contexts (Corrigan, 2003; Friedman, 2000).

Practice example 14.2

Informed consent problems can arise not only regarding clinical procedures but also through research activities in hospital settings. Research activities involve patients and their health providers in identifying potential research (patient) participants, recruiting patients for participation, and the delivery or measurement of a research intervention. Consider the following case study and how your own conduct during clinical practice may be implicated.

A young man falls off his bicycle and presents to a local emergency department for treatment. You treat him for his injury and he goes home. A week or so later, he receives a letter followed by a phone call at home from a research assistant who has been given his name by somebody at the hospital. The research assistant asks him if he would like to participate in a research study being undertaken by the nearby university. He queries the call, wondering how the university has obtained, not only his home telephone number but also his home address and details of his accident. He is told that staff members at the hospital gave the university the information. He indicates that he had not signed any consent form for his private details to be released, nor was he told about the research project. He tells the young research assistant that he would be happy to participate, but would need some further information about the project before proceeding.

He duly receives an email several days later telling him about the project, and informing him that someone would like to interview him for 20 minutes. He agrees and begins to answer questions. The questions require an answer scaled 1 to 10, estimating how he felt at the time of his treatment. Even though during the interview the questions are asked abruptly of him in a very quick manner, they run out of time to complete it. He is told that there are still more questions to be asked. They arrange another time and the same thing happens: the questions are asked too quickly, and without opportunity to discuss them. This time he says he is not emotionally capable of proceeding with the interview and the interviewer abruptly hangs up the phone.

He contacts the researchers at the university to outline a number of concerns in an email:

1. There was no initial consent for contact.
2. He experienced poor behaviour on the part of the research assistant who abruptly terminated the phone call when he decided to withdraw from the project.
3. He felt that the way emotions were explored during the interview was abrupt and unfeeling.

Neither the hospital nor the university appeared prepared to take responsibility for what occurred. Further, neither the hospital nor the university followed up on any of the concerns expressed, and neither offered an apology.

Reflective questions

1. What procedures should the hospital and the university each have followed to safeguard the patient's privacy before contacting the patient for participation?
2. In what ways could informed consent reduce risk to the patient in this incident?
3. How will you determine a patient's understanding of information in your professional discipline?
4. What are the most common ways to deliver information to patients for informed consent? What additional tools can you use to ensure good communication?
5. Have you ever been hospitalised, had surgery or had an invasive procedure? How did it feel to give or deny consent? What factors influenced your decision?

Further reading

These following sources provide bioethical, sociological and ethnographic insight into medical uncertainty and prognosis, and the difficult decisions patient families need to make in light of uncertainty. These sources highlight the social context that informs medical and family decision-making, and the role that technological intervention plays in making health care more ethically complex. These sources also explore medical uncertainty and the role of the health professional in communicating uncertainty to the family.

Guyer, R. (2006). *Baby at risk*. Herndon: Capital Books.
Kerr, A., & Franklin, S. (2006). Genetic ambivalence: Expertise, uncertainty and communication in the context of new genetic technologies. In A. Webster (Ed.), *New technologies in health care* (pp. 40–56). London: Palgrave Macmillan.
Mesman, J. (2008). *Uncertainty in medical innovation*. New York: Palgrave Macmillan.

Web resources

Australian Commission on Quality and Safety in Healthcare, *Shared decision making*: http://www.safetyandquality.gov.au/our-work/shared-decision-making
Australian Health Practitioner Regulation Agency (AHPRA), *Informed consent: guidelines for osteopaths*, (2013): http://www.osteopathyboard.gov.au/documents/default.aspx?record=WD13%2F10345&dbid=AP&chksum=v6H2tjB72bGXwCuEyW%2BJhw%3D%3D
National Health and Medical Research Council (NHMRC), *General guidelines for medical practitioners on providing information to patients*, (2004): http://www.nhmrc.gov.au/guidelines/publications/e57

References

American Academy of Pediatrics. (2012). Breastfeeding and the use of human milk. *Pediatrics*, *129*, e827–e841.

Beauchamp, T. L., & Childress, J. F. (1994). *Principles of biomedical ethics* (4th ed.). New York: Oxford University Press.

Belenky, M., Clinchy, B., Goldberger, N., & Tarule, J. (1986). *Women's ways of knowing.* New York: Basic Books.

Boardman, F. (2013). Knowledge is power? The role of experiential knowledge in genetically 'risky' reproductive decisions. *Sociology of Health and Illness, 36*(1), 137–150.

Brown, N, & Webster, A. (2004). *New medical technologies and society.* Cambridge: Polity.

Carroll, K. (2014). Body dirt or liquid gold? How the 'safety' of donated breast milk is constructed for use in neonatal intensive care. *Social Studies of Science.* doi:10.1177/0306312714521705

——. (forthcoming). The milk of human kinship: Donor human milk in the nicu. In C. Krolekke, I. Myong & S. Adrian (Eds.), *Critical kinship studies.* London: Routledge.

Carroll, K., & Waldby, C. (2012). Informed consent and fresh egg-donation for stem cell research: The case for incorporating embodied knowledge into ethical decision-making. *International Journal of Bioethical Inquiry, 9*(1), 29–39.

Cordasco, K. (2013). Obtaining informed consent from patients: Brief update review. In P. G. Shekelle, R. M. Wachter, P. J. Pronovost, K. Schoelles, K. M. McDonald, S. M. Dy, K. et al. (Eds.), *Making health care safer II: An updated critical analysis of the evidence for patient safety practices.* Rockville, MD: Agency for Healthcare Research & Quality.

Corrigan, O. (2003). Empty ethics: The problem of informed consent. *Sociology of Health and Illness, 25*(3), 768–792.

Egan, G. (2006). *The skilled helper: A problem-management and opportunity-development approach to helping.* New York: Brooks/Cole.

Ehrich, K., Williams, C., Farsides, B., Sandall, J., & Scott, R. (2007). Choosing embryos: Ethical complexity and relational autonomy in staff accounts of PGD. *Sociology of Health and Illness, 29*(7), 1–16.

Franklin, S., & Kaufman, S. (2009). Ethical and consent issues in the reproductive setting: The case of egg, sperm, and embryo donation. In R. Warwick, D. Fehily, S. Brubaker & T. Eastland (Eds.), *Tissue and cell donation* (pp. 222–242). Oxford: Wiley-Blackwell.

Friedman, M. (2000). Autonomy, social discruption, and women. In C. MacKenzie & N. Stoljar (Eds.), *Relational autonomy: Feminist perspectives on autonomy, agency and the social self* (pp. 35–51). Oxford and New York: Oxford University Press.

Guyer, R. (2006). *Baby at risk.* Herndon: Capital Books.

Held, Virginia. (1993). *Feminist morality.* Chicago: The University of Chicago Press.

Hoffmann, T., Legare, F., Simmons, M., McNamara, K., McCaffery, K., Trevena, L. et al. (2014). Shared decision making: What do clinicians need to know and why should they bother? *Medical Journal of Australia, 201*(1), 35–39.

Hundt, G., Green, J., Sandall, J., Hirst, J., Ahmed, S., & Hewison, J. (2006). Navigating the troubled waters of prenatal testing decisions. In A. Webster (Ed.), *New technologies in health care* (pp. 25–39). London: Palgrave Macmillan.

Jaggar, A. (1993). Taking consent seriously: Feminist practical ethics and actual moral dialogue. In E. Winkler & J. Coombs (Eds.), *Applied ethics* (pp. 69–86). Cambridge: Blackwell.

Jordens, C., Montgomery, K., & Forsyth, R. (2013). Trouble in the gap: A bioethical and sociological analysis of informed consent for high-risk medical procedures. *Bioethical Inquiry, 10,* 67–77.

Kerr, A., & Franklin, S. (2006). Genetic ambivalence: Expertise, uncertainty and communication in the context of new genetic technologies. In A. Webster (Ed.), *New technologies in health care* (pp. 40–53). London: Pagrave Macmillan.

Little, M. (2009). The role of regret in informed consent. *Bioethical Inquiry, 6*, 49–59.

Little, M., Jordens, C, McGrath, C, Montgomery, K, Lipworth, W, & Kerridge, I. (2008). Informed consent and medical ordeal: A qualitative study. *Internal Medicine Journal, 38*, 624–628.

McGrath, P., & Phillips, E. (2008). Western notions of informed consent and indigenous cultures: Australian findings at the interface. *Bioethical Inquiry, 5*, 21–31.

Mesman, J. (2008). *Uncertainty in medical innovation*. New York: Palgrave Macmillan.

Miracle, D., Szucs, K., Torke, A., & Helft, P. (2011). Contemporary ethical issues in human milk-banking in the United States. *Pediatrics, 128*, 1186–1191.

Mouce, G. (2013). An overview of information giving in fertility clinics. *Human Fertility, 16*(1), 8–12.

Murray, J. (2000). *Intensive care: A doctor's journal*. Berkeley: University of California Press.

Naffine, N, & Richards, B. (2012). Regulating consent to organ and embryo donation. *Bioethical Inquiry, 9*, 49–55.

Neu, J. (2011). Medical progress: Necrotising enterocolitis. *New England Journal of Medicine, 364*, 255–264.

Rid, A., & Dinhofer, L. (2009). Consent. In R. Warwick, D. Fehily, S. Brubaker & T. Eastland (Eds.), *Tissue and cell donation* (pp. 67–97). Oxford: Wiley-Blackwell.

Sullivan, S., Schanler, R., Kim, J., Patel, A., Trawo, R., Kiechl-Kohlendorfer, U. et al. (2010). An exclusively human milk-based diet is associated with a lower rate of necrotizing enterocolitis than a diet of human milk and bovine milk-based products. *Journal of Pediatrics, 156*, 562–567.

Swanson, V., Nicol, H., McInnes, R., Cheyne, H., Mactier, H., & Callander, E. (2012). Developing maternal self-efficacy for feeding preterm babies in the neonatal unit. *Qualitative Health Research, 22*(10), 1369–1382.

World Health Organization UNICEF. (2003). Global strategy for infant and young child feeding. Geneva: Author. Retrieved from http://whqlibdoc.who.int/publications/2003/9241562218.pdf

Note

1 Practice example 14.1 and Figure 14.1 are derived from ethnographic research conducted in an Australian NICU (UTS HREC 2011–117, chief investigator: Dr K. Carroll).

Communicating bad news: bad news for the patient

Jill Thistlethwaite

Learning objectives

This chapter will enable you to:
- define bad news in a healthcare context;
- discuss guidelines for breaking bad news;
- explain the patient-centred approach to difficult consultations;
- consider emotional responses to bad news;
- recognise and acknowledge patients' emotional cues.

Key terms

Bad news
Emotional cues
Empathic statement
Patient-centred care

Overview

Breaking **bad news** is a difficult and complex communication skill. This is partly because reactions to the same news may differ; for example, one woman may be happy to hear she is pregnant, whereas another may be devastated. So it is important that a health professional makes no assumptions about the quality of news without having an understanding of a patient's worldview and psychosocial factors. Of course, it is unlikely that a diagnosis of cancer, a confirmation of a sexually transmitted infection or news that a child has died will be anything other than unwanted. But even in these cases a professional should not make value judgments.

> **bad news**
> 'any news that drastically and negatively alters the patient's view of her or his future' (Buckman, 1984). It is only the patient, client or carer who can make the decision about whether news is welcome or 'bad'.

Despite the difficulties involved with determining and communicating bad news, it should not be considered in isolation from other skills required for patient–professional interactions. The professional needs to build rapport, explore the patient's ideas and concerns, adopt **patient-centred care** and be empathic. These strategies are central, too, to breaking bad news.

While every patient is different, there are certain strategies that should be learnt and adopted to help guide any consultation, including consultations that involve breaking bad news. These strategies include preparation, active listening, recognising and responding to **emotional cues**, and arranging follow-up as appropriate.

> **patient-centred care**
> care processes that are structured to benefit the patient.
>
> **emotional cues**
> cues that are commonly relayed through the body, by means of facial expressions, gestures, and so forth. Emotional cues may signal enjoyment, fear or distress.

This chapter considers the definition of bad news and uses examples of clinicians breaking bad news to the patient in relation to diagnoses of cancer and sexually transmitted infections. It highlights the importance of how information is given and the necessity of checking understanding. Health professionals also need to consider their own responses and emotions in dealing with difficult consultations, and ensure their own self-care.

Introduction

Communicating about bad news is not solely a task involving the giving of clinical information. It is a complex interaction, which may also comprise some or all of the following components:

- responding to a patient's and/or family member's/carer's emotional cues;
- dealing with the stress caused by a patient's expectation of cure;
- dealing with the involvement of family members;
- giving hope when the situation is bleak (Baile et al., 2000).

It is also important to be aware of the impact of breaking bad news on the informant (you as the health professional) as well as the recipient. Stress arising from frequent interactions such as these can cause reluctance in health professionals to deliver bad news in case of negative responses they cannot deal with appropriately (Tesser, Rosen & Tesser, 1971). Support from colleagues and debriefing following these difficult consultations are important.

In the past, doctors in particular were prone to be paternalistic and tried to shield their patients from upsetting diagnoses involving life-threatening conditions. The more acceptable approach today is patient- (or client-) centred (Stewart et al., 1995). Patient-centredness encourages health professionals to be collaborative and open with information sharing, and to involve patients and families in care management planning. Such collaboration, openness and involvement are important not just because patients increasingly expect them. They are important also because there is a legal requirement for patients to be given all relevant and appropriate medical information (see Chapter 22).

However, the legal dimensions of this communication should not cloud the health professional's expressions of sensitivity, empathy and compassion.

How to communicate bad news

A useful format for breaking bad news is the six-step approach known as SPIKES (Setting up, Perception, Invitation, Knowledge, Emotions, Strategy and summary; Baile et al., 2000). This is mainly used in the context of cancer diagnosis, with step 6 ('Strategy and summary') focusing on treatment options that may be outside the scope of the professional breaking the news. Considering complex tasks as a series of steps in this way is helpful, especially for learners. The protocol is evidence-guided; that is, research has evidenced its benefits (Baile et al., 2000). While SPIKES dates back 15 years, it is still widely used and referenced. We therefore refer to SPIKES here rather than other, comparable models that are also mainly focused on cancer diagnosis, communication and management.

SPIKES protocol

Step 1: Setting up the interview
- Arrange privacy and make sure there will be no interruptions.
- Involve significant others as appropriate.
- Sit down.
- Connect with the patient: eye contact, touch.
- Advise the patient of the time you have available.

Step 2: Assessing the patient's Perception
- Use open-ended questions: 'What have you been told about your condition so far?'
- Gather information to explore the patient's perception of the situation.
- Explore ideas, concerns and expectations.
- Correct misinformation as necessary.
- Try to determine whether the patient is in denial.

Step 3: Obtaining the patient's Invitation
- Find out how the patient would like to receive the information (this is a useful step at the time of ordering tests, so both doctor and patient are prepared for the ways the results should be communicated).
- Gauge how much information the patient wants.

Step 4: Giving Knowledge and information to the patient
- Warn the patient that bad news is coming: 'Unfortunately I've got some bad news to tell you.'

- Break information into small chunks.
- Use appropriate language and check for understanding of each chunk of information.

Step 5: Addressing the patient's Emotions with empathic responses
- Look out for the patient's emotional reaction.
- Identify the emotion (such as anger, sadness and disbelief).
- Identify the reason for the emotion, asking the patient about it if necessary.
- Make an **empathic statement** to acknowledge the emotion.

Step 6: Strategy and summary
- Present treatment options.
- Have shared decision-making.
- Reach consensus.
- Plan follow-up.

Depending on the context the health professional may already know the patient and perhaps have arranged the tests that are going to be discussed. However, this is not always the case in team-based care and it is important to check what the patient already knows, has been told and may be expecting. The patient record may not contain enough details about such important topics.

> **empathic statement**
> a statement that focuses on (and seeks to alleviate) the emotional state of another person.

Practice example 15.1

Below is an example of an initial consultation and then a follow-up interaction between a female patient and a male general practitioner (GP) which involves breaking bad news in relation to a diagnosis of breast cancer. This is a fairly common consultation as the risk of developing breast cancer during a woman's lifetime in one in eight (AIHW, 2012).[1]

Shelley Appleton is a 52-year-old woman consulting her GP. After the doctor asks her to sit down she begins by saying: 'I found a lump in my breast last night while showering and I'd like you to check it for me.' After asking about her symptoms (the lump is small and painless and in the lower part of the right breast) and family history (her grandmother died of womb cancer), the doctor examines Shelley's breasts. They then both return to their seats.

Doctor: Yes, you have a lump in the right breast. I can't tell you what it is at the moment. You will need to have a mammogram and possibly an ultrasound to check it out.

Shelley: [Looking anxious] Do you think it is cancer, doctor?

Doctor: At your age that is always a possibility, but I wouldn't worry until you have the tests. There's really no point in worrying. Have you had a mammogram before?

continued ›

Practice example 15.1 continued ›

Shelley: I've been meaning to get one but never got round to it, but I have heard it's painful.

Doctor: Not really. No more than an ordinary X-ray. You should really have had one at 50, you know.

Three days pass.

Doctor: Come in, Shelley. I have your test results. It's not good news.

Shelley: The other doctor at the X-ray centre said I should see you straight away. I guessed it is bad.

Doctor: Yes, I am afraid it very much looks like you have breast cancer. I will need to refer you to a specialist. Is there anyone you would like me to refer you to? Do you know any of the specialists?

Shelley: [Close to tears] It's our 25th wedding anniversary in five weeks. We've booked a holiday in Fiji. Will I still be able to go? What shall I tell Peter? Will I need an operation?

Doctor: I really can't answer any of those questions. You will need to discuss them with the breast specialist.

[Phone rings – doctor answers, says he is busy and asks the caller to ring back later.]

Doctor: Let me write you a referral letter. Dr Spencer is a good surgeon.

He turns to the computer and begins typing.

Analysis and reflection

The main failings of the doctor in the above consultation are a lack of empathy and a failure to respond to Mrs Appleton's cues in relation to her emotional state. The consultation is not wholly bad: the GP asks about Shelley's symptoms and family history to make an assessment of her risk of having cancer. He also examines her to confirm the presence of a lump. Finally, he makes the right management decision in referring her for diagnostic investigations.

The first part of the consultation seen above does not involve breaking bad news but, given Shelley's age and presentation, there is a high probability that she will have cancer. The doctor acknowledges her concern about this possibility, so telling her not to worry is unlikely to be reassuring. An empathic statement would have been more helpful – for example, 'Yes, cancer is a possibility, but I cannot be sure until you have some further tests. It is understandable that the tests and the wait will make you anxious, but it is very good that you have come in as soon as you noticed the lump, and I can get things moving quickly.'

Another issue that arises is whether this doctor indeed knows whether a mammogram is painful or not. His gender makes little difference, as only a proportion of female

GPs will have had the test themselves, depending on their age. Still, he will not have had the experience himself, and therefore should not claim to know whether a mammogram is painful or not. If Shelley does indeed find the mammogram uncomfortable, she may be less likely to trust this doctor in the future.

Next the doctor implies that Shelley has been remiss in not having had a screening mammogram at the recommended age of 50 years. This may make Shelley feel guilty, and it may lead her to blame herself in relation to the subsequent positive cancer diagnosis.

The second follow-up consultation focuses on breaking bad news. If we consider the doctor's performance in relation to the SPIKES protocol, we find there is a lot of room for improvement! Let us analyse the consultation bit by bit.

Step 1: The GP has seen the test results before he calls Shelley in but he had not advised the receptionist that he should not be interrupted during the consultation.

Step 2: It would have been better to ask Shelley if they had said anything to her after the tests. She has surmised 'it is bad'. The doctor could ask her what she is most concerned about rather than rushing into the news and then straight onto the management plan.

Step 3: Obtaining the patient's invitation is not so relevant in this case.

Step 4: Preparing Shelley for the diagnosis would have been helpful: 'Yes, I am afraid it is bad news.' Some doctors may use touch here to show empathy, perhaps holding the patient's hand. Eye contact should be maintained unless the client is obviously uncomfortable with this. The diagnosis is then given and allowed to sink in. How may the doctor then check that Shelley has absorbed this information? He could ask: 'Is there anything you don't understand at this point?' The doctor may have more information about the lump than just the diagnosis. He therefore needs to gauge about much information to give. Thus, he could have asked, 'Would you like me to go through the test results with you?'

Step 5: People react in different ways to bad news. The skilful health professional is able to use verbal and non-verbal cues to monitor emotions, and respond to them appropriately. This could involve offering a tissue if the patient begins to cry, acknowledging their anger, answering questions such as 'Why me?', 'Are you sure?' with empathetic responses and certainly not dismissing them.

Step 6: Even though the doctor is a GP and not a cancer specialist, he could have explored Shelley's ideas about the next steps, rather than immediately proposing that he should pass her on to another professional.

Theoretical links

Breaking bad news should be informed and guided by the theoretical underpinnings of good communication. How well bad news is communicated influences patients' psychological adjustment, their healing, and their subsequent ability to collaborate in making decisions about their treatment (Roberts et al., 1994). The literature distinguishes between:

1. patient-centred communication, where the patient's well-being, interests, preferences and understanding are skilfully interwoven with the relevant clinical and scientific facts;
2. disease-centred communication, where health professionals limit the amount of information based on their own value judgments rather than exploring patients' preferences, understandings and requirements;
3. emotion-centred communication, where patients' emotions are acknowledged and responded to while clinical and scientific information sharing is ignored (Schmid et al., 2005).

The patient-centred approach to communicating with patients appears to have the most positive outcome for patients at a cognitive, evaluative and emotional level, in comparison to disease-centred and emotion-centred communication (Schmid et al., 2005). Empathic health professionals help patients develop a greater capacity to cope with their condition and with clinical and scientific facts (Zachariae et al., 2003). Thus, cancer patients prefer receiving their diagnosis in an empathic way. Patients prefer retaining a degree of control; that is, they like to be reassured that their own behaviour plays a role in their own care and healing (Martins & Carvelho, 2013).

Further research is required to strengthen the evidence base for how bad news is conveyed in relation to patient outcomes. Much of the current research focuses on the provider and communication skills training, rather than on how to ensure communication promotes the patient's bio-psycho-social well-being (Paul et al., 2009). More research emphasis needs to be placed on clarifying the dynamics and effects of empathic communication. As one patient has written:

> There are words that hurt and there are words that heal. A lot of it has to do with the way your doctor relates to you as a human being. I want to see my doctor as a human being. (Dias, Chabner & Lynch, 2005)

Implications for practice

Standard communication skills include greeting the patient (and relative, if present) by name, inviting them to sit and maintaining appropriate eye contact. Breaking information into chunks and checking the patient's understanding regularly are important. Patients appreciate simple clear information (Barnett, 2002), delivered honestly (Girgis, Sanson-Fisher & Schofield, 1999). They retain information more successfully if it is tailored to their needs, rather than being given in a formulaic way (Roberts et al., 1994). A good start is a statement that signposts what is coming – for example, 'I'm afraid that the news isn't as good as we hoped' (Silverman, Kurtz & Draper, 1998).

It is difficult to assess the amount of information a patient wants. Evidence suggests that people want basic information about diagnosis, treatment options and common side effects of that treatment. But they may not want or take in all of this just after the initial bad news (Leydon et al., 2000). Health professionals tend to underestimate how much information patients would like, and they often ignore that a majority of patients want the truth (Fallowfied & Jenkins, 2004). Checking the patient's understanding frequently is important, as is not making assumptions based on age or other attributes. A patient's satisfaction correlates with their receiving the amount of information that matches their needs at a particular time (Schofield et al., 2003).

Patients may show a range of responses to the bad news, such as anger, denial, grief, distress and anxiety. Such feelings may not be openly expressed however, and the practitioner may need to ask how the patient is feeling in order to respond to the emotion. Techniques for recognising emotional cues include active listening, the use of open questions, and exploring concerns (Ryan et al., 2005).

Reflective questions

1. Have you ever been the recipient of bad news? This may not have been a health-related issue, but perhaps you were told you had failed an examination or your driving test, that you hadn't been successful in a job interview or you weren't picked to play on a team for an important sporting event. How did this make you feel? What can you remember about the way you were given the news? What constructive feedback might you have given the person delivering the news in order to reduce your feelings of, for example, anger, sadness, denial, lack of self-confidence or hopelessness?
2. Have you yourself ever had to break bad news? How did you prepare for this? Having read the previous sections of this chapter, how might you do this differently in the future?
3. Recognising and acknowledging a person's emotional cues is important. How do you feel about holding the recipient's hand? What are the potential advantages and disadvantages of using touch in this way? Particularly consider cross-cultural interactions.

Conclusion

Difficult consultations have an impact on both patients and health professionals. The feeling that a potentially difficult consultation has gone well helps reduce a practitioner's discomfort and obviously is of benefit to the patient. It is unlikely that you as a student will have to break bad news in relation to diagnoses and prognoses, but you may be in a situation of giving and explaining test results. You should also have the opportunity to conduct a simulated consultation and receive feedback on your performance.

Understanding, recognising and acknowledging patients' emotions and responses to bad news are important skills to learn and practise. The interaction may involve both verbal and non-verbal techniques, depending on the context. Patients may need to be invited to discuss their feelings: some people are reluctant to disclose these because they think the health professional is too busy to deal with them (Maguire, 1985).

Practice example 15.2

Read the following example, adapted from a real-life consultation, and reflect on Julie's story using the questions below.

Julie, a 22-year-old student, feels something is not quite right 'down below'. She explains to the nurse practitioner at the sexual health clinic that she just feels sore around her vaginal opening. The nurse asks her questions about her periods, use of contraception and sexual history. Julie has been with her current boyfriend for nine months. Both were tested for sexually transmitted infections eight months ago and the results were negative. As Julie is on the contraceptive pill they have not been using condoms since then. Julie has had no other sexual partners in this time and says she is sure her boyfriend would not have either. The nurse then examines Julie and finds a small break in the skin of her perineum. She takes swabs for chlamydia, gonorrhoea and herpes. She advises Julie that the clinic will ring her if any of the tests are positive. Three days later Julie has a voice mail message asking her to make an appointment for follow-up. She is very anxious, as she cannot get an appointment until the following week. The doctor she consults tells her that one of the tests shows she has herpes. Julie bursts into tears.

Reflective questions

1. What sort of information could Julie have been given at the initial consultation in order to better prepare her for the possible bad news?
2. What do you think about the manner in which Julie was contacted about the results? What are the options for patients who have investigations that may require follow-up? What are the advantages and disadvantages for both patients and practitioners in making an appointment for results?
3. Think how you would give Julie the news about the diagnosis. What would you do next?
4. Julie is now in the position herself of having to break bad news to her boyfriend, who is a sexual contact. How should Julie prepare to do this? What advice should she be given?
5. If you were Julie, how would you have liked this whole scenario to have been conducted? Do you think that people would vary in their responses to this question and, if so, why?

Reflective questions

1. Think of other examples of bad news. What are the similarities and differences in how you would communicate in each example? Is the SPIKES protocol useful in other situations such as informing about a positive diagnosis of HIV, an abnormal antenatal scan or the probability that a family member has dementia, for example?
2. Reflective practice is important for our professional development. How would you judge if a difficult consultation has gone well or badly?
3. If you yourself feel distressed after a difficult consultation, how will you debrief and deal with your own emotions?

Further reading

Buckman, R. (1992). *How to break bad news: A guide for health professionals*. Baltimore: John Hopkins Press.
This book is the seminal textbook on bad news communication.

National Breast and Ovarian Cancer Centre. (2007). *Breaking bad news: Evidence from the literature and recommended steps*. Surry Hills: National Breast and Ovarian Cancer Centre: http://canceraustralia.gov.au/sites/default/files/publications/nbocc-bbn-lit-review-and-next-steps.pdf[2]

References

AIHW (2012). *Cancer in Australia: An overview*. Cancer series no. 74. Cat. no.: CAN 70. Canberra: Author.

Baile, W. F., Buckman, R., Lenzi, R., Glober, G., Beale, E. A., & Kudelka, A. P. (2000). SPIKES – A six-step protocol for delivering bad news: Application to the patient with cancer. *The Oncologist, 5*, 302–311.

Barnett, M. M. (2002). Effect of breaking bad news on patients' perceptions of doctors. *Journal of the Royal Society of Medicine, 95*, 343–347.

Buckman, R. (1984). Breaking bad news: Why is it still so difficult? *British Medical Journal, 288*, 1597–99.

Dias, L., Chabner, B. N., & Lynch Jr, T. J. (2005). Breaking bad news: A patient's perspective. *The Oncologist, 8*, 587–596.

Fallowfield, L., & Jenkins, V. (2004). Communicating sad, bad and difficult news in medicine. *The Lancet, 363*, 312–319.

Girgis, A., Sanson-Fisher, R. W., & Schofield, M. J. (1999). Is there consensus between breast cancer patients and providers on guidelines for breaking bad news? *Journal of Behavioral Medicine, 25*, 69–77.

Leydon, G. M., Boulton, M., Moynihan, C., Jones, A., Mossman, J., Boudioni, M., & McPherson, K. (2000). Cancer patients' information needs and information seeking behaviour: In depth interview study. *British Medical Journal, 320,* 909–913.

Maguire, P. (1985). Improving the detection of psychiatric problems in cancer patients. *Social Science and Medicine, 20,* 819–823.

Martins, R. G., & Carvalho, I. P. (2013). Breaking bad news: Patients' preferences and health locus of control. *Patient Education and Counseling, 92,* 67–73.

Paul, C. L., Clinton-McHarg, T., Sanson-Fishter, R. W., & Webb, D. G. (2009). Are we there yet? The state of the evidence base for guidelines on breaking bad news to cancer patients. *European Journal of Cancer, 45,* 2960–2966.

Roberts, C. S., Cox, C. E., Reintgen, D., Baile, W. F., & Gilbertini, M. (1994). Influence of physician communication on newly diagnosed patients' psychologic adjustment and decision making. *Cancer, 74,* 336–341.

Ryan, H., Schofield, P., Cockburn, J., Butow, P., Tattersall, M., Turner, J., & Girgis, A. (2005). How to recognise and manage psychological stress in cancer patients. *European Journal of Cancer Care, 14,* 7–15.

Schmid, Mast M., Kindlimann, A., & Langewitz, W. (2005). Recipients' perspective on breaking bad news: How you put it makes a difference. *Patient Education and Counseling, 58,* 244–251.

Schofield, P. E., Butow, P. N., Thompsons, J. F., Tattersall, M., Beeney, L. J, & Dunn, S. M. (2003). Psychological responses of patients receiving a diagnosis of cancer. *Annals of Oncology, 14,* 48–56.

Silverman, J., Kurtz, S., & Draper, J. (1998). *Skills for communicating with patients* (pp. 83–84). Abingdon: Radcliffe Medical Press,.

Stewart, M., Brown, J. B., Weston, W. W., McWhinney, I. R., McWilliam, C. L., & Freeman, T. R. (1995). *Patient-centered medicine. Transforming the clinical method.* Thousand Oaks, CA: Sage.

Tesser, A., Rosen, S., & Tesser, M. (1971). On the reluctance to communicate undesirable messages (the MUM effect): A field study. *Psychological Reports, 29,* 651–654.

Zachariae, R., Pedersen, C. G., Jensen, A. B., Ehmrooth, E., Rossen, P. B, & von der Maase, H. (2003). Association of perceived physician communication style with patient satisfaction, distress, cancer-related self efficacy and perceived control over the disease. *British Journal of Cancer, 88,* 658–665.

Notes

1 This extract has been reproduced with permission from Cancer Australia. In 2011, Cancer Australia amalgamated with National Breast and Ovarian Cancer Centre to form a single national agency to provide leadership in cancer control and improve outcomes for Australians affected by cancer.

2 In 2011, Cancer Australia amalgamated with National Breast and Ovarian Cancer Centre to form a single national agency to provide leadership in cancer control and improve outcomes for Australians affected by cancer.

Communicating in an e-health environment

Vicki Parker, Douglas Bellamy and Deidre Besuijen

Learning objectives

This chapter will enable you to:

- become familiar with key terms associated with e-health;
- identify ways in which electronic and internet-based strategies are contributing to and changing the way health professionals communicate;
- learn how electronic information is gathered, stored and shared;
- analyse how e-health is contributing to better health outcomes for Australians and how it can contribute into the future;
- understand the benefits and barriers to adoption of e-health across a range of clinical and geographic contexts and with particular population groups;
- review and discuss examples of e-health strategies and their implications for staff and patients;
- reflect on how you will use e-health in your practice.

Key terms

E-health
Person Controlled Electronic Health Record (PCEHR)
Telecare
Telehealth

Overview

This chapter explores the development and application of **e-health** strategies and the way in which they contribute to effective health communication and improved health

e-health
information and communication technologies such as electronic health records, telemedicine and telecare, tele- and videoconferencing health and medical websites, and applications that enable tracking, measuring and recording of biophysiological parameters (World Health Organization, 2006).

outcomes. E-health aims to improve the safety and quality of health care by increasing access to services through tele-health and electronic consultations, enabling the collection and sharing of better quality information and resources, and empowering people to better manage their own health. It is envisioned that such strategies will also increase efficiency; reducing fragmentation and delay and reducing healthcare costs (Hillestad et al., 2005).

It is the responsibility of health professionals to become competent e-health practitioners. This means they need to develop familiarity with the e-health systems that support their practice and communicate effectively within them. Health professionals must know how to contribute to electronic clinical information and resources; use electronic information to inform clinical decisions; access information and professional development e-learning programs; and support the participation of consumers.

This chapter focuses on:

- how e-health strategies are incorporated into ways of communicating and working;
- the impact of e-health on consumers and their experiences of health care.

Introduction

The advancement of electronic technology has been significant over the last three decades. This has led to many opportunities and developments in e-health, including those that are designed to increase system efficiency and communication among health professionals as well as those that are more specifically consumer-oriented. The introduction of electronic repositories for the storage and sharing of health-related information about patients and the care they receive from health professionals has enabled a shift to a more streamlined approach where information accompanies patients as they move through the healthcare system. Consumer-oriented e-health connects patients with health information and services either as stand-alone services or integrated as an adjunct to existing resources (Norman, 2011).

Electronic information spaces, or portals as they are often called, make information available to health professions across disciplines, locations and sometimes organisations, enabling sharing of information and collaboration without the delays experienced previously. However, the usefulness of these systems depends on the interconnectivity of the various applications, the capacity of organisations to host the systems, and the capacity and tendency for staff to use them effectively (Goodwin, 2010).

The way in which clinicians engage with electronic systems depends on their role and the systems available to them within the organisation in which they work. Systems differ across contexts; some are relevant to all staff in an organisation and some are designed to meet the communication and information needs of particular services or sectors – for example, cancer services or community-based care.

Treating clinicians enter an electronic record of the results of their interaction with patients. Information entered by clinicians may include presenting signs and symptoms, medical and social history, clinical assessment findings, results of specific tests, treatments prescribed and any responses noted– for example, the effect of pain medication. Appointments and discharge summaries are also lodged by clinicians, care co-ordinators and discharge planners. Accurate, accessible, up-to-date information that is available to all treating clinicians helps to reduce duplication, overprescribing, and adverse events, thus ensuring patient safety (Hillestad et al., 2005).

The Person Controlled Electronic Health Record

Recent changes to the Australian healthcare system allow individuals to have an electronic health record that can be shared between healthcare providers. The idea is to reduce fragmentation and streamline care across primary and secondary sectors (van Dooren, Lennox & Stewart, 2013). The **Person Controlled Electronic Health Record (PCEHR)** gives individuals the opportunity to share their health information and to make clear their wishes about care they might receive in the future. The record alerts health providers to any allergies or significant health issues, and streamlines treatment by allowing new providers access to prescriptions and diagnostic test results. The PCEHR makes things simpler for patients and families by ensuring that the health professionals they consult have the information they need. While PCEHRs represent a valuable resource for continuity of care and patient safety, they are not compulsory; only those who register and provide permissions have records available.

> **Person Controlled Electronic Health Record (PCEHR)**
> a secure electronic record of a person's medical history electronically stored and shared through a network of connected systems. Consumers will have control over what information is accessible, and by whom, through consent and access permissions.

Telehealth

Telehealth enables wider distribution of health services through the utilisation of video-conferencing facilities and internet-based services across sites. Telehealth is particularly beneficial to those who live and work in rural communities. The benefits of telehealth can be divided into four areas: benefits to patients, benefits to health professionals, benefits to participating hospitals, and benefits to society (Moffatt & Eley, 2010). Patient benefits reported in the literature include increased access to services, reduced travel-related costs, reduced waiting time, constant connection with supportive

> **telehealth**
> the use of information and communication technology to provide healthcare services to people who are at a distance from the healthcare centre or the provider, and the administration and training that supports this service.

local networks, improved continuity of care and better quality services. Consumer-directed telehealth focuses on the consumer experience of the tools themselves and their influence on health knowledge, attitudes, behaviours and skills. Thus, telehealth bridges the gap between documenting information using traditional medical informatics and engaging the public in health care (Norman, 2011).

Telehealth is used to transmit voices, images, and information, reducing the need for people to travel to attend meetings and appointments:

> It encompasses diagnosis, treatment, preventive (educational) and curative aspects of healthcare services and typically involves care recipient(s), care providers or educators in the provision of these services directed to the care recipient. Video-conferencing is one of the main ways in which telehealth is improving access to healthcare services for patients who live in regional, rural and remote areas. (Australian Government Department of Health, 2012)

eHealth Benefits Framework

By increasing information transparency and sharing, the PCEHR system, eMedication Management, Secure Messaging Delivery and other eHealth initiatives will drive improvements in coordination of care, enhance patient satisfaction and ultimately save lives.

Research conducted both within Australia and internationally suggests the eHealth record system, eMedication Management and Secure Message Delivery can help reduce healthcare costs through increased quality, safety and access.

1. **QUALITY – supporting uninterrupted coordinated care across different healthcare providers at the right place and the right time**
   - Consolidation and reconciliation of patient information;
   - Improved continuity of care (healthcare information is consistent and easily shared between all relevant providers);
   - Increased levels of preventative care (such as immunisation).
2. **SAFETY – avoids or minimises situations which can harm or have the potential to harm patients during the course of care delivery**
   - Improvements in medication safety, leading to potential reductions in adverse drug events (ADEs);
   - Increased follow-up after an event (such as an abnormal test or hospitalisation).
3. **ACCESS – the ability of patients to obtain health care at the right place and right time irrespective of socioeconomic status, physical location and/or cultural background**
   - Control over who may view the consumer's information;
   - Geographic flexibility and mobility.

These three core benefits have the ability to translate into both healthcare system efficiencies and population health benefits.

1. **EFFICIENCY – achieving the desired results with the most cost-efficient use of resources**
    *   Timeliness of information;
    *   Reduction in duplicate testing.
2. **POPULATION – building a strong and resilient society through meeting the population's expectations regarding their health system**
    *   Increased consumer satisfaction with their healthcare delivery;
    *   Economic flow on effects through eHealth investments and a healthier population.

Source: http://www.nehta.gov.au/for-providers/about-ehealth-guidance/ehealth-benefits/ehealth-benefits-framework, retrieved December 26, 2014

Health professionals benefit from telehealth through access to videoconferenced education and participation in videoconferenced consultations and multidisciplinary meetings. Videoconferencing provides excellent learning opportunities for less experienced staff and for rural clinicians as they can discuss with other more experienced clinicians in spite of geographic distance. Telehealth saves hospitals money through reduced patient transfer costs (patient can be treated in their home town) and reduced travelling time for staff (staff do not need to travel to see patients). Figure 16.1 summarises electronic health information networks.

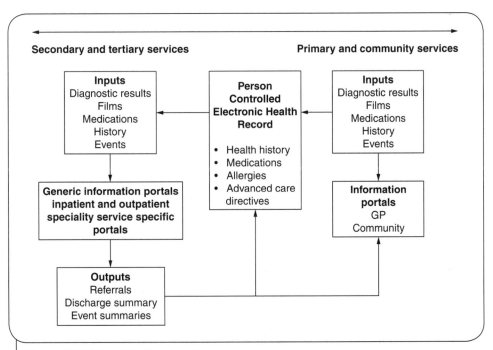

Figure 16.1 Electronic health information networks

In sum, the quality of the services provided is enhanced through the addition of telehealth clinics and multidisciplinary team consultations and videoconferencing. Interprofessional working is enhanced when telehealth is integrated into routine care. Communities benefit when access to services is increased and when there is greater opportunity for health promotion and education through electronic and internet-based information and events (Moffatt & Eley, 2010).

Practice example 16.1

Excerpt from a conversation with a cancer care coordinator (CCC) from a Local Health District (LHD).

Vicki: Mary, in your role as CCC, how do you communicate within an e-health environment?

Mary: The use of e-health technology has become embedded in the work we do as health professionals and my role as gynaecology CCC is no exception. Let me give an example. Recently I have been involved in the coordination of care for a 69-year-old woman with cervix cancer from a remote area within the LHD. To use this as an example I will describe the e-health technology and processes which were utilised to coordinate her care.

Following our unit receiving her faxed referral from a general gynaecologist in [regional centre], this information was immediately transferred to her digital medical record. As she was within our LHD she was already allocated a Medical Records Number (MRN). After talking with medical staff, the patient and rural CCC a videoconference appointment with one of our gynaecological oncologists was arranged. To confirm her diagnosis I faxed a request to the pathology company who reported on her biopsy to have her histopathology slides sent to our specialist pathologist for review. Review of this pathology was then added to our next multidisciplinary team (MDT) meeting which occurred just prior to our meeting her in clinic via videoconferencing (VC). The transfer of her scans, which were performed in [regional centre], was also arranged by entering this request into an online request system between hospitals. This allows them to be available for review at the MDT meeting or during her consultation. VC technology utilised in our MDT meeting enables treating staff in rural hospitals to link in, view pathology and imaging and be involved in the discussion regarding the patient's treatment plan.

Prior to her appointment we request that she completes a distress thermometer screening tool, which is faxed to the unit to assist us in supporting her needs at this time. At the consultation we arrange consent again via fax and admission for her to have a surgical staging procedure and further imaging – MRI and PET scans as an outpatient. As she has no family in [metropolitan centre], accommodation is arranged via email/phone for her during her stay. After this she is able to go home and when results of surgery and imaging

continued ›

Practice example 16.1 continued ›

are available her case is rediscussed at our next MDT meeting when the treatment plan for combined chemotherapy and radiation followed by brachytherapy is confirmed. I then contact her by phone and confirm this treatment and the appropriate referrals are arranged. I will send her written and online resources and information. She will need to travel to [regional centre] for the majority of her treatment, so a referral is done to the CCC in [regional centre] to continue support during treatment. As she will need to come to [metropolitan centre] for brachytherapy, I arrange a subsequent VC appointment with one of the radiation oncologists here to arrange. Again referral is arranged via email to assist with accommodation.

Documentation from her consultations, surgery and MDT review is available on her electronic medical record and within the CAP (clinical application portal). This, however, is only accessible by staff within our LHD. Some of the information especially regarding correspondence between oncology staff and units is entered into another system called ARIA.[1]

The electronic access of scans and imaging is in the general hospital or service-based but transfer of images can generally be arranged, though sometimes this is only possible by accessing a CD from the patient/service and having it downloaded. The inclusion of the general practitioner in all correspondence from consultations, hospital admissions and referrals is expected; however, the time delay for this to occur is variable.

. . . .

Analysis and reflection

From Mary's explanation in practice example 16.1 you can see how the various phases (events and interactions) of a patient's journey are chronicled within the electronic medical record (EMR) system and how inputs from each member of the multidisciplinary team can be made available to others. The result is that health professionals have the information they need to make decisions and to share with patients at critical times. The existence of the EMR does little on its own. Information within the portals needs to be managed and communicated in a systematic way. It is the way in which the information is retrieved and redirected at specific times and for a specific purpose that makes it an integral component of an integrated process of managing information and supporting patient care. A third essential component is the capacity to link professionals through videoconferencing or other telecommunication systems. These systems need to be reliable and ensure transmission of good quality sound and vision.

Mary's example is a good illustration of how complex cancer care involving many services across disciplines, sectors and distance is made possible through e-health innovations. These innovations have revised the nature of patient experiences, increasing their opportunity and capacity to participate in decisions about their care through improved communication and readily available information. E-health innovations have reduced disruption to patients and families, reduced the need to travel and live away from home in order to receive care, and improved the quality of health care by maintaining contact between healthcare visits.

It is also clear from the excerpt that there is more work to be done to alleviate duplication and connect systems more effectively. While e-health can reduce the impact of non-availability of services in rural areas, the sheer cost and cumbersome nature of some treatments (particularly in cancer care) means that comprehensive care will never be entirely available outside metropolitan centres. Hence, e-health remains of significant importance in ensuring the continuity of care as patients move from metropolitan- to rural-based services.

Implications for practice

The potential for e-health to improve health service delivery and health outcomes for patients is enormous, with many existing and emerging technologies changing the way health professionals communicate with each other, and the way in which consumers engage with health care and health information.

Face-to-face communication between patients and health professionals is an important aspect of any therapeutic relationship. It is important to consider how telehealth influences that relationship and the way in which non-face-to-face consultation is conducted and perceived by patients and their families. There is the potential to lose some of the connection that is achievable through eye contact and other non-verbal communication.

In a recent article, Sabesan, Simcox and Marr (2012) suggest a number of practical strategies for ensuring the effectiveness of telehealth consultations. These include:
- encouraging the presence of families, particularly where sensitive matters are being discussed;
- ensuring that the equipment is functional and that users are familiar with its operation;
- introducing and greeting all participating in the consultation;
- explaining that the level of service will be the same;
- positioning cameras and people to ensure eye contact;
- starting with a conversation about family, home and social matters;
- using visual aids;
- summarising the consultation and checking that the patient has understood the information at the end of the consultation.

An example of a community based e-health strategy is HealthPathways. It is a resource for anyone navigating the healthcare system in the Hunter New England region. It provides information about clinical specialists, diagnostic services, and so forth. HealthPathways is the first online health information portal of its kind in Australia.

Patientinfo (http://www.patientinfo.org.au) complements HealthPathways by providing helpful information recommended by local health professionals for patients with diagnosed conditions. The site reproduces patient information already in HealthPathways in a separate publicly available website that general practices and health professionals can recommend to patients. A collaboration between Hunter New England Health, Hunter Medicare Local, Little Company of Mary Health Care, and Kaleidoscope, the site is reviewed by health professionals and content approved by HealthPathways clinical editors.

Patientinfo provides:

- trusted and consistent information in easy to search categories, so patients can help manage their own health and reduce risk factors;
- culturally appropriate material for Aboriginal and Torres Strait Islander people, and people from culturally and linguistically diverse communities;
- opportunities for users to provide feedback.

Another emerging e-health trend is the use of electronic sensors and monitoring of environments, as well as wearable technologies. Applications include pervasive health monitoring, intelligent emergency management system and mobile telemedicine. These technologies have been used in the management of chronic disease and home-based care contexts, enabling people to remain and live safely in their own homes.

Theoretical links

E-health offers the opportunity for consumers to be empowered to actively manage their own health and to make evidenced-based choices. Health professionals are no longer the only source of health information, with consumers often already being well informed. However, there are concerns that some internet-based information is not of good quality and that some systems may not protect the confidentiality of consumers. Further, some consumers may not feel comfortable or able to engage with the technology (Wicks, Stamford, Grootenhuis, Haverman & Ahmed, 2014).

Studies that have examined satisfaction with telehealth have indicated overall satisfaction among users, but non-users may be resistant to change as they are concerned about a potential threat to the quality of communication and the quality of care (Brewster, Mountain, Wessels, Kelly & Hawley, 2014). This finding indicates that there is work to do on understanding such resistance and overcoming barriers in order to implement successful telehealth initiatives.

In a study conducted to examine the impact of telehealth and **telecare** on clients of a transition care program, Cartwright, Wade and Shaw (2011) reported significant benefits

telecare
technology that allows enables patients to stay safe and independent in their own homes, including communication and monitoring devices and systems.

to clients receiving post-acute care. These included improved personal well-being such as perceptions of health, safety and security. Older people who participated in the study were willing and able to use the technology reliably. Carers also reported that they felt that care was safer and that monitoring of the older person's health was improved. Other benefits included decreased use of personal care assistants. This study debunks the myth that older people are not comfortable using the available technology.

The uptake of telehealth has been slow in some areas, particularly those where the need for physical examination together with face-to-face consultation is considered essential. However, the 2010 introduction of the Medicare rebate for telehealth by the Australian government has created greater opportunity and acceptance of telehealth-enhanced models of care.

Conclusion

E-health strategies are wide ranging and are increasingly being integrated into the everyday business of health service delivery and health promotion. They are improving information availability and transfer, and changing relationships between consumers and health providers, and between health professionals. Telehealth is contributing to improved access to specialist services for people in rural communities, and significantly affecting the professional development opportunities available to rural clinicians. Although the greatest impact may be in rural areas, benefits accrue across all healthcare sectors, geographic and population jurisdictions.

The success of e-health applications is contingent on ensuring their suitability to context and populations, providing resources and education to support competency, reliability and uptake. E-health resources and communication strategies need to be incorporated into everyday ways of working for health professionals and presented in a way that respects, engages and empowers consumers.

Practice example 16.2 _ Malcolm's story

Malcolm, who is 87 years old, has been living in residential aged care for three years. His daughter Diane, who lives nearby, visits him often, but cannot manage to care for him in her own home. Malcolm has diabetes and mild dementia. Three months ago Malcolm fell over a fellow resident's walking frame and broke his arm. He also sustained wounds to his leg and forehead. Malcolm was taken by ambulance to the local hospital emergency

continued ›

Practice example 16.2 continued ›

department where his arm was X-rayed and a back slab applied to his fractured forearm. Since then he has returned to the hospital for follow-up care. The visits to the hospital, where he often has to wait several hours, increase his confusion and distress. He often doesn't know why he is there. As his dementia has worsened, so too has his diabetes. Due to his diabetes his wounds are not healing well; the one on his leg in particular is taking a long time to heal.

Diane doesn't understand why Malcolm's wound is not healing and is worried that he is not getting good care. She is particularly annoyed that he has to wait hours in the hospital corridor for his outpatient appointment. On these days he does not eat his regular meals and is hypoglycaemic (has a low blood sugar level) when he returns to the residential aged care facility. When Malcolm had realised some time ago that he was becoming forgetful, he made Diane promise that she would not allow anyone to perform 'heroics' if he were to become seriously ill (that is, Malcolm did not want doctors to operate on him to save him). Diane is concerned that she will not be able to fulfil his wishes and feels she has little control over what will happen to her father as his health deteriorates.

Reflective questions

1. What e-health strategies could be put in place to alleviate some of the problems experienced by Malcolm and Diane? Identify three problems and associated e-health solutions.
2. Identify how each of the strategies would benefit Malcolm and Diane, the health professionals involved in their care, and the two organisations (the hospital and the residential aged care facility).
3. How will these strategies influence Malcolm's and other residents' safety?
4. What are the logistical concerns associated with e-health/telehealth strategies in this context?
5. How does Medicare support such strategies? Who needs to be involved?
6. What other benefits can you see from the introduction of e-health for residential aged care residents?

Reflective activities

1. Register for your e-health record.
   a. Register here: http://www.ehealth.gov.au/internet/ehealth/publishing.nsf/content/home
   b. How easy it to register and use the site?
   c. What will you tell patients or potential users about the site?

2. Check out HealthPathways at http://hne.healthpathways.org.au.
Username: Medical
Password: Student
3. Review the following websites:
   a. http://www.medicareaustralia.gov.au/provider/incentives/telehealth
   b. http://www.aci.health.nsw.gov.au/resources/telehealth/telehealth-resource-package/telehealth
   c. http://www.nswrdn.com.au/site/index.cfm?display=289612
   d. http://www.canrefer.org.au
   e. http://www.nhsd.com.au

Further reading

Mair, F. S., May, C., O'Donnell, C., Finch, T., Sullivan, F., & Murray, E. (2012). Factors that promote or inhibit the implementation of e-health systems: An explanatory systematic review. *Bulletin of the World Health Organization, 90*(5), 357–364.
This paper describes the results a systematic review of factors that promote or inhibit the implementation of e-health systems.

Moffatt, J. J., & Eley, D. S. (2010). The reported benefits of telehealth for rural Australians. *Australian Health Review, 34*(3), 276–281.
These authors conducted a narrative review of existing literature to identify the reported benefits of e-health for rural Australians. The findings indicate that telehealth potentially reduces inequality and improves the health status of rural Australians, and also helps to overcome some of the problems associated with recruitment and retention of a rural workforce.

Rocchi, M., Pipa, D., & Lopatka, H. (2013). Preparing students for an e-health world: ICT competencies for entry-to-practice. *Canadian Pharmacists Journal/Revue des Pharmaciens du Canada, 146*(5), S1–S50. doi:10.1177/1715163513509067
This article describes an ICT competency framework that was developed following a literature search and review of existing validated, relevant, competency frameworks. Key pharmacy stakeholder groups were invited to validate the framework through an online survey.

Wicks, P., Stamford, J., Grootenhuis, M. A., Haverman, L., & Ahmed, S. (2014). Innovations in e-health. *Quality of Life Research, 23*(1), 195–203.
This is an overview of a number of e-health trends and initiatives presented at the ISOQOL Conference in Budapest, 2014. They illustrate how e-health can improve quality of life and quality of care across a range of chronic diseases, populations and contexts.

References

Australian Government Department of Health. (2012). *Telehealth*. Retrieved November 28, 2014 from http://www.health.gov.au/internet/main/publishing.nsf/Content/e-health-telehealth

Brewster, L., Mountain, G., Wessels, B., Kelly, C., & Hawley, M. (2014). Factors affecting front line staff acceptance of telehealth technologies: A mixed-method systematic review. *Journal of Advanced Nursing, 70*(1), 21–33.

Cartwright, C., Wade, R., & Shaw, K. (2011). *The impact of telehealth and telecare on clients of the transition care program (TCP)*. Southern Cross University Aged Services Learning & Research Collaboration. Retrieved from http://scu.edu.au/health-sciences/index.php/181

Goodwin, N. (2010). The state of telehealth and telecare in the UK: Prospects for integrated care. *Journal of Integrated Care, 18,*(6), 3–10.

Hillestad, R., Bigalow, J., Bower, A., Girosi, F., Meili, R., Scolville, R., & Taylor, R.(2005). Can electronic medical record systems transform health care? Potential health benefits, savings and costs. *Health Affairs, 24*(5), 1103–1117.

Moffatt, J. J., & Eley, D. S. (2010). The reported benefits of telehealth for rural Australians. *Australian Health Review, 34*(3), 276–281.

Norman, C. D. (2011). Consumer-directed telehealth. *Otolaryngologic Clinics of North America, 44*(6), 1289–1296.

Sabesan, S., Simcox, K., & Marr, I. (2012). Medical oncology clinics through videoconferencing: An acceptable telehealth model for rural patients and health workers. *Internal Medicine Journal, 42*(7), 780–785.

van Dooren, K., Lennox, N., & Stewart, M. (2013). Improving access to electronic health records for people with intellectual disability: A qualitative study. *Australian Journal of Primary Health, 19*(4), 336–342. doi:http://dx.doi.org/10.1071/PY13042

Wicks, P., Stamford, J., Grootenhuis, M. A., Haverman, L., & Ahmed, S. (2014). Innovations in e-health. *Quality of Life Research, 23*(1), 195–203.

World Health Organization. (2006). *Building foundations for e-health: Progress of member states*. Report of the WHO global observatory for e-health. Geneva: Author.

Note

1 ARIA is an oncology-specific electronic medical record. It is a complete medical record and can record all aspects of patient care, from diagnosis and staging through to treatment plans, medication prescribing, advanced directives and other aspects of a patient's cancer treatment.

17

Communicating for quality and safety in Aboriginal health care

George Hayden and Caris Jalla

Learning objectives

This chapter will enable to you to:
- understand holistic approaches to health and well-being, as being linked to not just physical, but also social, emotion and cultural well-being;
- describe the importance of Aboriginal and Torres Strait history and its impact on Aboriginal patient quality and safety;
- understand the diversity of Aboriginal and Torres Strait Islander groups;
- define cultural safety;
- define 'white privilege' and consider systematic racism;
- consider the differences in communication styles (for example, indirect and direct) and healthcare approaches (preventative and curative);
- reflect on your personal beliefs and values about Aboriginal and Torres Strait Islander people.

Key terms

Aboriginal worldviews
Communication
Cultural safety
Culture

Overview

This chapter provides a holistic approach to communicating for quality and safety in Aboriginal health care. It uses fictional case studies inspired by the authors' personal experiences and observations. The first practice example shares a story in the context of working across Aboriginal and non-Aboriginal groups. The second practice example emphasises how challenging health care can be for people in remote Aboriginal communities. Please note that the term 'Aboriginal' will be used here, but in doing so we acknowledge Torres Strait Islander people groups as part of Australia's Indigenous population.

Aboriginal perspectives on health

As are Aboriginal worldviews generally, Aboriginal perspectives on health have been described as 'holistic'. The term 'holistic' means that such perspectives take account of a wide variety of factors, including social, emotional, mental, physical and spiritual factors (Mussell, Nicholas & Adler, 1993). Put differently, a holistic approach considers 'upstream' (general socio-economic) factors, 'midstream' factors (contemporary socio-cultural practices and circumstances), and 'downstream' factors (people's unique lives). Al these factors are important to consider, particularly because they all play a role in explaining the current health status of Aboriginal people.

Aboriginal worldviews

Aboriginal worldviews are worldviews that emerge from Aboriginal culture. For example, Aboriginal worldviews include regarding family relationships and land ownership as central to Aboriginal identity.

A critical fact, too, is the British colonisation of Australia, compounded with racism, discrimination and social exclusion (Reading & Wien, 2009). All this has contributed to the loss of Aboriginal language, **culture** and self-determination, and this, in turn, has had negative impacts on Aboriginal people's health and disease patterns.

Our point of departure is that **communication** and relationship breakdown in health care is common, but avoidable, when working with Aboriginal patients (Campbell, 1995; Shannon, 1994). Creating culturally safe environments is vital – not only for patients and healthcare staff, but also within the staff team. This chapter focuses on working with Aboriginal and Torres Strait Islander (from now on, Aboriginal) patients and colleagues. The strategies highlighted in this chapter can also be used by those working with people from other non-Western cultures and with different worldviews.

culture
the values, norms and practices that groups of people have in common, and with which these people identify themselves.

communication
the process of people engaging in the exchange of knowledge, information, feelings and meanings. Communication can encompass spoken and written language, but it also includes many other kinds of meaning-making, including bodily gestures and the disembodied meanings of visual displays and architectural designs.

Introduction

Holistic health encompasses not just biophysiological well-being, but also social and emotional well-being. Holistic health is achieved and maintained by connections to land or country, culture, ancestry, family, community and spirituality (Department of Health and

Ageing Social Health Reference Group, 2004). Aboriginal health critically depends on connections to land, spirit, ancestry and country (the land to which family is connected), but this dependence is sometimes poorly understood by Western society (Garvey, 2008). In Western society, spirituality is often ignored in healthcare provision as it has been excised from the Western medical model. Western medicine operates according to the dictates of science, and dismisses aspects of our life world that are not framed in the discourse of scientific evidence as 'subjective', 'arbitrary' and 'ungeneralisable'. This creates a disregard for spirituality, and it downgrades Aboriginal people's priorities and concerns when having to cope with illness and when seeking health care.

Also well documented in literature are the worrying health disparities between the Aboriginal and non-Aboriginal populations (Alderete, 1999). Low life expectancy figures are often cited to emphasise Australian Aboriginal populations' health disadvantage. The 20-year gap in life expectancy between Caucasian Australian and Aboriginal peoples is in large part a result of mortality in Aboriginal adults from non-communicable disease and injury (Marmot, 2005). In response to this life expectancy gap between the two populations, however, policy and research commonly adopt a 'deficit perspective' – that is, a perspective that posits that Aboriginal peoples are not doing the right thing with regard to how to live and how to treat their health.

This chapter presents a different perspective, highlighting the strengths and positives that are evident in Aboriginal peoples' lives and approaches to their health. To capitalise on these strengths and positives, Aboriginal peoples need to play a central role in empowering healthcare workers, policy-makers and researchers to work effectively with them. Specifically, guidance from Aboriginal health professionals is critical to enable others to value an Aboriginal person's lived experience. Such guidance also emphasises that an Aboriginal person's 'worth' does not equate with their level of education attainment, their type of employment, or their income. Such guidance focuses on enabling people to acknowledge the uniqueness of an Aboriginal person's daily social and family activities, as a carer, a parent, an advocate or a mentor.

Understanding Aboriginal culture

Above all, what is valued in Aboriginal culture is the importance of family, cultural identity, community obligation and a connection to country (including ancestor and spiritual links). Virtues that are highly esteemed include an individual's sincerity, trustworthiness and helpfulness. Positive experiences in the health system are created by healthcare workers who know how communicate and to act according to these values. Genuine relationships between healthcare workers and patients can facilitate the informal reconciliation required for social and emotional well-being. To achieve this, we first and urgently need to overcome the historical legacy of mistrust between Aboriginal people and those working in the health sector in Australia (Garvey, 2008).

To project this challenge onto a broader canvas, 'upstream' factors must be considered when addressing these matters. Upstream factors are those that occur at a macro level.

Global forces such as world economics and industrialisation may affect local land use and destabilise cultural practices; think of how mining and natural gas projects are affecting Aboriginal–government relationships. Then there are federal government policies pertaining to education, employment, income, living and working conditions, many of which have challenged Aboriginal well-being since colonisation. It is noteworthy in this regard that the experiences for Indigenous peoples in other countries, such as New Zealand and Canada, have been quite positively influenced thanks to federal treaties, policies ensuring social and government recognition, and the incorporation of traditional Indigenous approaches to medicine in healthcare provision. Historically, Australia has a poor track record in addressing and accommodating these upstream factors (Marmot, 2005).

'Midstream' factors are intermediate; that is, they include health behaviours and psychosocial attitudes and beliefs. Midstream factors are intermediate in that they pertain to the habits and practices that define societies and cultures, and are at the same time enacted by individuals in the 'here and now'. Midstream factors are at issue when people seek health care, offering opportunities for public health education and health behaviour change.

'Downstream' factors operate at a micro level, including an individual's personal physiological and biological status, and their genetic make-up (Northern Territory Department of Health, 2012). When communicating with Aboriginal patients and families, each of these factors needs to be brought in view to ensure respectful and effective treatment.

The challenge we face, however, is that, in Australia, Indigenous groups make up only approximately 3% of the population, a low figure compared to other countries such as New Zealand. Not surprisingly, the percentage of Aboriginal health workers also remains small compared to that of the general population. As a result, Aboriginal health workers in systems such as hospitals and other services can be overburdened, faced with the challenge of dealing with the detrimental consequences of upstream factors, and the dual task of tackling midstream (socio-cultural) and downstream (individual) factors.

Sadly, the pressures on Aboriginal healthcare workers as representatives or consultants can have negative effects on their own health. These pressures and effects reverberate within their families and their community network, as the health of the individual is intrinsically linked to the health of their extended family and community, and vice versa. This may produce a vicious cycle, resulting in burnout on the part of members of the Aboriginal healthcare workforce, and greater isolation from the healthcare system.

As noted above, what adds to all these challenges is that Western health care and medicine embody a worldview that privileges material, scientific and technological values at the expense of social, relational and spiritual values. That is, the Western medical worldview is not just anchored in scientific evidence, but actively shuns extra-scientific knowledge, such as narratives, experiences, emotions and the like. Here, the term 'scientific' presupposes that we erase personal experiences and spiritual connections. The term 'scientific' encourages us to construe science as if it is somehow blessed with 'a view from everywhere'. Such a 'scientific' view, it is assumed, yields truths that naturally hold for everyone everywhere. If science fails to recognise its own limits, however, it risks becoming *unscientific* – a realisation that is now increasingly argued by contemporary philosophers of science (Prigogine, 1996).

Alternative healing practices, which have been shown to be beneficial, are often dismissed as unscientific, and sometimes even seen as detrimental to people's health. Nevertheless, it is not uncommon for people to have powerful spiritual experiences and healing outcomes that are not explained by science (Benedetti & Amanzio, 2011), and which are therefore not accommodated in existing healthcare communication and practice.

In our interactions with Aboriginal patients, families and staff, Aboriginal values, experiences and worldviews should shape our clinical care approach and our communication styles. By understanding similarities and differences between Aboriginal and non-Aboriginal perspectives, and by exploring these differences and keeping them in mind when communicating, we may be able to create 'culturally secure spaces' for Aboriginal patients and families. Achieving **cultural safety** means remaining attuned to and counterbalancing the potentially adverse effects of the 'power relationships between the service provider and the people who use the service' (Anderson et al., 2003). Here safety issues forth from Aboriginal people knowing that the health care they receive is anchored in a deep appreciation of their socio-economic circumstances, their socio-cultural practices, and their personal actions and values.

> **cultural safety**
> the fact (or the feeling) that I and my worldview are respected by the people with whom I interact.

Practice example 17.1

This practice example is about the challenges faced by an Aboriginal family when responding to the deterioration of their Aunt Mabel.

Geoffrey is a middle-aged Aboriginal man living in a metropolitan city in Australia. His older aunty, Mabel, who lives in a regional town, is very unwell. Mabel is a well-respected woman in her community and has been battling cancer for a number of years. Geoffrey, along with other family members around the state, make plans to drive to this town, some travelling as far as seven hours by car to be there. For this regional visit Geoffrey drives with his brother, sister, eldest son and niece to the town. He leaves his wife and youngest daughter in the city for this trip. Many members of the extended family make a considerable, but common effort, to visit her – taking time off work, and arranging for care of younger dependants where needed and travelling across the desert at the height of summer.

On arrival Geoffrey is united with extended family members from other regions. Some relatives have arrived outside of visiting hours and have been waiting in and around the hospital. Aunt Mabel's immediate family in the town is hosting a large number of visitors in their homes. Over the next week, most of the family members meet and congregate under a tree directly next to the hospital. Geoffrey comes to the hospital daily with an insulated drink cooler of cool drink and water, as midday summer temperatures are high.

A hospital staff member, Helen, has noticed this group converging over the last few days, and on the third day asks the group to disperse. Helen informs Geoffrey that

continued ›

Practice example 17.1 continued ›

patients and other community members are displeased with the group loitering and smoking. As Mabel's condition has worsened since his arrival, Geoffrey makes no apology for his family's presence and tells Helen they will be there as long as Aunt Mabel is in hospital. Helen leaves and informs the hospital's security guard Roger, who is a Torres Strait Islander. Roger approaches the group and notices the group, some smoking, and all drinking out of the cooler. He informs the group to move on or police will be called. Geoffrey is frustrated and tells Roger what he told Helen. Roger does not make any concession for the family, however, and there is a disagreement that leads to a fight. The police are called and three of the 12 family members present are arrested, including Geoffrey. During this time Aunt Mabel's health rapidly deteriorates and she passes away.

Analysis and reflection

It is not uncommon for Aboriginal families to travel to see sick relatives or attend funerals. Family kinships are strong and many aunties and uncles are considered close, as close as you might be to your mother and father. Similarly, many cousins are considered as brothers and sisters. Moreover, family obligations are non-negotiable.

Aunt Mabel might have had access to better health care in a city hospital, but for financial and family reasons remained in her town. Aunt Mabel always had a strong connection to her country (the land to which her family is connected). She was born into the region and raised her family in that town. Her funeral and burial must be conducted on her land, her country. Her late husband is buried nearby, and leaving her country would have significant effects on Mabel's and her family's spiritual and emotional well-being. Furthermore, with her negative prognosis, Mabel made a conscious decision to pass away in her country.

As can be expected, family members experienced heightened levels of stress with the news of Aunt Mabel's condition. Family members who smoked were smoking more intensely during this period. Aunt Mabel was considered one of the key family members who connected many of the extended family groups together. Her passing would create somewhat of a gap between the more distant family groups, due to the loss of a central, matriarchal elder. Other factors contributing to the stress included family separation (as not all family members accompanied the trip). This stress was further exacerbated by the family's reflections on the low life-expectancy of their Aboriginal people, nurturing a fatalistic view among them about hereditary diseases (such as diabetes and cancer), and social health conditions (such as suicide and alcoholism).

Geoffrey's father, Aunt Mabel's brother, passed away years earlier at a relatively young age, with the same cancer. Geoffrey is scared for his own health now, given these deaths. In general, he avoids health checks and healthcare appointments as he has not found a male doctor he feels comfortable with in the city he lives in. The conversations with Helen and Roger left Geoffrey frustrated. He knows that congregating inside the hospital in the waiting room would have been a problem, and that they would have been sent away straight away. Anyway, his family prefer to be outdoors. Geoffrey felt alienated and judged by the hospital staff, especially by the way they looked at him carrying the cooler. This experience affirmed his dissatisfaction with the health system and with government institutions.

Helen has had negative experiences with Aboriginal families in the four months that she has been working as a nurse in the town. In the city where she was raised, the only Aboriginal people she was exposed to were generally people in the city centre, some with antisocial behaviour. Since she started her new job, Helen has been verbally abused by an Aboriginal patient and feels insecure. She feels ill-equipped to work with Aboriginal families. In general she finds them rude (they don't make eye contact) and non-compliant (they miss appointments regularly). She has a fairly positive rapport with Roger so sends him to 'fix the problem'. Helen informs Roger that the group are smoking in the wrong area and that they are refusing to move.

Roger has had both positive and negative experiences with the local Aboriginal community. He has lived most of his adult life in the community and does not know Geoffrey and his visiting family members. When he sees the drink cooler, he wrongly assumed that the group were drinking alcohol. The individuals who were smoking were not aware of the no-smoking policy directly outside hospital entrances. Both Helen and Roger failed to mention this to the family.

As a result of the fight and arrest of family members, there is hostility between the family and the hospital staff. This contributes to Mabel's family's disengagement with the regional hospital over the week and subsequently. Some family members felt that the stress of the incident contributed to the passing of Mabel, and others felt the health care she received was poor. Yet others believed her passing was inevitable. The hospital was the main health service provider Mabel's family accessed. Her family generally avoided the local Aboriginal Medical Service in the region as confidentiality with Aboriginal staff had been compromised in the past.

What could have prevented this sad outcome? Better communication between Helen and Geoffrey, between Helen and Roger, and between Roger and Geoffrey could have prevented what happened. From commencing her new job, Helen could have asked her colleagues, both Aboriginal and non-Aboriginal, about some of her uncertainties and queries about with Aboriginal culture. She could have also asked for more information from her team manager about supports available to her regarding cultural awareness and safety. Roger could have clarified to Geoffrey the conversation he had with Helen and found out more about Geoffrey and his family's story. Geoffrey and family could have better shared their story with Helen and Roger. No-smoking policy signs could have been made clearer and communicated more respectfully by hospital staff. Regional hospitals should consider having a purpose-built and large waiting area for Aboriginal families to meet, separate from and different to isolated smoking sections.

Reflective questions

1. What are the main social, cultural and personal aspects of Mabel's story?
2. How has generational poverty affected Aunt Mabel's health and well-being (for example, education attainment, health literacy, financial literacy and ability to advocate for herself)?
3. What information would Geoffrey, Helen and Roger have needed to create a positive outcome to this story?
4. What impact will this experience have on Aunt Mabel's family members and their relationship with health services in the future?

Implications for practice

Reflect on your position and personal values. Aboriginal families, friends and colleagues have often shared their lived experiences of overt and covert racism. Crude generalisations, poor understanding of Aboriginal history and assumptions about individuals and their behaviour can be damaging to relationships from the offset. For example, a doctor or nurse speaking to a white spouse or partner of an Aboriginal patient but not to the patient themselves can cause frustration and anger. This creates an experience of disempowerment and is similar to situations where healthcare workers engage with a parent rather than with the child; with a carer rather than with the person with the disability; or with a translator rather than with a person with poor English skills. First impressions endure, and starting on the right foot, figuratively speaking, is critical to building rapport.

Rapport is best achieved by allowing the conversation to 'meander', rather than you taking charge and focusing directly on the issue that is *your* concern. Homing in on your concern means to favour Standard Australian English (SAE), which tends to involve 'direct communication'. Indigenous communication tends to set more store by 'feeling your way around the other person', and this is done through 'yarning'. Where SAE favours getting down to business, Indigenous communication revolves around others' being, their feelings, their mood, and their position in the world. Figure 17.1 schematises the difference between Indigenous 'yarning' and SAE's 'direct communication'.

Keep the context in mind. Consider the context that surrounds Aboriginal patients and families. That is, think about upstream, midstream and downstream factors when dealing with people from Aboriginal backgrounds. Can you see any political decisions, or policies and procedures in your healthcare systems, which create barriers for Aboriginal patients? Are their ways of service delivery that are more respectful towards Aboriginal values, and that do not assume the superiority of Western morality and Western medicine?

Figure 17.2 aims to remind you to pay close attention to what is involved with engendering effective communication, which is at the centre of the figure. The figure highlights

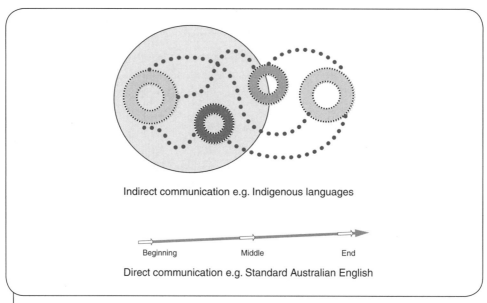

Indirect communication e.g. Indigenous languages

Beginning   Middle   End

Direct communication e.g. Standard Australian English

Figure 17.1 Direct and indirect communication

that effective communication requires trust, which emerges from your personal sensitivity towards the Indigenous person. Both effective communication and trust are again contingent on your strategic use of appropriate communication styles, and on your understanding of

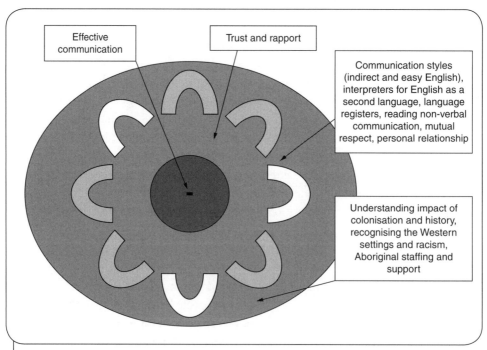

Figure 17.2 Communication in context (the picture symbolises Aboriginal Mob and non-Aboriginals sitting around a campfire)

the impact of relevant social and historical factors on the Indigenous person's position and condition.

Theoretical links

Holistic health, healing and fatalism

The central role of holism in Aboriginal health has been increasingly recognised since the 1970s (Hunter, 1999). It is defined by the National Aboriginal Health Strategy Working Party (1989) as physical as well as social, emotional and cultural well-being of both the individual and the community as a whole. It further encompasses both life and death.

In more recent studies, Shahid and colleagues (2009a, 2009b) investigated the beliefs and perspectives of Aboriginal people and cancer. Their findings emphasised paradigms uncommon to Western medicine with sickness being linked to spiritual causes. Excerpts from their research are highlighted below, highlighting the power of respectful relations:

> If you feel good inside regardless of your health, it will help you in any medical problems.

> Healing is not just physical; it's mental, emotional and spiritual as well.

> Aboriginal people have this notion of being sung [or cursed by another] … it's basically a bad magic put on somebody.

A broader perspective on 'the other'

Communicating with Aboriginal patients and families requires us to think about the broader context within which they live. One way of appreciating this broader context is to consider upstream, midstream and downstream factors. This parable explains what 'upstream', 'midstream' and 'downstream' mean:

> This is a parable of three friends. Imagine that you're one of these three friends who come to a river. It's a beautiful scene, but it's shattered by the cries of a child, and actually several children, in need of rescue in the water. So you do hopefully what everybody would do. You jump right in along with your friends. The first friend says, 'I'm going to rescue those who are about to drown, those at most risk of falling over the waterfall.' The second friend says, 'I'm going to build a raft. I'm going to make sure that fewer people need to end up at the waterfall's edge. Let's usher more people to safety by building this raft, coordinating those branches together.' Over time, they're successful, but not really, not as much as they want to be. More people slip through, and they finally look up and they see that their third friend is nowhere to be seen. They finally spot her. She's in the water. She's swimming away from them upstream, rescuing children as she goes, and they shout to her, 'Where are you going? There are children here to save!' And she shouts back, 'I'm going to find out who or what is throwing these children in the water.'

In health care, we have that first friend – we have the specialist, we have the trauma surgeon, the ICU nurse, the ER doctors. We have those people that are vital rescuers, people you want to be there when you're in dire straits. We also know that we have the second friend – we have that raft-builder. That's the primary care clinician, people on the care team who are there to manage your chronic conditions, your diabetes, your hypertension, there to give you your annual check-ups, there to make sure your vaccines are up to date, but also there to make sure that you have a raft to sit on and usher yourself to safety. But while that's also vital and very necessary, what we're missing is that third friend …

The upstreamists are the health care professionals who know that health does begin where we live and work and play, but beyond that awareness, is able to mobilize the resources to create the system in their clinics and in their hospitals that really does start to approach that, to connect people to the resources they need outside the four walls of the clinic. (Manchanda (2014); http://www.ted.com/talks/rishi_manchanda_what_makes_us_get_sick_look_upstream, retrieved January 12, 2015)

Cultural safety and racism

Considering the upstream, midstream and downstream dimensions of Aboriginal patients' and their families' lives may create *cultural safety*. The term 'cultural safety' was coined by nurses working with the Māori people in New Zealand (Ramsden, 1996). Cultural safety includes the knowledge of cultures' differences and the ability to accept them. Cultural safety counters racism – both covert and overt. Over time, cultural safety has expanded to emphasise improving relationships between health professionals and patients who differ by age and generation, gender, sexual orientation, socio-economic status, ethic origin, religious or spiritual beliefs, and disability (Ramsden, 1996).

Cultural safety is contingent on your communication style. Your communication style depends on the choices you make about language register (for example, medical versus everyday language) and tenor (for example, formal or informal language). Of course, health literacy training is vital for effective communication (Clifford, Stan & Lucinda, 2013; Payne, DeVol & Smith, 2006), but so is active listening (see Chapter 15). This is because cultural safety requires that we are sensitive to what register and tenor Aboriginal patients and families themselves prefer, and that we do not perpetuate 'white privilege' in our dealings with Aboriginal people (McIntosh, 1989).

> White privilege is like an invisible weightless backpack of special provisions, maps, passports, codebooks, visas, clothes, tools and blank checks… Power from unearned privilege can look like strength when it is in fact [a structure of institutionalised and taken-for-granted] permission … (McIntosh, 1989, p. 1, 4)

In summary, cultural safety emerges when healthcare workers become capable of relativising their own cultural attitudes and backgrounds, and recognise the value of Aboriginal behaviours and relationships.

Conclusion

Too often, communication between the healthcare professional and the Aboriginal patient falls short due to the privileging of Western values and judgments. It is not recognised that inequalities between majority and minority groups (such as Aboriginal people) continue to create multiple disadvantages for Aboriginal patients. Building effective relationships requires a foundation of mutual respect and trust, and this foundation is realised through appropriate, culturally safe communication.

For professionals who have had limited experiences with other cultures than their own, it is critical that they learn how to reflect on their own cultural backgrounds, and communicate in ways that do not take their own social and cultural judgments for granted. To understand and appreciate Aboriginal values and begin to enact cultural safety, health professionals should begin by asking questions about context and history, and by allowing Aboriginal patients to tell their full story. Only a respectful response to others' stories can break down initial barriers of mistrust.

Practice example 17.2

This vignette is about a Yolngu man from a village 500 kilometres from Darwin who suffers from renal (kidney) disease. Together with his mother and grandmother, he visits his doctor in the community health centre for an update. Due to their geographic isolation and limited access to schooling, their English is rudimentary.

The doctor they visit is from a white Anglo-Australian background himself, but he has extensive experience with working in Aboriginal communities. He has the task of communicating to the patient that his disease is getting worse, and that he is likely to have to move to Darwin for dialysis (a process of cleaning the blood using a special dialysis machine).

The doctor begins by stating that the patient's kidneys 'are working but they are not working normally'. He raises his hand to indicate poor liver function, using the hand's height from the desk to illustrate function as a percentage ratio. His overall aim is to convey that the patient is at risk of entering end-stage renal disease, that it is critical that he takes his medications, and that he may need to come in for dialysis because his chances of recovery are limited. Together, these messages are complex, and the interaction between the doctor and the family does not go well.

First of all, the messages turn out to be confusing for the patient and his relatives. This is not just because Yolngu language does not have equivalent expressions for technical devices and numerical percentages. It is also confusing because of the doctor's use of statements that appear to contradict one another: 'Your kidneys are working but they are not working normally.' Here, a familiar strategy for those from Western cultures – to soften the impact of bad news – backfires because it is heard by the Yolngu family as saying that 'the kidneys are working'.

continued ›

Practice example 17.2 continued ›

Second, in part because of this confusion and in part due to the unfamiliarity of the situation, the family's responses are minimal. The doctor therefore fails to register their acknowledgement in response to what he is saying, leaving him uncertain about whether or not his messages have been understood. He is therefore unable to know how to proceed in the conversation.

Third, because of the family's silence, the doctor does most of the talking. In fact, he talks for all of the quarter of an hour they are in the consultation. While the doctor is familiar with the Aboriginal practice of allowing for silences in the conversation, he is inclined to assume that their silences indicate understanding because this is a follow-up consultation.

Reflective questions

1. What assumptions did the doctor bring to the consultation, and were they justified?
2. What do you think the doctor could have done to make his messages clearer?
3. How could he have ascertained that his messages were understood by the Yolnu family?
4. Have you been in a situation where you assumed that your communication was clear, and you were made to realise that is was not well understood?
5. What is the Aboriginal term for the people group you may be working with?
6. Different regions in Australia have different clan groups. Do you know what they are called?

Further reading

Dudgeon, P., & Ugle, K. (2014). Communicating and engaging with diverse communities. In P. Dudgeon, H. Milroy, & R. Walker (Eds.), *Working together: Aboriginal and Torres Strait Islander mental health and wellbeing principles and practice*. Telethon Kids Institute. Retrieved September 30, 2014 from http://aboriginal.telethonkids.org.au/media/673984/wt-part-3-chapt-15-final.pdf

This resource provides a good overview of communication strategies that are critical for engaging with Aboriginal communities.

Web resources

Aboriginal and Torres Strait Islander social and emotional wellbeing: http://aboriginal.telethonkids.org.au/media/673974/wt-part-1-chapt-4-final.pdf

Communicating and engaging with diverse communities: http://aboriginal.telethonkids.org.
    au/media/673984/wt-part-3-chapt-15-final.pdf

How to name Aboriginal people?: http://www.creativespirits.info/aboriginalculture/people/
    how-to-name-aboriginal-people

References

Alderete, E. (1999). *The health of indigenous peoples.* Geneva: World Health Organization.

Anderson, J., Perry, J., Blue, C., Browne, A., Henderson, A., Khan, K. B., & Smye, V. (2003). 'Rewriting' cultural safety within the postcolonial and post-national feminist project: Toward new epistemologies of healing. *Advances in Nursing Science, 26*(3), 196–214.

Benedetti, F. & Amanzio, M. (2011). The placebo response: How words and rituals change the patient's brain. *Patient Education & Counseling 84*, 413–419.

Campbell, M. (1995). Communication with Aboriginal patients in the pre-hospital environment. *Australian Journal of Emergency Care, 2*(2), 24–27.

Clifford, C., Stan, H., & Lucinda, M. (2013). Health literacy practices and educational competencies for health professionals: A consensus study. *Journal of Health Communication, 18*(1), 82–102.

Department of Health and Ageing, Social Health Reference Group. (2004). *National Strategic Framework for Aboriginal and Torres Strait Islander People's Mental Health and Social and Emotional Well Being 2004–2009.* Department of Health and Ageing, Canberra: National Aboriginal and Torres Strait Islander Health Council and National Mental Health Working Group.

Garvey, D. (2008). *A review of the social and emotional wellbeing of Indigenous Australian peoples.* Perth: Australian Indigenous HealthInfoNet.

Hunter, P. (1999). Searching for a new way of thinking in Aboriginal health. *The Australian Health Consumer, 2*, 16–17.

Manchanda, R. (2014). *What makes us get sick? Look upstream.* TED discussion. Retrieved September 30, 2014, from http://www.ted.com/talks/rishi_manchanda_what_makes_us_get_sick_look_upstream/transcript?language=en

Marmot, M. (2005). Social determinants of health inequalities. *The Lancet 365*(9464), 1099–1104.

McIntosh, P. (1989). White privilege: Unpacking the invisible knapsack. Retrieved March 14, 2015, from http://www.isr.umich.edu/home/diversity/resources/white-privilege.pdf

Mussell, W. J., Nichols, W. M., & Adler, M. T. (1993). *Making meaning of mental health challenges in First Nations: A Freirean perspective.* Chilliwack: Sal'i'shan Institute Society.

National Aboriginal Health Strategy Working Party. (1989). *A national Aboriginal health strategy.* Canberra: Department of Aboriginal Affairs.

Northern Territory Department of Health. (2012). *Health Promotion Strategic Framework 2011–2015* [draft]. Retrieved September 30, 2014 from http://www.health.nt.gov.au/library/scripts/objectifyMedia.aspx?file=pdf/66/68.pdf

Payne, R. K., DeVol, P. E., & Smith, T. D. (2006). *Bridges out of poverty: Strategies for professionals and communities.* Highlands, TX: Aha! Process.

Prigogine, I. (1996) *The end of certainty: Time, chaos and the new laws of nature*. New York: The Free Press.

Ramsden, I. (1996). The Treaty of Waitangi and cultural safety. In *Draft guidelines for the cultural safety component in nursing and midwifery education*. Wellington: Nursing Council of New Zealand.

Shahid, S., Finn, L., Bessarab, D., & Thompson, S. (2009a). Understanding, beliefs and perspectives of Aboriginal people in Western Australia about cancer and its impact on access to cancer services. *BMC Health Services Research, 9*(1), 132. Retrieved September 30, 2014 from http://www.biomedcentral.com/1472–6963/9/132

Shahid, S., Finn, L., & Thompson, S. C. (2009b). Barriers to participation of Aboriginal people in cancer care: Communication in the hospital setting. *Medical Journal of Australia, 190*(10), 574–579. Retrieved September 30, 2014 from http://www.mja.com.au/journal/2009/190/10/barriers-participation-aboriginal-people-cancer-care-communication-hospital

Shannon, B. (1994). Social and cultural differences affect medical treatment. *Australian Family Physician, 23*(1), 33–35.

18

Communicating with culturally and linguistically diverse patients in cancer care

Phyllis Butow

Learning objectives

This chapter will enable you to:
- understand the need to be aware of the complexities of communicating in a cross-cultural health setting;
- appreciate the cultural, language and practical difficulties of communicating through interpreters with multilingual and multicultural populations in cancer care;
- recognise barriers to effective communication when working with multilingual and multicultural populations in cancer care.

Key terms

Cancer
Cross-cultural communication
Immigrants
Interpreters
Minority groups

Overview

With increasing immigration, many countries are multi-cultural. **Cancer** outcomes for **immigrants** and **minority groups** are known to be worse than for most of population. Communication barriers contribute to those disparities. Such barriers can stem from language deficits and poor health literacy; differing understandings of disease, treatment and

> **cancer**
> an illness that results from abnormal cell division in the body.
>
> **immigrants**
> people from countries other than Australia who have moved to Australia.
>
> **minority groups**
> groups of people from countries other than Australia who have immigrated to Australia.

interpreters
people who speak English and at least one other language. They are called in to attend doctor–patient consultations to translate technical and medical concepts for the patient.

patient and health professional roles; and mistrust between health professionals and patients. **Interpreters** are a partial but not complete solution to many of these barriers, and care needs to be taken to optimise doctor–interpreter–patient communication. Cultural advocates may be required to ensure patient needs are understood and addressed.

Introduction

Migration is increasing worldwide, with the number of people who do not speak the primary language of the country in which they live similarly increasing. For example, the 2013 census showed that 27.7% of Australians were born overseas, compared to 23.6% born overseas 10 years earlier in 2003 (Australian Bureau of Statistics, n.d.). Of those born overseas, 11.5% speak English poorly or not at all (Australian Bureau of Statistics, n.d.). Furthermore, Indigenous groups may also differ in language and cultural background from the population that now represents the majority.

Health care is challenging in a multicultural context, and this is particularly true of cancer care, due to the stigma and nihilism associated with this word and the high emotionality of many consultations. Thus it serves as a good exemplar of relevant issues, and will be the focus for this chapter.

Minority groups diagnosed with cancer have poorer cancer outcomes than mainstream groups, with lower screening and survival rates and higher rates of reported side effects (Chu, Miller & Springfield, 2007). A recent meta-analysis revealed significantly higher distress and depression in minority versus mainstream cancer patients. This finding is not wholly accounted for by differences in socio-economic status (Luckett et al., 2011). The finding was reinforced in a large registry-based study of migrants versus Anglo-Australian-born cancer survivors (Butow et al., 2013).

While many factors may contribute to such disparities, including poor health literacy, unfamiliarity with healthcare processes and differing beliefs and attitudes about illness, death and treatment, poor outcomes may also be due to language and communication barriers (Johnstone & Kanitsaki, 2007).

Language and communication barriers

Doctor–patient communication is a critical aspect of cancer care. Doctor–patient communication influences patient understanding and satisfaction with care, the quality of informed consent, adherence to agreed treatment regimens, psychological adjustment and coping in patients and families, and health professional burnout (Ong et al., 1995). In the cancer setting there are many issues which require careful and sensitive communication, including conveying bad news and discussing prognosis. Other such issues include facilitating informed decision-making, given the increasingly complex array of treatment options available. Then there are issues such as gaining patients' consent to participate in clinical trials, discussing expensive drugs, and advance care planning (see Chapter 7).

While communication can be challenging at any time, it is likely to be more so when health professionals and patients do not speak the same language or share a cultural heritage. Given the increasing rate of migration highlighted above, it is now an everyday experience for health professionals to treat immigrant patients and communicate with immigrant families.

Communication challenges between cultures can arise because of language difficulties (both verbal and non-verbal, as well as written), and can give rise to different illness explanations and role expectations. For example, in a study involving focus groups with 73 cancer patients and 18 caregivers who had migrated to Australia and spoke Chinese, Greek or Arabic:

> participants, especially those less acculturated, described feeling alone and misunderstood, failing to comprehend medical instructions, being unable to communicate questions and concerns and experiencing a lack of consistency in interpreters and interpretation. (Butow et al., 2007)

In another large study including over 250 immigrant cancer patients, it was found that the presence of an interpreter did not always compensate for language difficulties (Butow et al., 2013). Indeed, analysis of translated cancer consultations has shown that interpretation is often inexact, particularly of questions and answers about prognosis (Butow, Goldstein et al., 2011).

Patients have culturally determined beliefs about the causes of diseases, the way the body is structured and functions, and the efficacy of different complementary and alternative therapies (Tchen et al., 2003). Religious and spiritual beliefs and practices affect how patients respond to bad news, to offers of medical treatments such as transfusions, and to end-of-life family conferences.

Thus there is ample opportunity for miscommunication and confusion between health professionals and patients from different backgrounds. Patients from some cultural groups expect to be told what to do by health professionals, and they lose confidence in the expertise of their doctor if a shared decision-making approach is taken (Huang et al., 1999). Asian and Indigenous cultures often have a collectivist approach to health decision-making, and expect the family, or a trusted and respected elder in the community, to make decisions on the patient's behalf (Surbone et al., 2013), and the Western emphasis on the primacy of the doctor–patient relationship is at odds with this approach. These cultures may also believe it is better for patients to be spared knowledge of a cancer diagnosis, or a poor prognosis, to avoid them 'giving up' and losing hope. This, too, can be at odds with Western ethical standards of full disclosure and informed consent (Tan et al., 1993).

Cultures also differ in their expectations of non-verbal and emotional expression between health professionals and patients. In some cultures, an informal, warm and compassionate approach is expected of health professionals, and a more formal approach may be interpreted as cold and uncaring (Moore & Butow, 2005). On the other hand, a cultural tradition of silence and deference towards health professionals may lead some patients to be quiet and passive in consultations; this can be misinterpreted as reflecting misunderstanding or confusion (Janz et al., 2009).

Compounding all this, a patient's personal or historical experiences of discrimination, violence or institutionalised racism may reduce their trust in health professionals and institutions (Tan et al., 1993). For example, the ongoing impact of colonisation and subsequent socio-cultural and political isolation on Aboriginal Australians and their culture is felt throughout the health system (Treloar et al., 2014). Some Aboriginal people may delay seeing a doctor or choose not to take up active treatment for cancer because it would entail entering a hospital system where they are made to feel like second-class citizens (see Chapter 17). Thus, sensitivity to cultural issues; a flexible, enquiring, negotiative approach; and a particular effort to ensure that language and cultural barriers are overcome are often required.

Practice example 18.1

Below is an excerpt from an audio-recorded and translated consultation between a medical oncologist and an elderly Chinese woman, newly diagnosed with metastatic, incurable disease (Butow, Bell et al., 2011). Her husband was interpreting for her. She had just asked the oncologist how bad the cancer was.

[Excerpt 1:]

Doctor: [To the husband] I think it is better that she knows. Especially when she is asking the question, for her to know and to be very honest with her. She then knows that she can trust me to be honest and I will answer her questions.

Husband: Hmm, yeh, yeh.

Doctor: [Went on explaining that the disease – a stage 3A lung cancer – had spread throughout the body and was no longer curable]

Husband: [To the patient, his wife] She said it should be in its initial stage.

Below is an excerpt, again between a medical oncologist and a patient, newly diagnosed with metastatic, incurable cancer (Butow et al., 2013). The interpreter was a professional interpreter, present in the room.

[Excerpt 2:]

Patient: Ask the doctor if these are curable.

Interpreter: [To doctor] So the question is … how many in his situation, how many patients that his problem can be cured?

Doctor :   If you mean by cure that you will be completely cured that is very very unlikely.

Interpreter: If you mean to be cured completely, the possibility is not very high …

Doctor :   But you have a reasonably good chance to respond to the chemotherapy and therefore I should be able to control this cancer for … you know, for months and months.

continued >

Practice example 18.1 continued ›

Interpreter: But you have a great chance that if the chemotherapy works ... the disease should be under control and it [your life] should be able to be prolonged and prolonged.

In focus groups with interpreters who had experience in cancer consultations, one interpreter said the following:

[Excerpt 3:]   I mean, to the patients [it] is ... critical because in our culture it is really cruel to tell the patient that he is or she is diagnosed with cancer ... maybe it can cause him to be depressed or maybe diminish his ability or willingness to survive. So we ... can find some code word, like instead of saying you have cancer, we can use the word tumour ... and we're going to ... treat you for that tumour, but knowing that a tumour will be treated the same way as cancer would be treated. So we can get around that and use code words just to, you know, just to make it easier ... just to alleviate the situation and make it acceptable, more acceptable. (Butow et al., 2010)

The extract below comes from another oncology consultation at which several family members were present. The exchange was a side-exchange in English to the professional interpreter.

[Excerpt 4:]

Family: The doctor shouldn't let her know in fact ... *it just scare her!*

Can you please don't interpret this to her? Actually, she doesn't need to know. You can ask the questions for us, but you don't need to interpret to her. She doesn't need to know.

She now always says that she has pains ... she has no mood to eat ... we bring her out, go to yum cha with her ... before the doctor has told her that, she was very vital. She could even argue with me but *she becomes very frustrated after knowing that.* That's why we really don't want to let her know.

Analysis and reflection

In excerpt 1, the doctor tells the patient's husband beforehand that she intends to tell the patient the truth, with the rationale that truth and honesty would build trust between her and the patient. This is an approach that is often recommended in texts about **cross-cultural communication** (Butow & Baile, 2012). Doing this makes communication transparent, and respects patient autonomy.
The husband in this case appears to agree with this approach, but a clear negotiation does not take place to ensure there is agreement. In fact, it turns out the husband does not

> **cross-cultural communication**
> communication that takes place between people from different cultures.

agree, and goes on to falsify the interpretation, to ensure that his wife is not told the bad news. The doctor is not aware that her intended communication has not reached the patient.

In excerpt 2, it can be seen that the interpreter is not directly falsifying information, but is softening the oncologist's words in such a way that the patient may not fully understand the probable impact of his disease on his lifespan. As does this interpreter, interpreters generally may feel it is not culturally appropriate to be explicit about a bad diagnosis or prognosis.

The interview statement (excerpt 3) shows the pressure interpreters feel under to mitigate the bad news the doctor conveys. Excerpt 4 reveals that this pressure on the interpreter may come from the family insisting that bad news is not disclosed to the patient.

Thus, interpreting consultations where bad news is at issue can place the interpreter under considerable pressure. Without explicit training, and open discussion prior to the consultation between interpreter and doctor regarding how communication challenges should be handled, interpreters are poorly placed to interpret, relay and respond to critical information.

A related challenge inherent in many of the excerpts quoted above is the number of people in the room. Because of the importance placed on family involvement in many cultures, migrants may be more likely to bring family members to their consultation, and are also likely to bring a greater number of such family members. As noted by Surbone (2008), consultations involving family members or friends tend to be more lengthy and complex than with individual patients. Patients and family members are likely to have different information and support needs, there may be conflict within family members, and between family members and the patient, and generational differences in beliefs and approaches may be apparent. Health professionals may need to provide guidance and support or specific interventions to ensure families work together to the optimal benefit of the patient.

Implications for practice

Medical interpreting standards of practice developed by the International Medical Interpreters Association and Education Development Center (1995) state that interpreters must interpret accurately and maintain confidentiality, impartiality and professional distance at all times. However, interpreters experience difficulty trying to adhere to these standards, due to language and cultural differences in communication norms (Hsieh, 2006). These challenges may be further heightened in oncological settings because of the complexity of information and treatment options, cultural stigma related to cancer, and the frequency with which bad news is discussed.

Angelelli (2004) noted that interpreters actively grapple with these complexities. They influence the flow of consultations and attend simultaneously to structural, cultural, interactional and linguistic difficulties, with the aim of improving interactions. Hsieh (2007) termed these attempts as 'co-diagnostician behaviours', and identified five varieties: (1) assuming the provider's communicative goals, (2) editorialising information for medical emphases, (3) initiating information-seeking behaviours, (4) participating in diagnostic tasks, and (5) volunteering medical information to the patients.

Hsieh (2007) believes that co-diagnostician behaviours can be positive, but can also diminish the authority and control of the doctor, causing a rift between doctor and patient. She and others recommend a pre-consultation meeting when working with an interpreter, to discuss:
- who will be present, the tasks to be undertaken, likely technical words to be used, emotion and how this will be handled safely;
- roles, seating, and the role of touch;
- potential cultural issues in communication and how these will be approached;
- anxieties and uncertainties.

Similarly, post-consultation debriefing can be extremely helpful to identify any communication breakdowns, as well as to allow emotional expression.

Use of untrained interpreters, such as family members and members of the general public, can be highly problematic, although sometimes unavoidable. Untrained interpreters may have an emotional investment in the communication (such as protecting the patient from distressing news), a relationship which precludes discussion of certain topics (such as sexuality), a lack of linguistic skills in one or other of the languages being used, and a diffidence in questioning the doctor if they do not understand words or concepts. If an untrained interpreter is unavoidable, health professionals need significant skills in rapidly 'training' the interpreter to engage appropriately.

Theoretical links

The notion of culture is extremely complex. Good definitions are still lacking, since confusion persists about the interaction between place of birth, race, ethnicity and culture. Cross-cultural theories of communication in health care are small in number, and those that do exist tend to focus on very specific aspects of communication, such as emotional expression (Schere, Clark-Polner & Mortillaro 2011).

The language problem is often identified as one of the biggest challenges facing immigrant populations. More recently the wider role of health literacy has been emphasised. Health literacy concerns the development and application of knowledge and skills required in a specific health context (Nutbeam, 2009). Health literacy is commonly defined as the 'capacity to acquire, understand and use information in ways which promote and maintain good health' (Institute of Medicine of the National Academies, 2004; US Department of Health and Human Services, 2010). Yip (2012) proposed a cross-cultural model (Figure 18.1) emphasising the importance of assessing health literacy levels while taking into account different migrant groups' unique ways of enacting health literacy (for example, their unique ways of accessing or sharing healthcare information). Yip suggested that interventions to improve outcomes in multicultural health should focus on identifying individual strengths and weaknesses in each of the core skills to leverage patients' existing health literacy.

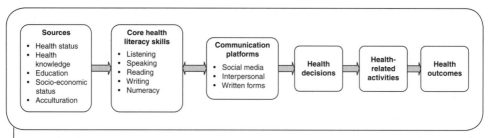

Figure 18.1 Health literacy model for limited English proficient populations (Yip, 2012). Reproduced with permission of Taylor & Francis Ltd, http://www.tandfonline.com.

However, this preliminary model lacks specificity to different healthcare settings, and does not consider the role of the interpreter. There is a clear need to further develop and test theoretical and empirical models of cross-cultural cancer health.

A recent report from the Ethnic Communities' Council of Victoria (2012) proposed a framework combining the linguistic competency and health literacy of the patient with the cultural competence of the service to affect health outcomes in migrant patients. System-level cultural competence can support communication through aspects such as the inclusion of minority group faces and experiences in patient literature, the settings in which communication occurs, signage and visiting arrangements. Thus, interventions at the patient, family, health professional and system level are required to fully and beneficially influence minority group outcomes.

Reflective questions

1. Talk to friends, family or colleagues who come from a different culture from you. How might your approaches to health and health care be different?
2. Find out what the policy is regarding family members interpreting for patients in your local hospital. Do you think it is ever reasonable to allow a family member to translate?
3. Given constrained healthcare dollars, is it realistic to spend the time with the interpreters recommended above to ensure effective consultations? Is it worth it?

Conclusion

Language, health literacy and cultural barriers can all influence effective communication in health care. Interpreters are an important but only partial answer to these barriers, and health professionals and systems need training and support to respond in culturally competent ways to multicultural clientele, interpreters and communities.

Practice example 18.2

A case study demonstrating some of these cultural challenges is presented below.

Francesca was a 74-year-old woman from Italy who had migrated to Australia to be with her son when her husband died five years ago. Francesca recently went to her GP with a lump in her breast and subsequently underwent a mammogram and biopsy. She attended her first surgical appointment with her son (Luigi) and his wife.

When the surgeon (Dr Barratt) came to get Francesca, Luigi rose quickly to his feet and asked if he could speak to the surgeon alone. His tone was urgent, and Dr Barratt took him in to his consulting room. Luigi, who spoke English well, asked Dr Barratt if his mother had breast cancer. Dr Barratt told him that this was indeed the case. Luigi was very distressed. He asked the surgeon not to tell his mother about her disease. Dr Barratt asked him why he felt that was the best course of action. Luigi said he was convinced his mother would give up and die, if she knew she had cancer. She had nursed her own husband through pancreatic cancer and had seen him suffer greatly. Dr Barratt listened carefully and validated his concerns. 'I can see that this is very hard for you and that you are very concerned about your mother. What do you think she already knows about her illness?' Luigi insisted that his mother did not know what was wrong with her – he had been present at all her appointments and had told her it was a benign growth. Dr Barratt acknowledged that he understood that in their culture families often do not disclose information about serious illness but also said that, in his experience, patients often know or suspect anyway. He also noted that Francesca's breast cancer appeared to be at an early stage, and could well be cured by surgery and chemotherapy. He suggested that Francesca may be imagining that things were much worse. He also said that if Francesca asked him a direct question he would have to answer her honestly as it would not be fair to her or him not to be truthful. He proposed that during the consultation, with the family present, he would ask Francesca what she knew about her disease and what she wanted to know. If she did not want to know anything he would also respect that. Luigi agreed with this approach.

During the consultation, Dr Barratt used an experienced Italian translator who quickly made Francesca feel at home. Dr Barratt asked Francesca what she thought was wrong with her, and she said she was worried she might have cancer. She said she was very worried about having to have chemotherapy, as her husband had suffered greatly with side effects and then died anyway. Luigi and his wife became teary and held Francesca's hands. Dr Barratt told Francesca that she did have cancer, but the lump was small, and it was likely that surgery and chemotherapy could cure her. He told her that the hospital team would support her in coping with the treatment, and that the chemotherapy she would receive was well-tolerated by most people. He then told her that her family loved her very much

continued ›

Practice example 18.2 continued ›

and had been worried she would not cope with the truth. Francesca said that indeed it was a relief to know the truth. Dr Barratt outlined the treatment plan. He turned to Luigi and his wife and said that he hoped they were comfortable with the way things had gone. They expressed gratitude for the care and support he had given them. Dr Barratt gave Francesca some written information about breast cancer in Italian, and a number to ring where she could speak to an Italian-speaking social worker if she would like more support.

Reflective questions

1. If you were Luigi, would you agree to the doctor asking your mother what her understanding of her illness was? What helped Luigi to agree to this approach?
2. Imagine you became ill in a country where you did not speak the language (perhaps while travelling). What would you do to ensure you got the best health care? What services do you think you should be offered in that country, to support you?

Further reading

Hsieh, K., & Gramer, E. M. (2012). Medical interpreters as tools: Dangers and challenges in the utilitarian approach to interpreters' roles and functions. *Patient Education and Counseling*, *89*(1), 158–162.

This article sets out some of the most common problems facing interpreters, and explains how a simple utilitarian view of the service that interpreters' provide risks ignoring these common problems.

Speigel, D. (Ed.). (2005). *Cancer, communication and culture*. New York: Kluwer Academic/ Plenum Publishers.

This book contains a number of chapters that delve into the various aspects of communicating with cancer patients.

Surbone, A., & Kagawa-Singer, M. (2013). Culture matters as well. *Journal of Clinical Oncology*, *31* (22), 2832–2833.

This article argues that engaging with patients' cultural background is critical to determining how we should communicate with them about cancer treatments, plans and prognoses.

Web resources

National Institutes of Health, *Cultural competency*: http://www.nih.gov/clearcommunication/ culturalcompetency.htm

NSW Multicultural Health Communication, *Service, Signs, symbols and communication tools*:
   http://www.mhcs.health.nsw.gov.au/publicationsandresources/signsandsymbols/pdf/
   sands/s-spdfs/s-s-catalogue.pdf

Queensland Health, *Multicultural clinical support resource*: http://www.health.qld.gov.au/
   multicultural/support_tools/mcsr.asp

....

References

Angelelli, C. V. (2004). *Medical interpreting and cross-cultural communication*. Cambridge:
   Cambridge University Press.

Australian Bureau of Statistics (n.d.) Migration, Australia, 2011–12 and 2012–13.
   Cat. no.: 3412.0. Retrieved from http://www.abs.gov.au/ausstats/abs@.nsf/
   Lookup/3412.0Chapter12011–12%20and%202012–13

Butow, P., Eisenbruch, M., Goldstein, D., Duggal-Beri, P., Jefford, M., Schofield, P. et al. Unmet
   needs in Chinese, Greek and Arabic speaking cancer patients in Australia. *Psycho-oncology*,
   16(9), S77–S78.

Butow, P., Aldridge, L. J., Bell, M. L., Sze, M., Eisenbruch, M., Jefford, M. et al. (2013). Inferior
   health-related quality of life and psychological well-being in immigrant
   cancer survivors: A population based study. *European Journal of Cancer*, *49*(8),
   1948–1956.

Butow, P., & Baile, W. (2012). Communication in cancer care: A cultural perspective. In
   L. Grassi & M. Riba (Eds.), *Clinical Psycho-Oncology: An International Perspective*.
   Chichester: Wiley-Blackwell.

Butow, P. N., Bell, M. L., Goldstein, D., Sze, M., Aldridge, L. J., Abdo, S. et al. (2011). Grappling
   with cultural differences; Communication between oncologists and immigrant cancer
   patients. *Patient Education and Counseling*, *84*(3), 398–405.

Butow, P. N., Goldstein, D., Bell, M. L., Sze, M, Aldridge, L. J., Abdo, S., Mikhail, M. et al.
   (2011). Interpretation in consultations with immigrant cancer patients. How accurate is it?
   Journal of Clinical Oncology, *29*(20), 2801–2807.

Butow, P. N., Sze, M., Dugal-Beri, P., Mikhail, M., Eisenbruch, M., Jefford, M. et al. (2010).
   From inside the bubble: Immigrant's perceptions of communication with the cancer team.
   Supportive Care in Cancer, *19*(2), 281–290.

Butow, P. N., Sze, M., Eisenbruch, M., Bell, M. L., Aldridge, L. J., Abdo, S., Tanious, M.,
   et al. (2013). Should culture affect practice? A comparison of prognostic discussions in
   consultations with immigrant versus native-born cancer patients. *Patient Education and
   Counseling*, *92*(2), 246–252.

Chu, K. C., Miller, B. A., & Springfield, S. A. (2007). Measures of racial/ethnic health disparities
   in cancer mortality rates and the influence of socioeconomic status. *Journal of the National
   Medical Association*, *99*, 1092–1100.

Ethnic Communities' Council of Victoria (ECCV). (2012). *An investment not an expense:
   Enhancing health literacy in culturally and linguistically diverse communities*. Carlton:
   Ethnic Communities' Council of Victoria.

Hsieh, E. (2006). Conflicts in how interpreters manage their roles in provider–patient
   interactions. *Social Science & Medicine*, *62*, 721–730.

—— (2007). Interpreters as co-diagnosticians: Overlapping roles and services between providers and interpreters. *Social Science & Medicine, 64*(4), 924–937.

Huang, X., Butow, P.N., Meiser, M., & Goldstein, D. (1999). Communicating in a multi-cultural society: The needs of Chinese cancer patients in Australia. *Australian and New Zealand Journal of Medicine, 29*, 207–213.

Institute of Medicine of the National Academies. (2004). *Health literacy: A prescription to end confusion*. Washington, DC: National Academies Press.

International Medical Interpreters Association and Education Development Center. (1995). Medical interpreting standards of practice. Boston, MA: International Medical Interpreters Association.

Janz, N. K., Mujahid, M. S., Hawley, S. T., Griggs, J. J., Alderman, A., Hamilton, A. S. et al. Racial/ethnic differences in quality of life after diagnosis of breast cancer. *Journal of Cancer Survivorship, 3*(4), 212–222.

Johnstone, M., & Kanitsaki, O. (2007). An exploration of the notion and nature of the construct of cultural safety and its applicability to the Australian health context. *Journal of Transcultural Nursing, 18*, 247–256.

Luckett, T., Goldstein, D., Butow, P.N., Gebski, V., Aldridge, L. J., McGrane, J. et al. (2011). Psychological morbidity and quality of life of ethnic minority patients with cancer: A systematic review and meta-analysis. *Lancet Oncology, 12*, 1240–1248.

Moore, R., & Butow, P. (2005). Culture and oncology: Impact of context effects. In D. Speigel (Ed.), *Cancer, communication and culture*. New York: Kluwer Academic/Plenum Publishers.

Nutbeam, D. (2009). Defining and measuring health literacy: What can we learn from literacy studies? *International Journal of Public Health, 54*(5), 303–305.

Ong, L. M. L, De Haes, J. C. J. M., Hoos, A.M. , & Lams, F.B. (1995). Doctor–patient communication: A review of the literature. *Soc Sci Med, 40*, 903–918.

Schere, K. R., Clark-Polner, E., & Mortillaro, M. (2011). In the eye of the beholder? University and cultural specificity in the expression and perception of emotion. *International Journal of Psychology, 46*(6), 401–435.

Surbone, A. (2008). Cultural aspects of cancer care. *Support Care Cancer, 16*(3), 235–240.

Surbone, A., Zwitter, M., Rajer, M., & Stiefel, R. (Eds.) (2013). *New challenges in communication with cancer patients*. New York: Springer.

Tan, T. K., Teo, F. C., Wong, K., & Lim, H. L. (1993). Cancer: To tell or not to tell? *Singapore Medical Journal, 34*(3), 202–203.

Tchen, N., Bedard, P., Yi, Q. L., Klein, M., Cella, D., Eremenco, S., & Tannock I. F. (2003). Quality of life and understanding of disease status among cancer patients of different ethnic origin. *British Journal of Cancer, 89*(4), 641–647.

Treloar, C., Gray, R., Brener, L., Jackson, C., Saunders, V., Johnson, P. et al. (2014). 'I can't do this, it's too much': Building social inclusion in cancer diagnosis and treatment experiences of Aboriginal people, their carers and health workers. *International Journal of Public Health, 59*(2),373–9. doi:10.1007/s00038–013–0466–1

US Department of Health and Human Services. (2010). Healthy people 2010:*Understanding and improving health*. Washington DC: US Government Printing Office.

Yip, M.-P. (2012). A health literacy model for limited English speaking populations: Sources, context, process and outcomes. *Contemporary Nurse, 40*(2), 160–168.

19

Communicating empathy in the face of pain and suffering

Catherine O'Grady and Aileen Collier

Learning objectives

This chapter will enable you to:
- define empathy as it plays out (and should play out) in clinical situations;
- understand the potential impact of empathic communication on the direction and outcomes of a clinical encounter;
- identify the actions of clinicians, patients and family members that can generate empathy;
- consider actions that can undermine the accomplishment of empathy;
- develop the ability to reflect on your own practice so as to effectively communicate empathy.

Key terms

Emotional resonance
Empathy
General practice
Palliative care
Professional judgment
Sympathy
Tender directiveness

Overview

This chapter examines the communication of **empathy** in two clinical contexts: **general practice** and **palliative care**. Drawing upon transcripts from these two settings, it illustrates how empathy can be accomplished in actual interactions with other people. The chapter demonstrates that empathy, once achieved, has consequences for relationship-building between practitioner and patient or family member. The chapter also demonstrates the effect of empathy on the type and quality of the medical and psycho-social information that the patient may offer. Empathy is shown to lead to more accurate sharing and perception of the patient's psycho-social state, more responsive therapies, improved outcomes, and better care.

The chapter highlights the collaborative basis of empathic communication. Through empathic collaboration between the health professional and the patient, the patient can more easily share overt as well as subtle clues about their underlying state. An empathic response on the clinician's part resonates with the patient's feelings, and tends to elicit a response from the patient to show that they feel understood.

> **empathy**
> a mental state whereby a person, experiencing compassion, shows they are affected by another person's suffering, and takes steps to alleviate that person's suffering.
>
> **general practice**
> that area of medicine that is available to us in the community when we have minor ailments, or ailments whose nature and severity are as yet unclear and need the attention of a general practitioner (GP).
>
> **palliative care**
> care that focuses on alleviating pain and suffering for patients who have no chance of ever being cured from their illness, and who face imminent death.

The chapter further outlines the dangers of a pre-learned, 'stock empathic' response from the clinician that fails to reflect and focus on the patient's feelings. The chapter illustrates how empathy may involve gesture, gaze and touch in concert with or in place of words. By bringing to light what makes for the effective communication of empathy, the chapter generates useful tools for reflecting on your own practice as a health professional.

Introduction

Within the healthcare world, empathy is regarded as a skill that is at the heart of caring and central to achieving patient-centred care (Frankel, 2009). The importance of empathy goes well beyond being friendly with people, or making people feel welcome. Indeed, empathy has real and significant outcomes for all involved in care.

Some studies of clinical communication link empathy to improved clinical outcomes (Hojat, 2007). These improved outcomes are the result of patients being encouraged – through the empathic attitude of health professionals – to provide more detailed information about their medical, social and emotional concerns (Beckman & Frankel, 1984). Where a clinician is empathic, patients are also more likely to adhere to treatments and to follow advice about how to manage their conditions (Squier, 1990). In addition, empathy leads not just to greater patient satisfaction and clinician–patient trust, but to improved health status (Stewart, 1995; Stewart et al., 2000) and enhanced quality of life (Ong, Visser, Lammes, & De Haes, 2000). Clearly, empathy has positive clinical and health effects. But what exactly is empathy and how is it conceptualised by practitioners?

Empathy has been defined as the ability 'to sense the client's private world as if it were your own, but without losing the "as if" quality' (Rogers, 1961, p. 284). The words 'as if' are significant in this definition, because they reflect an important distinction between *sympathy* and *empathy* (Barrett-Lennard, 1981). **Sympathy** is an affective state that involves sharing the other person's feelings. By contrast, empathy is an intellectual attribute that involves:

> **sympathy**
> an affective state that involves sharing the feelings and emotions of the other person. Sympathy may involve disclosure of similar experiences of one's own.

- a conscious awareness of the patient's emotions and situation;
- an ability to act on that awareness in ways that key in to the patient's feeling and concerns, while remaining clinically focused and appropriately therapeutic.

Yet empathy does not suggest detachment. To recognise a patient's situation and to respond to that patient in ways that resonate with their emotions implies 'awareness of the range and complexity of the patient's feelings and of the issues to which they relate'. To achieve this awareness 'involves seeking to understand what it would be like to be that person, living that person's life and feeling the way that he or she does' (Usherwood, 1999, p. 28).

Emotional resonance

In practice, empathy means maintaining 'a dual perspective' (Ruusuvuori, 2005, p. 205). A 'dual perspective' involves imagining oneself in the same situation as the one the patient is in, so as to achieve a sensitive and detailed understanding of their feelings. Such understanding is what we also refer to as **emotional resonance** (Halpern, 1993). Emotional resonance occurs when we are sensitised to others' feelings without forgetting that these feelings are not our own.

> **emotional resonance**
> a term introduced by Halpern (1993) to describe an empathic response that resonates accurately with the patient's emotions. This is because it is invested with the clinician's emotional engagement with the patient and informed by their detailed understanding of the patient's experience.

But how are emotional resonance and empathy actually accomplished between people, and what do they look and sound like? Neither emotional resonance nor empathy are simply attitudes or 'predispositions' that the clinician brings to their encounter with a patient. Rather, emotional resonance and empathy are developed *collaboratively* as patient and clinician engage with each other. As our practice examples illustrate, both emotional resonance and empathy are *activities* that patient and clinician or clinician and family member jointly achieve in practice and by way of interaction.

Practice example 19.1

Here is an extract from a type of general practice consultation that many clinicians consider to be particularly challenging. Such consultation is one where the patient's stated reason for coming to see the doctor masks other, often deeper psychological or emotional issues, or issues that are less easily openly expressed (O'Grady, 2011a). Empathy plays a crucial role in precisely such consultations. Empathy may generate an 'emotional resonance' through which the patient feels safe to bring underlying worries and issues into the open, so that these worries and issues can be discussed and addressed.

In the case study below, the patient is a 58-year-old woman who begins the interaction by asking for advice about ovarian cancer screening. She has had a single panic attack in the past and the doctor is aware of this. As the consultation unfolds, there are hints of a more pervasive anxiety and serious depression.

In the opening moments of the consultation, doctor (D) and patient (P) have discussed the abdominal symptoms that have led to the patient's request for cancer screening. The doctor has displayed sensitivity to the patient's concerns and has gone on to share the medical reasoning that would lead her to attribute the patient's symptoms to a pre-existing and benign condition. By the time the practice example begins, concern about ovarian cancer has been put to rest and the doctor moves to open up discussion about other issues.

D: All right, so how are you apart from that? That's one worry.

P: Um pretty good but you know when I came last time I told you I had ... you said I had, you thought I had a panic attack.

D: Yeah. [Sits back from the desk, takes hands off paper records and places them on lap, focuses gaze on the patient]

P: And I still sort of get that feeling ... inside. [Shrugs shoulders]

D: [Leans forward elbows on desk and hands cupping her face]

P: [Shrugs shoulders again]

D: It's a rotten thing ... rotten.

P: Hh.

D: Tell me about the feeling.

P   [Indicates chest] Um ... seem PK during the day.

D   Yeah.

P   But when I get into bed at night not relaxed ... it sort of goes chooooo. [Gestures to indicate fluttering feeling over chest and abdomen; slight shrug]

D   What's your head doing in that time?

P   That seems to be OK, just sort of [pats stomach and chest] in here sort of thing. [Shifts posture quickly in seat]

D   So is your heart beating strangely? [Enacts beating gesture across own heart]

P   A little bit yeah.

D   Mm.

Analysis and reflection

This part of the interaction has been selected for attention here as it is 'a critical moment' in the consultation (Candlin, 1987). It is a moment when emotionally sensitive and clinically significant information is being gingerly broached by the patient, and when an insensitive response on the doctor's part could have led to her retreat into silence. Note how the patient raises the matter of panic attack obliquely: '… you said I had, you thought I had a panic attack.' She appears reluctant to own such a diagnosis, presenting it as the doctor's assessment of her condition rather than her own.

At this point the doctor might have responded by providing reasons for this assessment. She might have gone on to ask a series of diagnostic questions in order to pursue the provisional diagnosis of panic attack. Instead, she chooses to be silent and attentive. This is important. The doctor's silence invites the patient to continue: 'Yeah. [Sits back from the desk, takes hands off paper records and places them on lap, focuses gaze on the patient]'. The doctor's silence, together with her focused gaze and attentive body language, encourages the patient to elaborate.

The patient responds tentatively, offering her symptoms in rather vague language: 'sort of'. Her apologetic shrugs, pauses, quavering voice and intake of breath all underline her discomfort as she attempts to talk about her experience. These subtle signs suggest feelings of disquiet. If the doctor reads these signs and responds to them with silence, inviting the patient to elaborate, she capitalises on those signs as offering an 'empathic opportunity' (Suchman et al., 1997). An empathic opportunity is offered by the patient by presenting a hint about or a clue to her emotional state. If the doctor responds to such a hint or clue, inviting more from the patient, the doctor shows empathy.

Critical to achieving empathy is acknowledging the patient's right to determine the direction of the conversation. Such acknowledgment is made apparent here by the doctor's attentive silence and interested gaze. By saying nothing, reorienting her body towards the patient, intensifying her gaze and looking interested, the doctor heightens her engagement with the patient. Then, as the patient shrugs apologetically once more, the doctor transforms the patient's understated, hesitant account of her experience with an utterance that seems to resonate with its true intensity: 'It's a rotten thing … rotten.'

With a small intake of breath the patient acknowledges this assessment of her state as 'rotten'. This assessment made by the doctor resonates with feelings that the patient was unable or unwilling to voice. It displays the doctor's awareness and emotional acknowledgment of the patient's experience. The patient's intake of breath indicates that the doctor's assessment acts as an empathic response: the doctor's assessment and the patient's response 'resonate'. Thus, here we have an example of how empathy results in 'emotional resonance' (Halpern, 1993).

For its part, the emotional resonance diffuses the patient's embarrassment and discomfort. The patient's experience of recurring panic attacks is now out in the open as a matter that can be talked about quite freely. The emotional resonance moves the conversation into a franker tenor. By asking the patient, 'Tell me about the feeling', the doctor confirms her personal engagement with the patient, while not losing sight of the patient's symptoms. This triggers a response from the patient in which she provides a more detailed, clinically useful description of her symptoms. It ushers in a series of more focused diagnostic questions and responses through which the character and intensity of her experience of debilitating panic attack begin to emerge.

Reflective questions

1. Why do you think the patient might not readily be open about her underlying worries with her doctor? Have you ever felt similarly unable to be open about specific things when attending your doctor?
2. Can you imagine a doctor choosing to respond differently to the patient's mention of a panic attack? What might a less empathic doctor have said?
3. What was the effect of the doctor's silence?
4. What if the doctor had responded differently, such as by elaborating upon her provisional diagnosis of panic attack or asking further diagnostic questions? How might these choices have altered the direction of the consultation?
5. What does this extract tell you about how empathy is achieved in interaction?
6. What does it tell you about the effects of empathy?

Implications for practice

Patients seldom raise emotional concerns without prompting (Beach & LeBaron, 2002; O'Grady, 2011a; Suchman et al., 1997). Rather, they tend to offer subtle verbal or nonverbal clues to signal any kind of underlying emotional distress. Such clues include indirect or 'oblique' references (for example, '… you thought I had a panic attack'), hesitations, quavering voice, and embarrassed shrugs such as we saw above. Sometimes a clinician may allow such clues to a patient's emotional state to pass without acknowledgment. Or the clinician might divert the consultation to a medical or scientific topic and expand on 'the evidence' or pursue the biomedical agenda through more diagnostic questioning. If these things happen, emotional and life-world matters of potential clinical significance are likely to remain hidden and unaddressed.

Clearly, in such contexts, the communication of empathy has important clinical work to do. A clinician's empathic response resonates with the patient's experience and confirms feelings that the patient has been unable to voice. As seen in practice example 19.1, such a response can put the interaction onto a new footing, allowing for franker discussion of the patient's personal experience. It should be clear now that empathic communication can alter the direction and outcomes of a consultation. A study that includes an analysis of the whole consultation from which practice example 19.1 is drawn reveals how the doctor's empathic responses accomplish a gradual transition from presenting problems that were biomedical in nature, such as abdominal bloating, to increasingly delicate matters, including debilitating panic attacks and, as emerges later in the consultation, serious clinical depression (O'Grady, 2011b).

More generally, empathy creates an interactional environment wherein patients are likely to talk more and more easily about their symptoms and concerns. This assists the clinician with collecting detailed information about all kinds of medical, life-world and emotional matters. In turn, this can lead to more accurate perceptions of the patient's medical and psycho-social state, more specific and responsive therapies, and ultimately, improved health outcomes (Neumann et al., 2009, p. 342).

Theoretical links

Empathy is sometimes seen as an intrinsic disposition or personality trait that a clinician might bring to their encounter with a patient. This chapter takes a different view of empathy. Here, *empathy is seen as a collaborative activity* that patient and clinician accomplish together. Such a view aligns with a model of empathy that has been very influential in clinical education (Suchman et al., 1997). In developing their theory of empathy, Suchman and his colleagues examined large numbers of recorded primary care consultations to locate sequences where patients expressed emotions, directly or indirectly, and where clinicians responded to or terminated these opportunities for empathy. From this analysis they generated a theoretical model that displayed those moves in an interactional sequence that led to the achievement of, or failure to achieve, empathy. Empathy emerged as an interactional activity involving a patient's implicit or explicit cue for emotional support, an empathic response from the clinician, and acknowledgement from the patient to indicate that their situation has been accurately perceived and responded to. As we also saw in practice example 19.1, empathy is thus an outcome of mutual engagement and responsive interaction.

In clinical contexts, however, effective empathy involves more than the ability to perceive, understand and respond to a patient's feelings. It also requires the capacity 'to act on that understanding with the patient in a helpful (therapeutic) way' (Mercer & Reynolds, 2002, p. 11). In light of this, recent models of empathic communication have expanded beyond the empathic sequence to encompass the effects and consequences of empathy. The 'effect model of empathic communication' (Neumann et al., 2009) demonstrates that empathy has immediate positive effects not only on relationship-building, but also on the direction and trajectory of a consultation, as illustrated in practice example 19.1.

Conclusion

This chapter has provided you with the opportunity to reflect upon empathic communication as it plays out in a challenging general practice consultation involving a patient with underlying emotional and psychological concerns. You will have noted the mechanisms for achieving empathy that involve not just words but also bodily actions including gaze, gesture and shifts in body orientation. These actions function in concert with words to heighten engagement with the patient at critical moments. You will have seen the impact of an empathic response that resonates accurately with the patient's feelings at a particular moment to display the doctor's understanding of the patient's experience. Perhaps you have contrasted such a response with the stock expressions of empathy that are sometimes provided in clinical communication training. Such standardised, decontextualised phrases might not be appropriate in a particular interactional context and so need to be used judiciously. Where a clinician's response fails to reflect the patient's feelings at a particular moment of interaction, it may be perceived by the patient as a sign that the clinician is not attending and has not grasped their true state of mind. Routine and rehearsed phrases can suggest 'the detached physician'; they can undermine 'emotional resonance', and run counter to the achievement of empathy (O'Grady, 2011a, p. 87).

While practice example 19.1 has given you clues about how to achieve empathy in interaction, the example is not intended to provide you with a script to follow. Empathy is accomplished through responsive, collaborative interaction, and each clinical encounter is unique. Language and behaviours that are effective at a specific moment in one clinical encounter may not readily apply in another. Nevertheless, engaging with practice examples enables you to see, appreciate and critique what experienced colleagues do to accomplish empathy. Such engagement expands the repertoire of resources available to you as you reflect in and on your own practice. It assists you to develop **professional judgment** (Schön, 1983), a faculty that can be relied upon to inform your own choices as you develop empathy with your own patients.

> **professional judgment**
> a faculty that practitioners develop over time as they build up a repertoire of experiences, actions and examples that guide and inform their actions and choices in subsequent situations (Schön, 1983).

With this in mind, we will now turn to a second practice example, which will examine how empathy is accomplished in another clinical context, that of palliative care.

Practice example 19.2

Here is a field-note extract from an observation of an interaction between a dying patient, her daughter and the hospital palliative care nurse. Again, empathy plays a crucial role in the interaction by generating an interactional environment wherein care and possible symptom issues can be addressed and the daughter of a dying person feels supported.

We (the researcher[1] and the palliative care nurse) enter the four-bed bay where the elderly patient whom the palliative care nurse (PCN) has come to see is in the corner bed, beside the window. The curtain between her and the next patient is closed. It is clear to me that she (the patient) is dying. The patient's daughter is sitting at the table beside the window. The PCN introduces me (the researcher) and asks permission for me to be present during the consultation. The patient's daughter responds affirmatively, stressing,

continued ›

Practice example 19.2 continued ›

'I would be lost without [she names the PCN]'. The nurse sits down alongside the patient's daughter, asking how both she and her mother are. She carefully listens as the patient's daughter, choked with tears, expresses that she feels her mother's condition is deteriorating. The nurse, reaching forward, nods in response. She (the daughter) conveys to the nurse that she is particularly concerned that her mother is thirsty and that her mouth seems very dry. The nurse moves towards the bedside followed by the patient's daughter, the nurse positioning herself at one side of the bed while the daughter is on the other. I watch on as the nurse gently sprays some water into the patient's mouth explaining what she is doing while gently stroking her (the patient's) head. There is what I would describe as a **tender directiveness** in the interaction: the nurse takes the lead, but does so in a tender way.

> **tender directiveness**
> the ability to take direct action in a warm, sensitive manner and in empathic response to a person's concerns.

The patient obviously appreciates the water. Yet she (the patient) also appears agitated, trying to remove the bed covers. Her daughter expresses concern. The PCN nods, proposing that she (the patient) may just be too hot, and at the same time removes the blanket. The patient's daughter interjects: 'I think her legs might be itchy.' 'If she is itchy then we can use this,' replies the PCN, reaching for the bottle of moisturiser. I watch on as she (the nurse) dispenses some cream into her hand passing the container across the bed to the patient's daughter to do the same. In mirror image they stand at either side of the bed rubbing the cream gently into the dying woman's arms. I feel 'touched' as I watch the actions of the patient's daughter and the nurse in what appears a moment of intimacy.

Reflective questions

1. How is empathy generated in the interaction between the nurse, patient and her daughter? What does the nurse 'do' as well as 'say'? Consider the role of the nurse's positioning, bodily actions, shifts in body orientation and gestures.
2. How does the patient's daughter respond?
3. What other characteristics does the nurse demonstrate during the empathic encounter with the patient and her daughter?
4. What does this extract tell you about how empathy is communicated?
5. What does it tell you about the effects of empathy?

Further reading

Beach, W., & Dixson, C. (2001). Revealing moments: Formulating understandings of adverse experiences in a health appraisal interview. *Social Science & Medicine, 52*(1), 25–44.

This study of a single health encounter focuses on the role of empathy in bringing to light a patient's hidden concerns. Using conversational analysis the researchers show how empathic formulations, deployed collaboratively by patient and interviewer, accomplish the gradual transition from presenting problems that are biomedical in nature to delicate life-world issues, including abuse.

Bikker, A., Cotton, P., & Mercer, S. (2014). *Embracing empathy: A universal approach to person-centred empathic healthcare encounters.* Oxford: Radcliffe Health.
Based on a broad definition of relational empathy in clinical contexts, this book, which includes exercises and videoclips, focuses on understanding the patient's situation, perspective and feelings, and communicating and acting on this understanding in a beneficial way.

O'Grady, C. (2011). Teaching the communication of empathy in patient-centred medicine. In B. Hoekje & S. Tipton (Eds.), *English language and the medical profession: Instructing and assessing the communication skills of international physicians.* Bingley: Emerald Group Publishing.
Drawing upon close analysis of the discourse of a challenging general practice consultation, this book chapter describes how clinically effective empathy is accomplished by interaction. With reference to this analysis, it illustrates a learning approach that makes use of authentic discourse data to enhance the ability of clinicians to communicate empathy.

Sobel, R. (2008). Beyond empathy. *Perspectives in Biology and Medicine, 51*(3), 471–478.
This engaging essay focuses on the individual ingredients of a successful patient–clinician encounter, including empathy. These ingredients encompass scientific competence, imagination as the basis for empathy, care, and attentive, non-judgmental listening.

Web resource

The power of empathy, a lecture conducted by Helen Riess, Associate Professor of Psychiatry, Harvard Medical School: http://www.youtube.com/watch?v=baHrcC8B4WM

References

Barrett-Lennard, G. (1981). The empathy cycle: Refinement of a nuclear concept. *Journal of Counseling Psychology, 28,* 91–100.
Beach, W., & LeBaron, C. (2002). Body disclosures: Attending to personal problems and reported sexual abuse during a medical encounter. *Journal of Communication,* September, 617–639.
Beckman, H., & Frankel, R. (1984). The effect of physician behaviour on the collection of data. *Annals of Internal Medicine, 101,* 692–696.
Candlin, C. (1987). Explaining moments of conflict in discourse. In R. Steele & T. Threadgold (Eds.), *Language topics: Essays in honour of Michael Halliday.* Amsterdam: John Benjamin.
Frankel, R. (2009). Empathy research: A complex challenge. *Patient Education and Counseling, 75,* 1–2.

Halpern, J. (1993). Empathy: Using resonance emotions in the service of curiosity. In H. Spiro, M. Curnen, E. Perscel & D. St James (Eds.), *Empathy and the practice of medicine*. New Haven: Yale University Press.

Hojat, M. (2007). *Empathy in patient care. Antecedents, development, measurement and outcomes*. Berlin: Springer.

Mercer, S., & Reynolds, W. (2002). Empathy and quality of care. *British Journal of General Practice, 52*, S9–S12.

Neumann, M., Bensing, J., Mercer, S., Ernstmann, N., Ommen, O., & Pfaff, H. (2009). Analyzing the 'nature' and 'specific effectiveness' of clinical empathy: A theoretical overview and contribution towards a theory-based research agenda. *Patient Education and Counseling, 74*(3), 339–346.

O'Grady, C. (2011a). The nature of expert communication as required for the general practice of medicine – a discourse analytical study. Unpublished doctoral thesis, Department of Linguistics, Macquarie University, Sydney.

—— (2011b). Teaching the communication of empathy in patient-centered medicine. In B. Hoekje & S. Tipton (Eds.), *English language and the medical profession: Instructing and assessing the communication skills of international physicians*. Bingley: Emerald Press.

Ong, L., Visser, M., Lammes, F., & De Haes, J. (2000). Doctor–patient communication and cancer patients' quality of life. *Patient Education and Counseling, 41*, 145–146.

Rogers, C. (1961). *On becoming a person. A therapist's view of psychotherapy*. Boston: Mifflin.

Ruusuvuori, J. (2005). 'Empathy' and 'sympathy' in action: Attending to patient's troubles in Finnish homeopathic and general practice consultations. *Social Psychology Quarterly, 68*(3), 204–222.

Schön, D. (1983). *The reflective practitioner. How professionals think in action*. New York: Basic Books.

Squier, R. (1990). A model of empathic understanding and adherence to treatment regimens in practitioner-patient relationships. *Social Science & Medicine, 30*, 325–329.

Stewart, M. (1995). Effective physician-patient communication and health outcomes: A review. *CMAJ, 152*(9), 1423–1433.

Stewart, M., Brown, J., Donner, A., McWhinney, I., Oates, J., Weston, W. et al. (2000). The impact of patient-centred care on outcomes. *Journal of Family Practice, 49*(9), 796–804.

Suchman, A., Markakis, K., Beckman, H., & Frankel, R. (1997). A model of empathic communication in the medical interview. *JAMA, 277*(8), 678–682.

Usherwood, T. (1999). *Understanding the consultation*. Buckingham: Open University Press.

Note

1 The researcher/observer is the second author of this chapter.

Taking the heat in critical situations: being aware, assertive and heard

Benn Lancman and Christine Jorm

Learning objectives

This chapter will enable you to:
- explain why health care operates with significant uncertainty;
- discuss the responsibility of all team members to strive for best patient outcomes;
- articulate why good followers communicate their knowledge and understanding fully and openly to the leader;
- define 'graded assertiveness' as a powerful communication strategy that ensures any conflict remains patient-centred and is more likely to be constructive;
- argue that good leaders encourage their team to enact graded assertiveness and thereby contribute to everyone's situation awareness.

Key terms

Conflict
Graded assertiveness
Hierarchy
Situation awareness
Uncertainty

Overview

Communication in health care is often undertaken under pressure, in conditions of considerable **uncertainty**, and in circumstances where mistakes have significant consequences. The more complex and dynamic the situation, the more difficult it is to have knowledge of all the variables at play. Being aware of context variables is referred to as **situation awareness**. Complex circumstances demand situational awareness, and a commitment to effective, intelligent communication practices.

Increasingly, health care is delivered by teams with members from different specialties. Each team member may bring a unique perspective, skill set and expertise. Each team member has a moral and ethical responsibility to advocate the best outcomes for the patient using their individual expertise and experience. Too often, however, team members lack the communication skills to be effective. Their communication and agency may be impaired by rigid patterns of **hierarchy** and authority.

This chapter explores the challenges of communication in critical situations. It presents an example of care provided to a severely injured motor vehicle accident patient, and of an intraoperative surgical complication. We discuss the technique of **graded assertiveness** to facilitate communication that encounters different kinds of hierarchical constraints.

> **uncertainty**
> the sense of not knowing what will happen next.
>
> **situation awareness**
> the kind of awareness that a person may have of their surrounding context, including people, processes and objects.
>
> **hierarchy**
> different levels of power that people have in formal organisations.
>
> **graded assertiveness**
> assertiveness that becomes stronger and more insistent depending on others' responses.

The chapter claims that graded assertiveness should be seen as a communicative act that all team members have a responsibility to be able to undertake. Indeed, graded assertiveness is presented as critical to enhancing any leader's situation awareness.

Introduction

Health practitioners are required to make a multitude of decisions throughout the day. Each decision requires a combination of knowledge, clinical experience, and awareness of the unique clinical context for that patient. 'Situation awareness' is a concept that refers to a person's or team's understanding of the past, present, and potential futures of a complex situation.

Unlike formal knowledge or expert skills, situation awareness requires ongoing investment to maintain awareness and understanding of a complex situation. Think about driving a car – the skills and knowledge needed to drive are acquired early in your driving experience, but each time you drive you are constantly scanning the mirrors and looking out the windows to maintain your situation awareness.

When there is a rapidly evolving clinical scenario, maintaining situation awareness becomes a major task for team leaders. Any decision a practitioner makes can only be as good as the information upon which it is based. In a team environment, all members contribute information, and this creates 'group situation awareness'. Effective team leaders establish a shared and explicit expectation about team relationships and communication. This ensures that team members will be effective. Effective team members are better at communicating changes in the clinical status of a patient (or other pertinent environmental information) when it matters (Gillespie et al., 2013; Wacker & Kolbe, 2014). This effectiveness manifests as bidirectional communication: it ensures that care is coordinated and that decisions are based on the most up-to-date and accurate information. Too often, however, hierarchy creates communication barriers.

'Speaking up'

Because modern health care is becoming increasingly complex, it needs to be delivered by collaborative and multidisciplinary teams. This means that the quality of how teams function has a significant impact upon the quality and safety of clinical care delivered. Despite our increasing appreciation that all team members play a role in creating safe and high-quality care, there is still reluctance from many practitioners to speak up; even when they do so, sometimes they aren't heard. Admittedly, emergency departments and operating theatres are noisy and highly interruptive environments (Coiera et al., 2002; Grundeiger & Sanderson, 2009; Rivera-Rodriguez & Karsh, 2010; Weigl et al., 2011). But not hearing another team member may be more commonly due to power differentials in the healthcare team than to circumstantial noise. Indeed, the severity of this problem of not hearing another person is likely to be proportional to the importance accorded to people's status in the hierarchy, or the 'hierarchy gradient' that prevails in the organisation.

Organisations that have a steep hierarchy gradient tend to display rigid modes of communication and inflexible decision-making. For example, imagine a ward nurse has a question for the medical team about her patient. She speaks to the nurse in charge, who speaks to the intern, who speaks to the registrar, who speaks to the consultant. Decisions are communicated in an equally linear and hierarchical way. This kind of hierarchical approach to communication and decision-making is often evident in the operating theatre, an environment where communication frequently 'fails' (Lingard et al., 2004; McDonald, Waring & Harrison, 2005).

In organisations that have a less hierarchical approach to communicating and decision-making (that is, a low hierarchy gradient), there are fewer practical, psychological and physical barriers between front-line workers and senior staff. In a ward with a low hierarchy gradient, the same ward nurse would feel comfortable asking her question or communicating her perspective to the consultant directly. Ward practice would routinely accommodate such communication, and there would be fewer psychological barriers (such as fears) and physical barriers (such as closed office doors or junior doctors surrounding the senior consultant) obstructing such communication.

That said, a disadvantage of a low hierarchy gradient can be confusion about who is responsible for taking decisions and a degree of disorganisation during non-routine or dynamic situations such as emergencies. Emergencies do not leave adequate opportunity for dynamically negotiating decision-making roles. Effective teamwork during emergency situations requires clear pre-established leadership roles and lines of authority (Klein, 1998). By the same token, if these roles and lines of authority become *too rigid*, they will diminish the dynamics of team member's responses, and a degree of flexibility is always needed to adequately deal with emerging circumstances. Before going into greater detail about these issues, let us consider practice example 20.1.

Practice example 20.1

This dialogue is between members of a trauma team managing a patient with complex needs following a motor vehicle accident.

'John Doe' is a male in his sixties. He was a front seat passenger in a sedan that was struck by another car at 80 km/hour, the impact on the passenger-side door. He was trapped in the vehicle for about 30 minutes before emergency services could extract him. On arrival at the hospital he was met by the trauma team. His clinical condition was extremely unstable. He required ongoing blood transfusion to maintain a low normal blood pressure. An ultrasound scan of his abdomen identified free fluid (suggestive of internal bleeding). Discussion occurred between anaesthetist and surgeon about the most appropriate place for this patient to go – the operating theatre or the angiography suite.

Anaesthetist: So what's the plan?

Surgeon: Let's get this guy into the scanner and work out what's going on. Probably need to embolise his spleen.

Anaesthetist: Look, I'm needing to pump in a fair bit of blood at the moment. Should we just take him to theatre?

Surgeon: Why should he go to theatre?

Anaesthetist: I think he's quite unstable. Don't we take unstable patients to theatre first?

Surgeon: I don't think he's unstable. I don't really believe those numbers. We are taking him to CT [computed tomography].

Anaesthetist: [Under his breath] What do you classify as unstable then? Full arrest? There's a hospital protocol for this.

The patient is transferred to CT and subsequently to angiography for embolisation of a ruptured spleen. Before the embolisation procedure can begin the patient has a cardiac arrest.

Surgeon: [Swears] What's going on with this guy? There must be something we are missing.

Anaesthetist: No. He's just bleeding to death from his spleen. Now can we take him up to theatre?

Surgeon: If we get him back, then yes.

Analysis and reflection

The practice example demonstrates a clear disconnect between the surgeon's and the anaesthetist's clinical priorities. The surgeon failed to incorporate the anaesthetist's assessment into his own planning, while at the same time the anaesthetist did not make sufficient effort to communicate his impression of the clinical situation.

The correct course of action seems clear in hindsight, but is often not obvious during an uncertain and chaotic trauma scenario. Usually there is little information available about the patient or their injuries upon their arrival to the emergency department. Each clinician in this context is required to make the best of a bad situation.

How could this have been done better? First, in any uncertain situation it is paramount for the team leader to make the best use of the resources available. In this example the surgeon, as team leader, should have placed greater weight on the concerns of the anaesthetist about the patient's instability. Rather than being dismissive of another's concerns, further enquiry ('Why do you think he is unstable?') would have allowed adequate exploration of the issues and a more informed decision about the most appropriate treatment location. There was also the opportunity to involve the team in the surgeon's thinking. Explaining the requirements for the CT scan and negotiating a time for reassessment would have helped maintain a cohesive team and enhanced group situational awareness. For example, questions that could have been asked are: 'Do you think he would cope with a 15-minute CT scan? At the end of the scan we can reassess before going further.'

While the anaesthetist in this scenario identified a clinical concern, he was a poor advocate for the patient, and a poor team member. Rather than muttering under his breath when his concerns were not appreciated at the first communication, there was an opportunity to use hints, probes and the like to ensure that their impression was incorporated into the clinical management. This is referred to as 'graded assertiveness'. Examples might be: 'I am very concerned the patient may arrest soon if we don't take them to theatre'; 'I think this patient meets criteria for urgent surgery. Is there a reason you don't want to operate?'; 'This patient meets the criteria for theatre based on the hospital policy. I am taking the patient to theatre now.'

> **conflict**
> feelings of dislike, disagreement or animosity between people.

Muttering concerns or disagreement is an example of destructive **conflict** and undermines the team leader to the entire team. Such comments are often made to more junior staff and set a very poor example for a highly functioning team. It is not surprising that other trauma team members didn't offer relevant opinions to help with decision-making.

Theoretical links

Despite the centrality of teamwork in health care (see Chapter 1), our teams are more likely to perform poorly compared with those in other industries. Healthcare teams are often formed at a moments' notice, with minimal planning, and with many members who may not even know each others' names and roles, let alone their skills and experience. Edmondson has recently introduced the concept of 'teaming' (Edmondson, 2012) to describe the behaviours necessary for successful function in situations with dynamic, ad hoc teams and multiple team memberships (such as the group of people caring for the trauma patient). The core processes of teaming are 'speaking up', collaboration, experimentation and reflection (Edmondson, 2012).

However, communicating questions and suspicions is difficult for anyone, especially for novice health professionals (Klein, 2006). And yet it is critical that team members ask questions in situations of uncertainty. Novices often have more questions because they 'lack a sense of the dynamics of the situation. They have trouble explaining how the current state of affairs came about and how it will play out' (Klein, 1998, p. 156). They are understandably wary about publicising any uncertainty and anxiety, and may err on the side of silence. This is in no small measure due to the constant social assessment by more senior team members of juniors (Spitzberg, 2013).

When detection of a problem comes from a team member with low credibility, others need to assess whether to ignore or support the query (Klein, 2006). Despite potentially low credibility, junior team members' questions and comments may have significance for enhancing team effectiveness. In effect, their questions and comments are central to enabling decision-makers and team leaders to broaden their situation awareness; such questions and comments enable them to take account of unnoticed and alternative perspectives (Fioraou et al., 2010). To act effectively in complex situations, team members need to pay attention to all possible sources of information, and integrate that information into team action. To promote such expansion of existing perspectives and known information, strategies have been proposed that invite members' questions and comments, including 'self-talk', 'closed-loop communication' and 'leader-inclusiveness' (Gillespie et al., 2013; Wacker & Kolbe, 2014).

Teaming is now a health professional education priority. That is, health professional educators need to develop students' 'followership', leadership and dynamic communication skills. Given the need for dynamic communication and questioning, health professional training without a collaborative focus makes little sense, particularly when it comes to leadership training (Jorm & Parker, 2014).

Pre-registration health-professional education needs to become more interprofessional, to ensure that health professionals, besides commanding adequate expert knowledge and techniques, are also capable of relationships that allow for safe and effective team collaboration. Such relationships are no longer optional: '[T]he increasing complexity of work in hospitals has increased the level of *ad hoc* negotiation that resists formal structure' (Bleakley, 2014, p. 150). Besides formal structures, effective relationships are key to improving the quality, efficiency and success of care in the face of rising uncertainty and complexity (Iedema, Mesman & Carroll, 2013).

Implications for practice

Good communication in critical situations is often equated with strict compliance with predetermined checklists and protocols. Thus, there is much recent enthusiasm for checklists (Gawande, 2009). The basis of this enthusiasm is the assumption that, irrespective of the situation in which professionals find themselves, communicative acts will be both perfect and effective if these acts rigidly adhere to checklists and pro formas. Since protocols followed too strictly may create new and unexpected safety risks, this assumption is highly contestable (Bosk et al., 2009; Rydenfält, Ek & Larsson, 2013). Admirable compliance with checklists may in fact mask ineffective teamwork, fear of conflict, and problematic knowledge gaps (Whyte et al., 2008).

If someone becomes angry because they interpret a novice's question as a challenge to their hierarchical status, their response will further discourage lower-status team members from commenting on what appear to them to be unsafe acts. Particularly 'in confined work areas, such as the operating theatres, even watching rudeness that occurs between colleagues may impair team members' thinking skills' (Flin, 2010). Lower-status professionals may then opt for silence in the face of problematic and unsafe situations to avoid expected conflict (Lingard, 2012).

Silence was found to be the preferred option for 26% of Scottish anaesthetic assistants who said they would not 'speak up' if they disagreed with a decision in theatre. For the remaining 74%, 'speaking up' was limited to asking for the logic behind a decision (Rutherford, Flin & Mitchell, 2012). Implicit in these findings is that 'speaking up' is expected by around a quarter of trainees to incur a negative assessment of their competence, knowledge or intentions (Sutcliffe, Lewton & Rosenthal, 2004).

Here, 'graded assertiveness' offers a method for limiting the chance of conflict while questioning others' actions. Using the 'probe, alert, challenge, emergency action' or PACE approach, our questioning of the actions of higher-status people can be varied from 'low assertiveness' to 'high assertiveness'. The PACE approach provides a structure for junior team members to disguise an important question as a request for education or as curiosity. By avoiding a direct challenge to the team leader the social cost of supporting the problem solving activities is reduced.

The PACE approach has the benefit of informing the team leader about perhaps previously unrecognised or under-appreciated issues, and thereby enhancing the situation awareness of both leader and the team as a whole:

- *Probe:* This is sometimes referred to as a 'hint'. This is a non-confrontational way to open up a dialogue about what appears to be an abnormality. A *probe* is usually framed as a question from the perspective of the person asking another (here for simplicity we will refer to the other as the team leader). The probe may afford the leader an opportunity to either explain what is happening and justify it, or correct their own actions with minimal to no embarrassment, without 'loss of face'. 'I thought we try and keep the blood pressure higher than that...'

'I usually aim for a blood pressure of more than 90 systolic. What targets do you aim for?'

- *Alert:* The next level is to provide the leader with a more direct alert or alternative. Attention is explicitly drawn to the perceived abnormality. It should be coupled with an offer to help solve the problem. This may include getting additional help. An alert assumes that the person in authority has not noticed the problem or is busy dealing with more pressing concerns. 'Did you notice that blood pressure is very low? Would you like me to give some fluid?'. 'The patient's oxygen saturations are low. Would you like me to put some oxygen on?'

- *Challenge:* This is the level that articulates the question as a demand for attention and action. In the authors' experience most issues are dealt with at one of the previous two levels. A *challenge*, however, goes further. It quite directly asks for an explanation for and action in response to a perceived deviation. 'Is there a reason you are happy with such a low blood pressure for this patient?'. 'Can you explain to me why you don't want to treat this low blood pressure?'

- *Emergency action:* When prior attempts to address concerns have failed and the patient remains at what is perceived as an immediate risk, assertive communicative action must be taken. This can be very difficult and intimidating. It is important for the questioner to maintain the focus on the patient, to be clear about their justification for intervening, and framing that justification in a patient-centred manner. 'The blood pressure is dangerously low. I am going to treat it now.' 'In the interest of the patient's safety, you must listen to me now.'

Reflective questions

1. Have you ever noticed something but the person you were trying to tell wouldn't listen or you didn't feel comfortable telling them? This issue could relate to anything: forgetting an ingredient while baking a cake, leaving a door or window open at home, or directions when driving or walking at the shops. How did you handle that? What can you remember about the way that person responded? Did they listen or argue? What constructive feedback would you give them to improve the way they treated you as a 'team member'?

2. Have you ever witnessed conflict between two people about an appropriate course of action? Can you think of an example of constructive conflict and destructive conflict? What things were done well? What could have been done better?

3. Graded escalation is a difficult tool to use at those final stages of assertiveness. How would you feel about 'putting your foot down'? Would you feel comfortable taking control of the situation if the person you were interacting with was your supervisor? What about someone you are supervising? Or a different craft group all together (nursing, medical, allied health)?

Conclusion

Teamwork is challenging at the best of times and, given the rising complexity of contemporary care, is becoming increasingly central to what health professionals do.

Good teamwork involves opportunities for junior health professionals to ask questions and make comments about what is happening, particularly when what is happening is perceived to be wrong or unsafe. Healthcare environments are often busy and chaotic, and this means that all team members need to act as 'eyes and ears' for one another and the team leader. It requires 'moral courage' to speak up, particularly when the workplace atmosphere does not encourage open and constructive dialogue (Bleakley, 2014).

The importance of creating a trusting and engaged atmosphere cannot be overstated. Such an atmosphere encourages questions and thoughtful responses. This chapter has described a technique that will help those who want to ask questions and make comments to become more effective team members. Graded assertiveness is a communication approach that provides a range of communication options for ensuring that patient safety concerns are effectively voiced in a way that also incurs the minimum possible social cost and personal risk.

Practice example 20.2

Read the following example and reflect on the story using the questions below.

Justine is a 28-year-old female who going to have a laparoscopic cholecystectomy (removal of gall bladder via keyhole surgery) for management of an infection due to gallstones. Aside from being overweight she is otherwise medically well. The surgery was booked as an emergency case.

The surgical registrar (SR) has almost finished his training and recently completed a rotation with the upper gastrointestinal surgical service. He informs his consultant (Mr Jones) he feels confident he can complete the operation unassisted and he will call when it is finished.

The surgery commences uneventfully, but due to the patient's weight and the significant number of stones in the gallbladder the operation is technically difficult. The SR makes a decision to pierce the gallbladder and remove the stones. As he is attempting to puncture the gallbladder his instrument slips and causes a significant laceration in the liver, which starts to bleed profusely. The following conversation followed between the SR, anaesthetic registrar (AR) and scrub nurse (SN).

SR: [swears]
AR: What happened?
SR: Nothing. Diathermy up to 120.

continued ›

Practice example 20.2 continued ›

[The SR attempts to stop the bleeding with the electrocautery.]

SN: I don't think that's working.

SR: Give me a second.

SN: Do you want to call Mr Jones?

SR: I said give me a second.

AR: It doesn't look like its stopping. I'm going to call blood bank.

SN: I think Mr Jones would open the abdomen.

SR: I can do this. Is the diathermy up? Why isn't it stopping? Are you sure the diathermy is working? I can't see anything. Give me the suction.

AR: 900 mLs in the sucker. How are you going over there?

SR: ...

Reflective questions

1. Whose responsibility is it to call for help when a situation becomes overwhelming? What happens when a team member is resistant to calling for help? What strategies could you use to overcome that resistance?

2. How could the AR or SN have communicated more effectively to the SR? How would a graded escalation approach be applied to this example?

3. Why do you think the SR was resistant to calling for help? What factors outside the operating theatre (for example, ego or pride) could play a role?

4. The SR was extremely focused on fixing the bleeding complication. What would his situational awareness have been like? What are the consequences of poor situational awareness in this case?

Reflective questions

1. Think of some examples of conflict within a group. How are they similar or different to healthcare communication? Would techniques such as graded assertiveness be helpful in those contexts? What about within a family? A sports team? School or university?

2. Some teams perform well, some teams perform poorly. How can you tell the difference? How would you work to improve future team performance?

3. Health care is an emotionally charged environment. How do you manage destructive conflict behaviour being directed towards you? What steps can you take to protect yourself and your patients from bad communicators?

Further reading

Edmondson, A. (2012). *Teaming: How organizations learn, innovate, and compete in the knowledge economy.* Hoboken NJ: Jossey Bass.
This book provides a broad multi-industry and commercial perspective, most relevant for managers.

Jorm, C. (2012). *Reconstructing medical practice – engagement, professionalism and critical relationships in health care.* Farnham: Ashgate.
This book sets out the prevailing priorities of doctors and describes how these priorities prevent them from acting as effective team members and thus from engaging with 'systems issues'.

Klein, G. (2006). The strengths and limitations of teams for detecting problems. *Cognition, Technology & Work, 8*(4), 227–236.
This article draws from a range of disasters to discuss how teams contribute to appropriate 'sensemaking' and when and how teams can also become sources of distraction.

Spitzberg, B. H. (2013). (Re) Introducing communication competence to the health professions. *Journal of Public Health Research, 2*(3), e23.
This is a thoughtful article focused on understanding the ways communication affects others, in particular patients and families.

Web resource

The silent treatment: http://www.silenttreatmentstudy.com/silencekills

References

Bleakley, A. (2014). Theorizing team process through a foucauldian perspective: Gaining a voice in team activity at the clinical coalface. In A. Bleakley, *Patient-centred medicine in transition* (pp. 149–162). New York: Springer.

Bosk, C., Dixon-Woods, M., Groeschel, C., & Pronovost, P. (2009). The art of medicine: Reality check for checklists. *The Lancet, 374,* 2–3.

Coiera, E. W., Jayasuriya, R. A., Hardy, J., Bannan, A., & Thorpe, M. E. C. (2002). Communication loads on clinical staff in the emergency department. *Medical Journal of Australia, 176,* 415–418.

Edmondson, A. C. (2012). *Teaming: How organizations learn, innovate, and compete in the knowledge economy.* Hoboken NJ: Jossey Bass.

Fioraou, E., Flin, R., Glavin, R., & Patey, R. (2010). Beyond monitoring: Distributed situation awareness in anaesthesia. *British Journal of Anaesthesia, 105,* 83–90.

Flin, R. (2010). Rudeness at work: A threat to patient safety and quality of care. *BMJ, 341,* 212–213.

Gawande, A. (2009). *The checklist manifesto: How to get things right.* New York: Metropolitan Books.

Gillespie, B. M., Gwinner, K., Fairweather, N., & Chaboyer, W. (2013). Building shared situational awareness in surgery through distributed dialog. *Journal of Multidisciplinary Healthcare, 6*, 109.

Grundeiger, T., & Sanderson, P. (2009). Interruptions in healthcare: Theoretical views. *Int J Med Inform., 78*, 298–307.

Iedema, R., Mesman, J., & Carroll, K. (2013). *Visualising health care improvement: Innovation from within*. Oxford: Radcliffe.

Jorm, Christine, & Parker, M. (2014). Medical leadership is the new black: Or is it? *Australian Health Review*. Retrieved from http://www.publish.csiro.au/paper/AH14013

Klein, G. (1998). *Sources of power: How people make decisions*. Cambridge and London: MIT Press.

——. (2006). The strengths and limitations of teams for detecting problems. *Cognition, Technology & Work, 8*(4), 227–236.

Lingard, L. (2012). Productive complications: Emergent ideas in team communication and patient safety. *Nursing leadership (Toronto, Ont.), 25*, 18–23.

Lingard, L., Espin, S., Whyte, S., Regehr, G., Baker, G. R., Reznick, R. et al. (2004). Communication failures in the operating room: An observational classification of recurrent types and effects. *Quality and Safety in Health Care, 13*(5), 330–334.

McDonald, R., Waring, J., & Harrison, S. (2005). 'Balancing risk, that is my life': The politics of risk in a hospital operating theatre department. *Health, Risk & Society, 7*(4), 397–411.

Rivera-Rodriguez, A. J., & Karsh, B. T. (2010). Interruptions and distractions in healthcare: Review and reappraisal. *Qual Saf Health Care, 19*, 304–312.

Rutherford, J. S., Flin, R., & Mitchell, L. (2012). Teamwork, communication, and anaesthetic assistance in Scotland. *British Journal of Anaesthesia, 109*(1), 21–26.

Rydenfält, C., Ek, Å., & Larsson, P. A. (2013). Safety checklist compliance and a false sense of safety: New directions for research. *BMJ Quality & Safety, 23*(3), 183–186.

Spitzberg, B. H. (2013). (Re) Introducing communication competence to the health professions. *Journal of Public Health Research, 2*(3), e23.

Sutcliffe, K., Lewton, E., & Rosenthal, M.. (2004). Communication failures: An insidious contributor to medical mishaps. *Academic Medicine, 79*, 186–194.

Wacker, J., & Kolbe, M. (2014). Leadership and teamwork in anesthesia-making use of human factors to improve clinical performance. *Trends in Anaesthesia and Critical Care, 4*(6), 200–205.

Weigl, M., Muller, A., Zupanc, A., Glaser, J., & Angerer, P. (2011). Hospital doctors' workflow interruptions and activities: An observation study. *BMJ Quality & Safety, 20*(6), 491–497.

Whyte, S., Lingard, L., Espin, S., Baker, G. R., Bohnen, J. Orser, et al. (2008). Paradoxical effects of interprofessional briefings on or team performance. *Cognition, Technology & Work, 10*(4), 287–294.

Part **4**

Regulation and law

21

Communicating about how the safety and quality of care are regulated

Donella Piper, Luke Slawomirski and Rick Iedema

Learning objectives

This chapter will enable you to:

- define the terms 'regulation', 'regulatory entity', 'regulatory mechanisms', 'responsive regulation' and 'professional conduct';
- identify the main entities charged with regulating and communicating safety, and quality in health care;
- discuss and analyse the different regulatory mechanisms aimed at communicating and improving safety and quality;
- reflect on what motivates people to adhere to or contravene regulatory interventions;
- understand the potential regulatory consequences of poor communication on health professionals;
- reflect on what regulatory mechanism you would utilise to respond to a colleague's poor communication and conduct more generally.

Key terms

Professional conduct
Regulation
Regulatory entities
Regulatory mechanisms
Responsive regulation

Overview

The quality and safety of health care in Australia is carefully prescribed and monitored, or, to put this in one word, healthcare quality and safety are *regulated*.

Regulation involves the use of a variety of approaches to steer the flow of events and to control risk (Ayers & Braithwaite, 1992; Healy, 2011). Thus, regulation draws on everything from persuasion (for example, best practice advice: 'It is best to …') to coercion (that is, mandatory practice: 'You must …'). Regulation is therefore a tool for communicating with health professionals about how patient safety can be or must be achieved. Regulation also has special relevance to and consequences for how health professionals and health services communicate with one another, and how they communicate with their patients.

> **regulation**
> the rules and procedures which are issued by government to ensure care is provided in ways that conform with the standards and evidence that are accepted in Australia as defining best practice.

Why does health care need to be regulated, and why can't we rely on healthcare professionals to regulate themselves? The main reasons why patient safety is regulated are to protect the public from harm occasioned by professional practices that fail to meet national standards, to align health professional behaviours with developments and changes in healthcare systems, and to ensure the health professions constantly improve their performance and that of health service providers (Healy, 2011).

A number of **regulatory entities** and regulatory mechanisms have been put in place to improve patient safety and enforce national professional standards. Regulatory entities consist of members from the professions, government, the market and society (Healy, 2011; Runciman, Merry & Walton, 2007). Regulatory entities include professional boards; councils and authorities; departments of health; safety and quality commissions; and institutes, insurance funds and consumer groups.

> **regulatory entities**
> organisations formed to regulate health professional behaviour using regulatory mechanisms.

The **regulatory mechanisms** adopted by these entities to communicate, facilitate and enforce safe, high-quality care range from persuasion through to 'voluntary strategies': continuing education, conferences, improvement projects, and the like. Regulatory mechanisms also include 'command and control' strategies: criminal and civil penalties for lack of adherence to standards and best practice, and boards where licences to practise may be revoked (Ayers & Braithwaite, 1992; Healy & Braithwaite, 2006; Runciman, Merry & Walton, 2007). Success of these mechanisms depends on a combination of factors. Depending on the issue at hand, workplace culture and the nature of the risk, persuasion may be appropriate; at other times, coercion may be needed.

> **regulatory mechanisms**
> the strategies used to regulate health professional behaviour.

This chapter provides an overview of the regulation of safety and quality and how this influences how healthcare professionals communicate with each other and with their patients. The chapter discusses the main regulatory entities and presents three case studies. Overall, the case studies highlight the relevance and impact of regulation on patient safety and professional behaviour and communication. The first two (in practice example 21.1) provide examples of specific regulatory mechanisms that were employed to regulate health professionals' clinical behaviour. They highlight the impact of pre-existing organisational culture and human behaviour on the success (or not) of regulatory mechanisms. The third example (in practice example 21.2) focuses more specifically on how poor health professional communication is regulated, and makes reference to the potential disciplinary consequences of poor communication for health professionals.

Introduction

According to Healy (2011) the main regulatory entities in the Australian health sector are government, civil society, the market and the professions.

In relation to *government*, intergovernmental bodies with responsibilities for safety and quality in health care include the Council of Australian Governments (COAG) and the Standing Council on Health, which comprises health ministers of the states, territories and the commonwealth.

The relevant Commonwealth agencies include the Australian Health Practitioner Regulation Agency (AHPRA), the Australian Commission on Safety and Quality in Health Care (ACSQHC), the Independent Hospital Pricing Authority (IHPA) and the National Health Performance Authority (NHPA). The functions and powers of these agencies is set out in the *National Health Reform Act 2011*.[1]

AHPRA is the national organisation responsible for implementing the National Registration and Accreditation Scheme for health providers across Australia. AHPRA works in partnership with the relevant national boards, such as the Medical Board of Australia. AHPRA and the national boards work to regulate the health professions, and they do so in the public interest.

ACSQHC was initially established in 2006 by the Australian, state and territory governments to lead and coordinate national improvements in safety and quality. It became an independent, statutory authority on 1 July 2011. ACSQHC is not a regulatory body, but its legislated functions include developing health service accreditation standards, as well as clinical standards.

IHPA determines the National Efficient Price (NEP) and the National Efficient Cost (NEC) for public hospital services. These price signals ensure that public hospitals receive funding based on 'unit costs' – the standard costs of a specific treatment. From 1 July 2012, the Australian government has been using the NEP and NEC to determine its funding contribution to local hospital networks (LHNs; also referred to as 'local health districts').

NHPA's responsibility is to report on the performance of public and private hospitals, primary care networks and community care services right across Australia. These reports can be found on the MyHospitals and MyHealthyCommunities websites (see the 'Web resources' section at the end of this chapter).

The Commonwealth Department of Health is the government agency with responsibility for health and health care at a national level. State government agencies include the six state and two territory health departments as well as the various jurisdictions' safety and quality commissions and councils who advise the department of health.

Coroners, healthcare complaints commissioners, the ombudsman and law courts also have a role in communicating and regulating aspects of safety and quality. The coroner may become involved when there is an unexpected death in a health service that falls within the coroner's jurisdiction. Complaints commissioners and the ombudsman become involved when there is a formal complaint about a health professional or health service provider. Law courts become involved when there are allegations that the law has been breached. These entities are discussed in more detail in Chapter 23.

The medical professions' commercial or *market* behaviour is regulated by the Australian Competition and Consumer Commission (ACCC). The ACCC ensures that health professionals' commercial interests do not operate in conflict with their professional duties to their clients and the public (Healy, 2011). In the past, the *health professions* self-regulated via their specific professions council, board and/or college. Because health professional self-regulation was seen to fall short, the professions are now regulated via the federal entity AHPRA. The various professions' councils, boards and/or colleges still conduct **professional conduct** hearings and advise the AHPRA.

Outside of governmental agencies and entities, many non-government *civil society* entities, such as the Consumers Health Forum and interest groups like the Medical Error Action Group, seek to influence and improve how safety and quality are communicated and regulated from a consumer perspective. Most states and territories have local healthcare consumer advocacy bodies.

> **professional conduct**
> all-round proficiency and good conduct.

Responsive regulation

Each of the various entities mentioned utilises a variety of different *regulatory mechanisms*. Adopting a distinction proposed by John Braithwaite and colleagues (2005), Runciman, Merry & Walton (2007) describe regulatory mechanisms as ranging from 'soft' (persuasive) to 'hard' (coercive). 'Soft' strategies are aimed at encouraging certain behaviour and are voluntary in nature. 'Hard' strategies demand and enforce certain behaviour via command and control.

Braithwaite and colleagues (2005) themselves argue that regulatory strategies should be thought of as hierarchical, as depicted in Figure 21.1. Their hierarchy moves from persuasive mechanisms at the bottom of the pyramid to coercive strategies at its top.

Figure 21.1 depicts the responsive regulatory pyramid developed by Braithwaite, Healy & Dwan (2005) and Healy & Braithwaite (2006). According to Healy & Braithwaite (2006), regulatory mechanisms should be responsive to the context, conduct, and culture of those being regulated. This is referred to as **responsive regulation**.

> **responsive regulation**
> the use of mechanisms, strong and weak, such that regulation can be sensitive to the specific contexts and activites that are regulated. This suggests that, rather than issuing only mandatory policies or advisory guidelines, a wide range of regulatory mechanisms whose strength and impact vary is used.

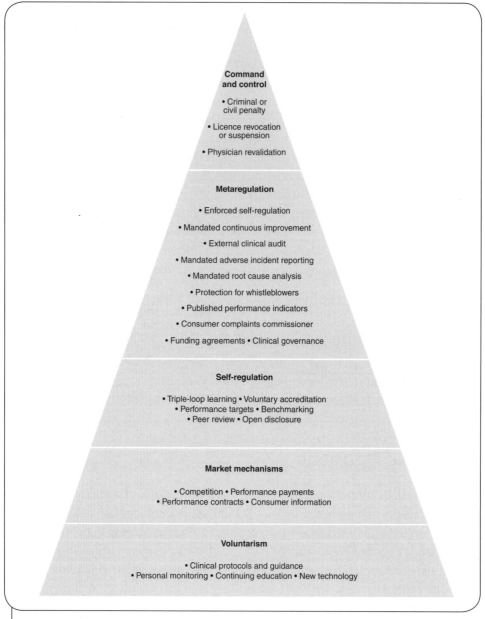

Figure 21.1 The regulatory pyramid and healthcare safety and quality mechanisms (Healy & Braithwaite, 2006)

According to Healy and Braithwaite (2006), the key elements of responsive regulation are:

- the regulator first chooses a mechanism from the base of the pyramid using persuasion;
- a single regulatory mechanism is seldom sufficient as the weaknesses of one mechanism must be complemented by the strengths of another;

- there must be the capacity for regulatory escalation to coercion if persuasion fails (Healy & Braithwaite, 2006).

For Braithwaite, Healy & Dwan, responsive regulation means that 'regulators are more likely to succeed by using [a range of] mechanisms [because] [e]scalating sanctions can be invoked; that is, soft words before hard words, and carrots before sticks' (2005, p. vii). The authors note that:

> The base of the pyramid represents a dialogue-based approach for securing compliance with a just rule or standard where rewards rather than sanctions apply ... As we move up the pyramid, more demanding and punitive strategies are invoked. Persistent infractions elicit a formal request to remedy problems, and possibly entail repeat inspections and the public disclosure of failure to meet standards. Closure or removal of license are a last resort, and signal the failure of both the regulator and the regulatee (the person/organisation being regulated) to ensure that the public is well served. (Braithwaite, Healy & Dwan, 2005, p. xi)

Let us now explore how responsive regulation manifests in healthcare practice. As part of our practice example, we explore two UK case studies that mobilised similar regulatory mechanisms but which produced different effects.

Practice example 21.1 — Communicating about practice regulation

Part 1: Deploying a 'ward level medication safety scorecard'

This example is based upon research conducted by Ramsay and colleagues (2014) in two UK hospitals. The researchers developed and implemented two ward-level medication safety scorecards in conjunction with staff at two English hospitals. The aim of 'scorecards' was to present a visual communication tool to remind staff about safety concerns as outlined on the scorecard. The first scorecard (Scorecard A, Table 21.1) contained medication safety indicators. Non-compliance was coded in red on the scorecard (strikethrough used in table below), and compliance was coded in green (italics). Scores were presented on a weekly basis to staff and each week's performance was compared with the previous week.

Table 21.1 Scorecard A used in Hospital A

XXX ward – medication safety	Target	Previous	Performance	Change
		DD/MM	DD/MM/YYYY	↑=↓
Allergy documentation				
Patients whose allergy documentation was completed	100%	**Z%**	*X/Y (Z%)*	↑=↓

(cont.)

continued ›

Practice example 21.1 continued ›

(Table 21.1 (*cont.*)

XXX ward – medication safety	Target	Previous	Performance	Change
Patients whose allergy symptoms were documented	100%	Z%	X/Y (Z%)	↑=↓
Patients whose allergy documentation was signed	100%	Z%	X/Y (Z%)	↑=↓
Patients whose allergy documentation was dated	100%	Z%	X/Y (Z%)	↑=↓
Patient identification band				
Patients who had an ID band	100%	Z%	X/Y (Z%)	↑=↓
Patients who had an appropriately coloured ID band	100%	Z%	X/Y (Z%)	↑=↓
POD lockers				
Total no. drugs in POD lockers	–	X	Y	
No. drugs labelled for incorrect patient in POD lockers	0%	Z%	X/Y (Z%)	↑=↓
No. unlabelled drugs in POD lockers	0%	Z%	X/Y (Z%)	↑=↓
No. patients whose POD locker contained drugs labelled for incorrect patient	0%	Z%	X/Y (Z%)	↑=↓
No. patients whose POD locker contained unlabelled drugs	0%	Z%	X/Y (Z%)	↑=↓
Drug omissions				
Total drugs prescribed	–	X	Y	
Drug omissions (percentage of drugs prescribed)	0%	Z%	X/Y (Z%)	↑=↓
Unexplained omissions (percentage of omissions)	0%	Z%	X/Y (Z%)	↑=↓

(*cont.*)

continued ›

Practice example 21.1 continued ›

(Table 21.1 (*cont.*)

XXX ward – medication safety	Target	Previous	Performance	Change
Patients who experienced any drug omission	0%	Z%	~~X/Y (Z%)~~	↑=↓
Trigger drugs				
Patients administered Vitamin K	0%	X	X	
Patients administered Octaplex	0%	X	X	
Patients administered FFP	0%	X	X	
Patients administered Naloxone	0%	X	X	
Patients administered Flumenazil	0%	X	X	
Patients administered Glucagon	0%	X	X	
Patients administered any trigger drugs	0%	X	X	
Secure drug storage				
Badge entry to ward required?	Y	Y/N	Y/N	↑=↓
Clinical room locked?	Y	Y/N	Y/N	↑=↓
Drug cupboards locked?	Y/NA	Y/N/NA	Y/N/NA	↑=↓
ID challenged?	Y/NA	Y/N/NA	Y/N/NA	↑=↓
Access to secure drugs				
Morphine ampoules	N/NA	Y/N/NA	Y/N/NA	↑=↓
Midazolam ampoules	N/NA	Y/N/NA	Y/N/NA	↑=↓
Oral diazepam	N/NA	Y/N/NA	Y/N/NA	↑=↓
Oral codeine	N/NA	Y/N/NA	Y/N/NA	↑=↓
Insulin (from fridge)	N/NA	Y/N/NA	Y/N/NA	↑=↓
Safety notices				
Penicillin traffic light poster present	Y	Y	Y/N	↑=↓
Medication safety bulletin present	Y	N	~~Y/N~~	↑=↓
SureMed information present	Y	Y	Y/N	↑=↓

(*cont.*)

continued ›

Practice example 21.1 continued ›

(Table 21.1 (*cont.*)

XXX ward – medication safety	Target	Previous	Performance	Change
	SUMMARY	Indicators that improved	↑	X
		Indicators that stayed the same	=	X
		Indicators that got worse	↓	X

Source: Reproduced from Ramsay et al. (2014)

Based on feedback from staff at both hospitals, the content of the scorecard A was amended for implementation in the second hospital. Scorecard B contained fewer overall indicators, but more indicators in relation to prescribing medication were added. Thus performance for the previous week was coded red for non-compliance (strikethrough used in table below) and green for compliance (italics), as well as being coded amber for part compliance (underline).

Table 21.2 Scorecard B used in Hospital B

XXX ward	Target	Previous	Performance	Change
		DD/MM	DD/MM/YYYY	↑=↓
Allergy and ID bands				
Patients whose allergy status was completed: symptoms documented, signed and dated	100%	X/Y (Z%)	*X/Y (Z%)*	↑=↓
Patients with ID band	100%	X/Y (Z%)	~~X/Y (Z%)~~	↑=↓
Appropriate ID band (if allergy)	100%	X/Y (Z%)	*X/Y (Z%)*	↑=↓
ID bands on same wrist (if allergy)	100%	X/Y (Z%)	~~X/Y (Z%)~~	↑=↓
POD lockers				
Drugs for correct patient in POD locker	100%	X/Y (Z%)	~~X/Y (Z%)~~	↑=↓
Drug omissions				
Doses omitted over the last 24 hours (except code 6)	0%	X/Y (Z%)	~~X/Y (Z%)~~	↑=↓
Unexplained omissions (% of omissions)	0%	X/Y (Z%)	~~X/Y (Z%)~~	↑=↓
'Drug not available' (code 7) for two consecutive omissions (% of omissions)	0%	X/Y (Z%)	*X/Y (Z%)*	↑=↓

continued ›

Practice example 21.1 continued ›

(Table 21.2 (*cont.*)				
XXX ward	**Target**	**Previous**	**Performance**	**Change**
Prescribing				
Prescriptions without prescriber's signature	0%	X/Y (Z%)	X/Y (Z%)	↑=↓
Doses administered without prescriber's signature	0%	X/Y (Z%)	X/Y (Z%)	↑=↓
Once-only prescriptions without drug start time	0%	X/Y (Z%)	X/Y (Z%)	↑=↓
Unacceptable abbreviation of units	0%	X/Y (Z%)	X/Y (Z%)	↑=↓
Brand prescribing (excluding exceptions)	0%	X/Y (Z%)	X/Y (Z%)	↑=↓
	SUMMARY	Indicators that improved	↑	X
		Indicators that stayed the same	=	X
		Indicators that got worse	↓	X

Source: Reproduced from Ramsay et al. (2014)

The scorecards were deployed in both hospitals as part of unannounced visits. Performance on medication safety indicators was measured against the number of times patients were subjected to mis-medication or a medication risk. The researchers found that many patients experienced medication safety risks. Overall, neither hospital saw significant improvement in medication safety as a result of the feedback using the scorecards.

The researchers conducted interviews with staff to try to explain these results. They found that scorecards were not always shared with staff, and feedback meetings did not always take place as planned. Ward managers and leading clinicians did not always engage in the project because of competing priorities. Staff thought the project needed to run for a longer period of time and that there were staffing, hospital reorganisation and resource issues that limited the effect of the scorecards. In addition, there were professional differences in the approach to the scorecards: nurses used the scorecards more consistently than did doctors.

The researchers concluded that ward level medication safety risks are frequent. Communicating evidence of medication errors using scorecards may encourage awareness of medication safety risks, but it has limited effect on service performance. The main reason for this is that organisational processes, context and professional cultures play a very big role in how health professionals behave, and to what they decide to respond. Regulatory mechanisms must take these organisational, contextual and cultural factors into account if they are to be successful in changing behaviour.

continued ›

Practice example 21.1 continued ›

Part 2: Reduced mortality with hospital pay for performance

This example is based upon research conducted by Sutton and colleagues (2012), also in the UK. The researchers evaluated Advancing Quality (AQ), a financial incentive scheme to improve care across hospitals in northern England. AQ is an example of a pay-for-performance program – a program that awards services funding on the basis of their performance on quality and safety measures. Pay-for-performance programs have been adopted internationally, despite equivocal evidence that they improve patient outcomes.

The researchers analysed 30-day in-hospital mortality among 134 435 patients admitted for pneumonia, heart failure, or acute myocardial infarction to 24 hospitals covered by the pay-for-performance program. They compared mortality rates for 18 months before and 18 months after the introduction of the program.

AQ resulted in a significant reduction in patient mortality at 18 months after implementation.

One of the reasons put forward by the authors for this result was that the size of the incentive payment was slightly larger than in previously reported schemes. Other non-financial reasons included the approach to implementation and the context in which the programs were introduced and communicated. While hospitals were competing with one another, collaboration was encouraged via a 'tournament style' approach. Collaboration was facilitated by staff from all participating hospitals meeting face to face at regular intervals to share problems and learning. Participation of all hospitals within a region rather than a select few and the smaller size of the program were also cited as factors of success.

Although a follow-up evaluation indicated that these improvements were not maintained at 42 months post-implementation, a significant fall in patient mortality for conditions not covered by the AQ initiative was observed at 42 months in participating hospitals, raising the possibility of a positive spill-over effect of the scheme to other clinical areas (Kristensen et al., 2014).

Analysis and reflection

The implementation of the medication scorecards and the AQ initiative are both examples of voluntary activities that sit at the base of the responsive regulation pyramid. They are regulatory activities designed to influence health professionals' behaviour. They do so by facilitating greater staff awareness in the case of part 1, and via praise and incentives in part 2. However, part 1 presents an example of failure to influence behaviour to improve care outcomes, and part 2 presents a successful one. This difference highlights the need to reflect on a broader issue: how does the regulation attempted through these kinds of projects affect the conduct of clinicians who are targeted in this way?

Quick (2011) conducted a scoping study to address this very question, and found there is a shortage of studies asking it. One of the reasons for the lack of research into how regulatory projects affect health professional behaviour is that it is very difficult to identify the impact that a regulation initiative has on behaviour. This is because of the myriad things that influence behaviour in health care, such as professional and organisational cultures, processes and resource issues. Quick (2011) concluded that *factors internal to the organisation*, and *not* regulatory design, mostly determine the effect of and compliance with the regulation initiative.

While it can be reasonably assumed, based upon the research to date, that regulation influences how clinicians behave, we are not really clear about how this influence works *in situ*. Put differently, research remains uncertain about how regulation affects what clinicians do and how they work.

Quick (2011) concluded clinicians are more likely to change their behaviour when different regulatory mechanisms are utilised. Not surprisingly, if mechanisms with varying regulatory strengths all guide health professionals to conduct themselves in the same particular ways – such as job contracts, guidelines, professional codes of conduct, education, and financial incentives – regulation has a better chance of succeeding.

Finally, Quick (2011) stated that there is increasing interest in the question about whether attempts to regulate practice are necessarily always justified. Of special interest here is the tension between individuals' clinical judgment and professional or bureaucratic regulation. Research suggests that professionals give greater priority to their own judgments and those of colleagues than to regulation and advice coming from 'experts elsewhere'. Regulation therefore struggles to gain acceptance by professionals and result in compliance. At the least, regulation, whether through guidelines, protocols, codes of conduct, checklists or laws, needs the commitment and skills of effective and well-regarded clinical leaders to communicate and achieve its aims, objectives and benefits.

Implications for practice

A lot of communication in health care pertains to how to improve the quality and safety of health care. Some of this occurs through targeted 'redesign' projects, and some of it occurs through policies issued by health departments, or guidelines promulgated by medical or nursing bodies. This means that healthcare professionals are no longer responsible for being adequately trained, skilled and certified. They also need to stay abreast of new regulatory initiatives, and what these mean for their specific ways of working.

In practice this means that the contemporary healthcare professional is expected to be involved in some kind of improvement activity. The focus of such activity may be purely professional (such as how to improve their surgical techniques), or they may be organisational (such as how to ensure confused hospitalised older people are cared for appropriately by all teams and specialties involved). The more complex health care becomes, the more pressing, too, becomes health professionals' involvement in these kinds of regulatory and improvement activities.

Because of the complexities of care, many of these activities centre on communication – communication with colleagues, and with other stakeholders in specific domains of care. Increasingly, therefore, we witness health professionals becoming involved in *clinical networks*: groups of people who meet to address pressing issues together, and work with regulatory agencies to promote new practices beyond their own teams, organisations, or services, to those of the rest of the state. You will be expected increasingly to network – and communicate about the work you do and how – with other stakeholders: colleagues, patients, bureaucrats, and other health professionals. The New South Wales Agency for Clinical Innovation is a unique example of a government initiative that is oriented towards regulating healthcare practice through convening healthcare interest groups, with the purpose of getting those groups to deliberate about how to 're-regulate' their practices.

··

Theoretical links

The question about what makes health professionals ignore or comply with regulatory mechanisms is complex. Drawing on 'practice theory', researchers have analysed projects seeking to regulate complex clinical practices. Practice theory posits that people identify with specific practices and the resources that come with them. In addition, practice theory suggests that people's choices in this regard need not always be reasoned, logical or even beneficial.

Further, practice analyses reveal numerous challenges to do with how regulation applies to, and fits in with, complex *in situ* practices. That is, an initiative may promote certain kinds of behaviour, but the behaviour has little 'fit' with existing practices. Often, it appears that professionals trying to meet regulatory projects' ideals have to cope with unavoidable constraints (such as a lack of suitably trained staff), numerous confounders (such as uncertainties about patients' diseases and treatments), and competing imperatives (such as several patients needing care at the same time). Such constraints, confounders and imperatives may defeat the improvement aims of the most appropriately designed regulatory projects.

For example, one recent study focused on how professionals attempted to meet the demands of a project that sought to measure and reduce central line infections. The project attempted to regulate practice through requiring professionals to identify and report central line infections. But the project failed to recognise already existing infection control skills and achievements, and this made it difficult to standardise the project's improvements. The project further glossed over challenges associated with identifying infections in the first place (Dixon-Woods et al., 2012).

To clarify the effect of regulation on practice, then, practice theory considers the totality of complex tasks that occupy professionals at any one time. While one particular aspect of practice may be targeted by the new regulation, it is impossible to consider that aspect in isolation from what goes on more broadly *in situ*. While the priority for regulators may be to isolate and count infection events, professionals are more likely to face uncertainty about whether a particular infection has occurred, how and whether to inform the patient, how to control the patient's behaviour, and how to ensure all staff members are consistent in what they do.

Inevitably, professionals are embroiled in practice in ways that make categorical identification of infections not just difficult, but also often unnecessary. Their principal priorities are to treat infections, make patients better and move patients along, rather than classifying, counting and reporting their occurrences (Dixon-Woods et al., 2012). It is clear, too, that the ways in which and extent to which professionals communicate about their practices assists in regulating – 'making regular' – their practices. This communication about their daily work enables practitioners to formulate shared agreements about how their practices are to be identified, valued and improved (Iedema, Mesman & Carroll, 2013).

Reflective questions

1. Reflect on what motivates you to behave a certain way: are you more likely to adhere to rules no matter what those around you are doing, or are you more likely to go along with what those around you are doing? Also reflect on what role the nature of healthcare work plays here: to what extent do complex situations prevent you or encourage you to understand and comply with regulations?

2. In the Ramsay et al. (2014) medication scorecard study summarised in part 1 of practice example 21.1, nurses engaged with the scorecards more than doctors did. One of the reasons suggested as to why this was so was the perceived likelihood of sanction (a regulatory activity at the top of the responsive regulation pyramid) imposed upon nurses at the two hospitals. Nurses believed that if they committed a medication error they would be 'removed from their responsibilities' whereas doctors would not. How might this influence their commitment to regulation? How might it influence your commitment to regulation? What could have potentially increased doctors' engagement with the scorecard?

3. Identify some different regulatory mechanisms aimed at improving medication safety in Australia. What level of regulation do they occupy in Braithwaite's regulatory pyramid?

4. What do you think are the two main reasons for the failure of the scorecards in part 1 and the success of the AQ program in part 2? Would a regulatory strategy higher up the regulatory pyramid have improved the outcome in part 1? Why? Why not?

Conclusion

Regulation is defined as the systems put in place to improve practice and performance. The goal is to influence the behaviour of providers and improve systems of care to ensure good patient outcomes. A hierarchy of potential schemes exists, ranging from voluntary and implicit to punitive. Their success depends not only on design but also on the complexity of practice, the context, the professional culture and the method of implementation of the regulatory strategy. A range of practice factors influences the behaviour of providers and clinicians. Where practice theory and research enquire into the complexity of care practices, responsive regulation tries to focus on what best affects provider motivation and behaviour.

Practice example 21.2

Nursing and Midwifery Board of Australia v Halliday [2013] NTHPRT 1

This practice example is based upon the facts set out in the legal case, *Nursing and Midwifery Board of Australia v Halliday* [2013] NTHPRT 1. It presents an example of a regulatory mechanism towards the top of the regulatory pyramid: regulation through discretionary punishment. It highlights how poor communication can become a professional conduct issue with regulatory consequences that can restrict your ability to practise. It also highlights the need to reflect on how you would appropriately respond if you witnessed unprofessional behaviour in the workplace setting.

The *Health Practitioner Regulation National Law Act 2010* (NT) mandates how registered health professionals must behave in its professional conduct provisions (detailed below). Similar provisions exist in all Australian jurisdictions. These provisions allow regulators to impose serious penalties and conditions upon registered health professionals when they fail to behave at the standard expected of them. The case study highlights how regulation attempts to direct behaviour in relation to how health professionals communicate with patients and regulators, and the consequences for professionals when their conduct falls below the standard expected. In this instance, the tribunal found that the nurse was guilty of professional misconduct because of the way she communicated with her patient *and* because she failed to communicate a change in employment to the regulator as required. These findings highlight the impact of lack of adherence to regulators' decisions both personally and professionally.

Defining professional misconduct as set out in the *Health Practitioner Regulation National Law Act 2010* (NT)

Professional misconduct is the most serious of the breaches envisaged by the *Health Practitioner Regulation National Law Act 2010* (NT) ('the Act'). Section 5 of the Act

continued ›

Practice example 21.2 continued ›

defines the terms 'unprofessional conduct' and 'unsatisfactory professional performance' as follows:

> **professional misconduct**, of a registered health practitioner, includes—
>
> (a) unprofessional conduct by the practitioner that amounts to conduct that is substantially below the standard reasonably expected of a registered health practitioner of an equivalent level of training or experience; and
>
> (b) more than one instance of unprofessional conduct that, when considered together, amounts to conduct that is substantially below the standard reasonably expected of a registered health practitioner of an equivalent level of training or experience; and
>
> (c) conduct of the practitioner, whether occurring in connection with the practice of the health practitioner's profession or not, that is inconsistent with the practitioner being a fit and proper person to hold registration in the profession.
>
> **unprofessional conduct**, of a registered health practitioner, means professional conduct that is of a lesser standard than that which might reasonably be expected of the health practitioner by the public or the practitioner's professional peers and includes—
>
> (a) a contravention by the practitioner of this Law, whether or not the practitioner has been prosecuted for, or convicted of, an offence in relation to the contravention;
>
> (b) a contravention by the practitioner of—
>
>   (i) a condition to which the practitioner's registration was subject; or
>
>   (ii) an undertaking given by the practitioner to the National Board that registers the practitioner; and …

The facts of the case are as follows. On 9 December 2011, Nurse Dianne Elliot Halliday (the practitioner), while working as a registered nurse at the surgical ward, Ward 2B at Royal Darwin Hospital (RDH):

- yelled at a patient to 'shut up';
- pushed the patient onto the patient's bed;
- placed her hands around the patient's neck;
- pushed the patient into the back of the bed, choking the patient with her hands;
- yelled at the patient again to 'shut up';
- after retrieving the remote for the bed from the floor and giving it to the patient, said to the patient words to the effect of, 'We're not slaves, you can do it yourself'.

The first issue was whether the conduct described was in breach of conduct statement 8 of the Australian Nursing and Midwifery Council's *Code of professional conduct for nurses in Australia* (2008) because the practitioner failed to promote and preserve the trust and privilege inherent in the relationship between nurses and people receiving care. The second issue was whether her conduct constituted unprofessional conduct under The *Health Practitioner Regulation National Law Act 2010* (NT) in respect of a condition

continued ›

Practice example 21.2 continued ›

placed upon Nurse Halliday's registration immediately following the assault. That condition required her to report a new nursing position prior to commencing the position and to provide adequate details of the position after a request from the board. The third issue was whether the conduct was unprofessional or substantially below the standard reasonably expected of a registered health practitioner of an equivalent level of training and experience.

Nurse Halliday was found guilty of unprofessional conduct and professional misconduct. She had her registration suspended for three months and conditions imposed on her registration including requirements that she be supervised (to be reviewed after 12 months), report the name of each employer and nominated supervisor to the board, and have her nominated supervisor provide reports to the board every three months.

Reflective questions

1. Imagine you are a practitioner working with Nurse Halliday. Reflect on how you would respond to this inappropriate behaviour in the workplace setting. What organisational and regulatory mechanisms are available to you assist you in responding? For example, would you report Nurse Halliday's behaviour? If so, to whom? Should you confront her directly about her behaviour? Why or why not? How would you feel if you witnessed Nurse Halliday's behaviour and were asked to appear as a witness at the tribunal?
2. Identify the stakeholders relevant to this fact situation. How well do you think the tribunal balanced the different stakeholders' arguments and needs in reaching its decision?
3. What other regulatory entities might be involved in this fact situation? Why?
4. What are some additional regulatory mechanisms that could be put in place to prevent fact situations similar to the case study happening again?

Further reading

Bismark, M., Spittal, M., & Studdert, D. (2014). Mandatory reports of concerns about health, performance and conduct of health practitioners, *MJA 201*(7) 399–403.
This study describes the frequency and characteristics of mandatory reports made to the Australian Health Practitioner Regulation Agency (AHPRA).

Etienne, J. (2010). The impact of regulatory policy on individual behaviour: A goal framing theory approach. Discussion paper no. 59. London: Centre for Analysis of Risk and Regulation, London School of Economics.

This paper presents a theoretical framework for analysing how people respond to regulation. It identifies how best regulatory policy can influence behaviour.

Healy, J., (2011). *Improving health care safety and quality reluctant regulators.* Farnham and Burlington VT: Ashgate Publishing.
This book analyses the healthcare systems of different countries. The result of the analysis is the presentation of a conceptual framework for responsive regulation.

Runciman, B., Merry, A., & Walton, M. (2007). Ethics, professional behaviour and regulation. In B. Runciman, A. Merry & M. Walton (Eds.), *Safety and ethics in healthcare: A guide to getting in right* (pp. 157–177). Farnham and Burlington VT: Ashgate Publishing.
This chapter defines the concepts of ethics, ethical frameworks and decision-making, professional behaviour and regulation. In addition it provides case studies and problem questions to enable the reader to apply the definitions and questions to fact scenarios.

Tingle, J., & Bark, P. (Eds.). (2011). *Patient safety, law policy and practice.* London and New York: Routledge.
This book explores the impact of law as a regulatory tool on patient safety. It examines the different ways that legal systems are being used as well as what alternative regulatory mechanism should be used to facilitate patient safety.

Web resources

Commonwealth

Australian Commission on Safety and Quality in Health Care (ACSQHC): http://www.safetyandquality.gov.au
Australian Competition and Consumer Commission: http://www.accc.gov.au
Australian Government Department of Health: http://www.health.gov.au
Australian Health Practitioner Regulation Agency (AHPRA): http://www.ahpra.gov.au
Council of Australian Governments (COAG): http://www.coag.gov.au
Council of Australian Governments Health Council: http://www.ahmac.gov.au/site/home.aspx
Independent Hospital Pricing Authority (IHPA): http://www.ihpa.gov.au/internet/ihpa/publishing.nsf
MyHospitals: http://www.myhospitals.gov.au
MyHealthyCommunities: http://www.myhealthycommunities.gov.au
National Health Performance Authority (NHPA): http://www.nhpa.gov.au/internet/nhpa/publishing.nsf/Content/home-1
National Health Reform Act 2011 (Cth): http://www.comlaw.gov.au/Details/C2011C00952

Australian Capital Territory

ACT Health: http://www.health.act.gov.au
Coroner's Court: http://www.courts.act.gov.au/magistrates/courts/coroners_court
Health Services Complaints Commissioner: http://www.healthcomplaints.act.gov.au

New South Wales

Clinical Excellence Commission: http://cec.health.nsw.gov.au
Coroner's Court: http://www.coroners.lawlink.nsw.gov.au/coroners/index.html
Health: http://www.health.nsw.gov.au/Pages/default.aspx
Health Care Complaints Commission: http://hccc.nsw.gov.au

Northern Territory

Coroner's Office: http://www.nt.gov.au/justice/courtsupp/coroner/index.shtml
Department of Health: http://www.health.nt.gov.au
Health and Community Services Complaints Commission: http://www.hcscc.nt.gov.au

Queensland

Coroners Court: http://www.courts.qld.gov.au/courts/coroners-court
Health Quality and Complaints Commission: http://www.hqcc.qld.gov.au
Patient Safety Unit: http://www.health.qld.gov.au/psu
Queensland Health: http://www.health.qld.gov.au

South Australia

Coroners Court: http://www.courts.sa.gov.au/OurCourts/CoronersCourt/Pages/default.aspx
Health and Community Services Complaints Commissioner: http://www.hcscc.sa.gov.au
Quality & Safety Unit: http://www.sahealth.sa.gov.au/safetyandquality
SA Health: http://www.health.sa.gov.au

Western Australia

Coroner's Court: http://www.coronerscourt.wa.gov.au
Council for Safety and Quality in Healthcare: http://www.safetyandquality.health.wa.gov.au/
    home/wacsqhc.cfm
Department of Health: http://www.health.wa.gov.au/home
Health and Disability Services Complaints Office: http://www.hadsco.wa.gov.au/home

Tasmania

Department of Health and Human Services: http://dhhs.tas.gov.au
Health Complaints Commissioner: http://healthcomplaints.tas.gov.au
Magistrates Court of Tasmania, Coronial Division: http://www.magistratescourt.tas.gov.au/
    divisions/coronial

Victoria

Coroners Court: http://www.coronerscourt.vic.gov.au
Health: http://www.health.vic.gov.au
Office of the Health Services Commissioner: http://www.health.vic.gov.au/hsc
Quality Council: http://www.health.vic.gov.au/qualitycouncil

Others

Consumers Health Forum of Australia: http://www.chf.org.au

Medical Error Action Group: http://www.medicalerroraustralia.com

References

Australian Nursing and Midwifery Council. (2008). *Code of professional conduct for nurses in Australia*. Melbourne: Author.

Ayers, I., & Braithwaite, J. (1992) *Responsive regulation: Transcending the deregulation debate*. New York: Oxford University Press.

Braithwaite, J., Healy, J., & Dwan, K. (2005). *The governance of health safety and quality*. Canberra: Australian Council for Safety and Quality in Health Care.

Dixon-Woods, M., Leslie, M., Bion, J., & Tarrant, C. (2012). What counts? An ethnographic study of infection control data reported to a patient safety program. *Milbank Quarterly*, *90*(3), 548–591.

Healy, J. (2011). *Improving health care safety and quality reluctant regulators*. Farnham and Burlington VT: Ashgate Publishing.

Healy, J., & Braithwaite, J. (2006). Designing safer health care through responsive regulation. *Medical Journal of Australia*, *184*(10), S56–S59.

Iedema, R., Mesman, J., & Carroll, K., (2013). *Visualising healthcare improvement: Innovation from within*. Oxford: Radcliffe Publishers.

Kristensen, S.R., Meacock, R., Turner, A. J.Boaden, R., McDonald, R., Roland, M., & Sutton, M. (2014). Long-term effect of hospital pay for performance on mortality in England. *New England Journal of Medicine*, *371*, 540–548.

Quick, O., (2011). *A scoping study on the effects of health professional regulation on those regulated: Final report submitted to the Council for Healthcare Regulatory Excellence*. London: Council for Healthcare.

Ramsay, A., Turner, S., Cavell, G., Oborne, C., Thomas, R., Cookson, G., & Fulop, N. (2014). Governing patient safety: Lessons learned from a mixed methods evaluation of implementing a ward-level medication safety scorecard in two English NHS hospitals. *BMJ Quality & Safety*, *23*, 136–146. doi:10.1136

Runciman, B., Merry, A., & Walton, M. (2007). Ethics, professional behaviour and regulation. In B., Runciman, A. Merry & M. Walton, *Safety and ethics in healthcare: A guide to getting in right* (pp. 157–177). Farnham and Burlington VT: Ashgate Publishing.

Sutton, M., Nikolova, S., Boaden, R., Lester, H., McDonald, R., & Roland, M., (2012). Reduced mortality with hospital pay for performance in England. *New England Journal of Medicine*, *367*, 1821–1828. doi:10.1056/NEJM sa1114951

Note

1 The federal government, in its 2014–15 budget papers released on 12 May 2014, outlined plans to consult states and territories on amalgamating these agencies into a single organisation: see http://www.budget.gov.au/2014–15/index.htm

22

Communicating bad news: when care goes wrong

Rick Iedema, Kate Bower and Donella Piper

Learning objectives

This chapter will enable you to:
- describe the main components of incident disclosure communication including an apology, an explanation about what went wrong, an opportunity for the patient and/ or their family to provide an account, a plan of care for what needs to be done for the patient, and a strategy for improving care so that the failure or error does not happen again;
- understand the importance of incident disclosure for patients, and for clinicians and health services, and be able to explain that it is important that problems in care are talked about and their causes are understood, that mutual respect is shown, and that it is acknowledged that care processes must be improved to prevent them from causing more avoidable harm;
- identify and apply the principles of the 2013 *Australian Open Disclosure Framework* to examples from real-life healthcare incidents, taken from recent research on open disclosure.

Key terms

Apology
Incident
Incident disclosure
Open disclosure
Patient safety

Overview

Analyses of medical records, incident reports, observations and interviews have revealed that care may at times go wrong. The frequency of such failures and errors is difficult to establish, mainly due to a lack of reliability of relevant docu-mentation. Errors and failures are not always reported and are not always immediately evident. Reported **incident** rates have varied between 6% and 16% (Wilson et al., 1995), with some commentators putting incident rates as high as 25–30% (Classen et al., 2011). A small proportion of these incidents involve death and permanent disability (Vincent et al., 2008).

> **incident**
> an unplanned event that results in an undesirable outcome for the patient.

When a patient experiences harm as a result of an incident, it is now mandatory in most Australian health services that they are told what went wrong and why, a practice referred to as incident disclosure or 'open disclosure'. The policy that mandates inci-dent disclosure is the *Australian Open Disclosure Framework* (Australian Commission on Safety and Quality in Health Care, 2013). This framework is a component of the National Safety and Quality Health Service Standards against which most health services (includ-ing hospitals, day procedure clinics and dental services) are to be accredited (Australian Commission on Quality and Safety in Health Care, 2012). Open disclosure is part of Standard 1: 'Governance for safety and quality in health service organisations'. This chap-ter discusses the kind of communication that takes place when things go wrong in care. It discusses the requirements set out in the framework and presents research findings about clinicians' understandings and uptake of open disclosure.

Introduction

Open disclosure refers to open communication about unex-pected outcomes in health care. Open disclosure should be initiated when an incident that causes harm to the patient comes to the attention of health service providers, the patient or other stakeholders. Open disclosure involves (1) the clinician(s) communicating to the patient an explanation for what happened, (2) an **apology**, (3) an opportunity for the patient to recount their experience, (4) a plan for the patient, and (5) a practice improvement plan (Australian Commission on Safety and Quality in Health Care, 2013). Each of these five elements is equally central to open disclosure.

> **apology**
> a statement of regret that includes the word 'sorry'. There is a difference between 'We are sorry that this happened' and 'We are sorry that we did the wrong thing'. The latter expression is admissible in some states' courts of law as constituting an acknowledgement of liability (all states except New South Wales and the Australian Capital Territory).

The open disclosure policy was first formulated in Australia around 2001. At this time there were many pressures on stakeholders in health care to improve the quality and safety of treatment processes. In part, pressure resulted from the publication of the

Quality in Australian Health Care (QAHC) study in 1995 (Wilson et al., 1995). This study revealed that between 6% and 16% of acute healthcare episodes involve healthcare incidents: errors and failures attributable to the care process or to clinicians. On the basis of its findings, the QAHC study estimated that 18 000 patients might be dying or be permanently disabled due to incidents across the whole of Australia each year.

The QAHC study obliged policy-makers to broaden their attention from achieving budget efficiency to raising the quality and safety of health care. When a large Australian healthcare insurer (HIH) collapsed in the late 1990s (due to financial mismanagement – not due to exorbitant compensation payouts to harmed patients), this collapse produced sudden rises in clinicians' and services' insurance premiums. To keep clinicians' and services' insurance payments in check and to reduce the frequency of clinical incidents, a number of policy steps were taken. One of these was the introduction of the open disclosure policy. If clinicians are open and honest about clinical incidents, the policy reasoned, they will be better able to learn from mistakes, and patients will be less likely to sue. The introduction of the open disclosure policy was a radical strategy: it acknowledged the importance of consumers' right to error- and failure-free health care, and the need for clinicians to be transparent about service shortcomings and to be serious about service improvement.

The 2003 publication of the Australian Open Disclosure Standard (Australian Council for Safety and Quality in Health Care, 2003) resulted from an initiative of the then Australian Council for Quality and Safety in Health Care (now the Australian Commission for Quality and Safety in Health Care). The council convened a group of clinicians, consumers, policy-makers, insurers and lawyers, asking them to draw up principles to provide guidance to those charged with communicating 'unexpected outcomes'

> **incident disclosure**
> the practice of communicating to patients about what went wrong and why, when an incident has occurred.

(that is, incidents) to patients. Then, in 2013, the Australian Commission on Quality and Safety in Health Care issued an updated version of the standard: the *Australian Open Disclosure Framework* (Australian Commission on Safety and Quality in Health Care, 2013). This framework integrates several years of research conducted in Australia on the desirability, success and effectiveness of **incident disclosure** communication, particularly for patients and their families (Iedema, Allen, Britton, Grbich et al., 2011; Iedema et al., 2008).

Research findings indicated that patients and families often had different views to clinicians about what constitutes an incident, or which aspect of an incident is most important. The revised framework has incorporated this research by adding the opportunity for a patient to relate their experience of the incident as an essential component of incident disclosure, equal in importance to the factual explanation provided by clinicians. This framework forms part of the National Safety and Quality Health Service Standards (NSQHS) (Australian Commission on Quality and Safety in Health Care, 2012). This means that most healthcare services, including hospitals, day procedure clinics and dental services, must be formally accredited for their adherence to and performance on healthcare incident

Australian Open Disclosure Framework

Better communication,
a better way to care

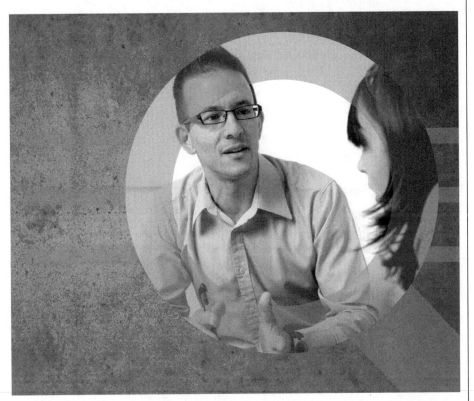

AUSTRALIAN COMMISSION
ON SAFETY AND QUALITY IN HEALTH CARE

NSQHS
STANDARDS

Australian College of Nursing   The Royal Australasian College of Physicians

Figure 22.1 *Australian Open Disclosure Framework* document

disclosure. Although **open disclosure** discussions are unique, based on the specifics of the incident, they share the key components set out in the 'Key components of open disclosure discussions' feature below. Note that these elements may be discussed in one or more meetings between the health service and the patient, family and carers.

> **open disclosure**
> a nationwide policy that requires clinicians to be open and honest with patients about incidents and health service-caused harms.

Key components of open disclosure discussions

1. Introductions

The patient, their family and carers are told the names and roles of everyone attending the meeting, and this information is also provided in writing.

2. Saying sorry

A sincere and unprompted apology or expression of regret is given on behalf of the healthcare service and clinicians, including the words, 'I am' or 'We are sorry'.

3. Factual explanation: providers

A factual explanation of the adverse event is provided, including the known facts and consequences of the adverse event, in a way that ensures the patient, their family and carers understand the information.

4. Factual explanation: patient, family and carers

The patient, family and carers have the opportunity to explain their views on what happened, contribute their knowledge and ask questions.

5. Personal effect of the adverse event

The patient, family and carers are encouraged to talk about the personal effect of the adverse event on their lives.

6. Plan agreed and recorded

An open disclosure plan is agreed on and recorded, in which the patient, their family and carers outline what they hope to achieve from the process and any questions they would like answered. This is to be documented and filed in the appropriate place and a copy provided to the patient, their family and carers.

7. Pledge to feed back

The patient, their family and carers are assured that they will be informed of any further reviews or investigations to determine why the adverse event occurred, the nature of the proposed process and the expected time frame.

8. Offer of support

An offer of support to the patient, their family and carers should include:

    a. ongoing support including reimbursement of out-of-pocket expenses incurred as a result of the adverse event;

    b. assurance that any necessary follow-up care or investigation will be provided promptly and efficiently;

    c. in the relevant settings, clarity on who will be responsible for providing ongoing care;

    d. contact details for any relevant service they wish to access;

    e. information about how to take the matter further, including any complaint processes available.

9. Support for patients and staff

The patient, their family and carers engages in open disclosure with staff. Staff are supported by their colleagues, managers and health service organisation, both personally and professionally.

10. Other health service organisations

In cases where the adverse event spans more than one location or service, relevant clinicians and staff will ensure, where possible, that all relevant staff from these additional institutions are involved in the open disclosure process.

Practice example 22.1

This case study is derived from an excerpt from an interview conducted with the daughter of a 71-year-old female patient in 2009. The patient suffered from atrial fibrillation, and was found to have some abnormality on her lungs. She was not informed about the nature of this abnormality. She developed pleural fusions requiring a number of attendances at the hospital. She was anxious because she was under the care of the respiratory, cardiology and general medicine departments, with no one appearing to take direct responsibility for her care. Clinicians from these three departments were not communicating with each other, often resulting in lengthy treatment delays.

The patient continued to deteriorate, suffering from weight loss and rising lethargy. Finally, to drain the liquid around her lungs, a 'pleurodesis' was performed under the care of the respiratory department, after which she was discharged. Further deterioration led to her being readmitted, but this time as a cardiac patient. The cardiologist, when asked by the patient's daughter whether 'there was anything more sinister to worry about', reassured her that there was not. He explained the problem was that her mother's heart was not working properly. The patient, however, fearing she had cancer, was very anxious, so much so that her family, worrying that she was depressed, persuaded her to see a counsellor.

Fourteen months after the pleurodesis, the lung specialist recommended and performed a thoracotomy, and diagnosed mesothelioma. This was the first time the family had heard of this diagnosis. As she became even more unwell the patient was nursed at home supported by the palliative care team. At this time family members discovered that the cytology report from the pleurodesis had already suggested that she had mesothelioma. In the 14-month period since the pleurodesis none of the clinicians had informed them of this. At this stage it was too late for treatment by an oncologist and the patient died not long after. This is how the daughter tells the story:

> The person that performed the operation at [major hospital]... the pleurodesis in 2008, didn't tell us, or didn't tell Mum. The private cardiologist who was communicating with that person who did the pleurodesis, he didn't tell us, even though I'd asked him if there was anything more sinister. And her GP never said anything either. So, as a result of getting that cytology report, I rang the GP, and asked if he knew. And he said no, he'd never seen that report. I then rang the private cardiologist [and asked] if, in her file, there was any of that information. And the receptionist got Mum's file out and said, yes, didn't you know?

> And I said, no, I didn't know. And I said, could you be so kind as to fax me all the relevant documentation from that pleurodesis. And she said she couldn't fax it to me, but she could fax it to the GP, and I could request it. So I did that, and once I requested it from the GP, he then admitted that he had looked back on his emails, and he had failed to read the email that told him, in 2008, that Mum had suspicions of mesothelioma, and mesothelioma cells. So there's three sort of different people within the whole system that didn't divulge that information, and continued to treat her from a heart perspective, when that didn't seem to be the issue at all.

continued ›

Practice example 22.1 continued ›

Family members believe that if the patient had seen the oncologist earlier, she might have lived longer with an improved quality of life. Her husband feels his wife 'was robbed of [14 months] because she wasn't given the choices'. She didn't have the choice of treatment because she wasn't told just how sick she was.

Encouraged by the palliative care team the family decided to make a complaint to the hospital about the fact that they had not been informed of the patient's mesothelioma for 14 months. They contacted the patient consumer relations department. On legal advice the daughter wrote a letter explaining that the family was not seeking compensation but wanted a personal meeting with the people involved. She asked for an apology and wanted to know what changes the hospital was planning to implement to ensure errors like this one were not repeated. She requested this because family members were left with many unanswered questions. They still do not understand why none of the three main clinicians knew of or told them about the mesothelioma diagnosis.

After repeated phone calls to the hospital, the hospital finally responded four months after the daughter sent the letter of complaint. There was no offer of a disclosure meeting and no apology, and the hospital informed them that they were not planning any improvement in their system. The family was very angry and disappointed with this response. The patient's daughter wrote again and has never had a reply from the hospital. She had been led to believe that her complaint was being taken seriously and now feels she was lied to. Now the family do not ever expect an apology, believing that fear of litigation has prevented this. They are left feeling very angry.

Reflective questions

1. Imagine you are a clinician charged with arranging an open disclosure meeting for the family. What conversations would you have with your colleagues before the meeting with the family, whom would you invite to the meeting, and what would you say to the family at the meeting? Refer to the key components of open disclosure discussions box above.

2. Again imagine you are a clinician taking part in the open disclosure meeting. How would you respond to the patient's daughter's concerns about the poor communication during the incident? Would you try to justify what happened? Would you accept blame for what happened?

3. Imagine you are a member of the patient's family. Describe how you would feel about the incident and what would be of most concern to you. Do you agree with the patient's daughter's judgment that the clinicians were treating the patient for a disease problem that was not relevant, mainly because they did not communicate appropriately with one another and did not pay sufficient attention to what in fact was wrong with the patient? What would you like to express in the open disclosure meeting with the hospital?

Analysis and reflection

Practice example 22.1 offers an example of a patient with 'co-morbidities' (multiple diseases), which meant she was not under the care of a single medical department. Perhaps because of this, a critical diagnosis of mesothelioma was allowed to 'fall through the cracks': none of her care providers took full responsibility for managing her care, or for communicating test results. On top of this, the daughter had to pursue the hospital for critical information, and only thanks to this did the general practitioner become aware of the missed diagnosis. The daughter's requests to the hospital for a meeting were ignored, even though she reassured the service that she was not seeking to sue. The family never received an apology, nor an explanation about why the mesothelioma was missed, nor reassurance that similar disasters would not befall other patients and that the hospital would look into its processes and procedures.

It is precisely to avoid these situations that open disclosure policy stipulates that all Australian health services must disclose errors and invite harmed patients (and/or their families) to a meeting to discuss problems openly and honestly.

If we consider what open disclosure might mean in a context such as the case in practice example 22.1, we realise that it cannot simply be about clinicians deciding to provide the relevant technical and clinical information to the harmed patient or the family. Instead, open disclosure accommodates the possibility that the patient or their family identifies a problem that they want to discuss with the service. Thus, open disclosure also provides an opportunity for the patient and the family to raise questions about the care that was provided. This may involve challenging clinicians about their version of events and their understandings of what went wrong, and making clear to clinicians that it is *they* who are to accept that a healthcare incident may have occurred without noticing anything. Open disclosure also encompasses the duty that is now placed on clinicians to 'hear' patients and their families, and to demonstrate that they are capable of improving their ways of working and outcomes in ways that satisfy those harmed.

Further, how we think about open disclosure depends on whose perspective we take. Do we take the perspective of the clinicians, and accept their profession-specific and scientifically delineated notions of what constitutes an incident? The case in practice example 22.1 was not recorded as an incident and thus does not 'formally' rate as one. Therefore, open disclosure also asks health professionals to take the perspective of the patient. Framed this way, open disclosure is much more than the service providing clinical and technical information following the reporting of an incident. Open disclosure should be conducted as two-way dialogue, as is stipulated in the *Australian Open Disclosure Framework* referred to previously.

Implications for practice

Keeping in mind that open disclosure is a two-way dialogue between the health service and the patient and their family, there are several key actions that can contribute to a successful open disclosure:

- When a patient or family asks to discuss what they think may be a problem in care, acknowledge the possibility that an incident that escaped the attention of the service and health professionals may have occurred.
- When an error or unexpected event is found or claimed to have occurred, inform all stakeholders (the patient, the family and the health professional stakeholders involved in the care) as soon as possible that further investigation is required. Most health services will have specific people, such as patient safety officers and open disclosure coordinators, to assist you in communicating about an incident.
- Try to understand the incident from the patient's perspective, and ask yourself how you would like to be treated. Always be respectful, empathic and compassionate when communicating with patients or their families.
- Acknowledge that the patient's experience of the incident is of equal importance to the medical explanation of the incident, remembering that sometimes patients may place emphasis on one aspect of an incident which from your perspective may seem insignificant.
- See open disclosure as an opportunity to improve your practice as a clinician and to learn from your colleagues and patients. Open disclosure can also be healing for clinicians who have been involved in a serious incident; it enables them to talk about issues they need to understand themselves, too.
- Ultimately, open disclosure is also a way of supporting your colleagues and contributing to a safer environment for all patients.

Theoretical links

Incident disclosure or open disclosure represents a practice that is informed by a number of theoretical orientations, including but not limited to, theories of patient safety, pedagogy, restorative justice, apology and narrative ethics. These theoretical orientations also play a prominent role in the analysis of disclosure practices.

Patient safety is a bundle of theories about how the safety of clinical practices can or should be enhanced (Vincent, 2010). One patient safety theory pertains to learning from errors and mishaps, and incident reporting is regarded as an important means for initiating such learning, as incident reports enable clinicians to reflect on what went wrong. *Pedagogic theory* pertains to how we learn. In health, it has been found that openness about incidents is critical for learning from problems (Vincent, 2004).

---

patient safety
a set of theories that specifies the risks that patients experience in health services as well as the risk minimisation strategies that clinicians can deploy to keep their patients safe.

Openness is an important component also of *restorative justice theory* – a theory that regards sincerity and openness among those who erred and those who suffered harm as a result of central importance to mutual healing (Braithwaite, 2002). By bringing all stakeholders together to talk openly about their roles in what went wrong, all are better enabled to understand the other, and more inclined to learn.

Another theory that is important in this context is one that addresses the communicative dimensions and effects of an *apology* (Tavuchis, 1991). Of particular interest are apologies articulated by people in positions of authority for the benefit of citizens, clients or patients. For many people with power and authority, apologising is notoriously difficult (Lazare, 2004).

Finally, *narrative ethics* is a theoretical orientation that sets great store by people's right to tell or *narrate* their experiences. Here, narration is a means to ensuring that the story-tellers become involved in decision-making through the power of their story. The objective of narrative ethics is to make people's stories count as evidence alongside other kinds of evidence that tend to be regarded as more important and powerful (Berlinger, 2005).

Conclusion

Incident disclosure is critical for reassuring patients and families that clinicians fully understand and have comprehensively thought through the care that they provide. It is critical for inspiring trust among patients and consumers generally in clinical expertise and professionalism, and in clinicians' commitment to self-initiated improvement.

Research shows that open disclosure does not always happen when it should (Iedema, Allen, Britton, Grbich et al., 2011; Iedema et al., 2008). Not being offered open disclosure following unexpected outcomes is very difficult for patients and their families. It ties them up in the process of seeking explanations, and it denies them the opportunity to grieve about what happened and come to terms with their harm or their loss. Research also suggests that people start legal proceedings when they suspect they were not told the full story about their incident (Vincent, Young & Phillips, 1994). Also, non-disclosure limits patients' and families' confidence about subsequent treatment needs and decisions.

Finally, patients and relatives have been shown to be more informed about inappropriate care and incidents than clinicians are willing to admit and acknowledge (Iedema, Allen, Britton & Gallagher, 2011). Patients and families knowing about inappropriate care means that they could play an important role in incident investigation and practice improvement. Not surprisingly, some services have begun to move towards involving patients in precisely such processes (McDonald et al., 2010). Here, 'disclosure' may no longer be the appropriate term, and another, more collaborative concept is needed.

Indeed, to ensure healthcare improvement and learning, incident management necessitates two-way dialogue involving clinicians, patients and their families, and health service managers.

Practice example 22.2

Richard's 85-year-old mother is in a low-care aged care facility, suffering from Parkinson's disease. Here he tells the story of a medication error that happened to his mother. Read his story and then reflect using the questions below.

My mother is in a low-care aged care facility. She has Parkinson's disease. She's been there for about 12 months and recently my brother and I felt that her condition was going downhill and that it was likely related to her medication. We've come to realise that the quantity and timing of medication is particularly important in treating Parkinson's. Usually my mother self-medicates and even though sometimes she is a bit forgetful, there is nothing wrong with her mentally and it works. But her specialist recently added a dose of the main Parkinson's medication, Sinemet, to be taken at 4:00 a.m. So during the day she self-medicates but obviously she is sleeping at 4:00 a.m. so needs to be woken by one of the aged care staff and given that dose.

Mum is one of the few patients in the facility that self-medicates. Most of the residents are medicated by the nurses. So I arranged with the head nurse there to have someone wake Mum up at 4:00 a.m. and give her the half-tablet. I would check in with Mum on my visits and ask if she had the tablet and also I kept the week's worth of tablets by her bed and replaced them each week so I could keep an eye on the numbers. So everything went ok for a while, but then for some reason Mum wasn't getting woken up for that dose.

So I spoke to the head nurse again and said, 'Would you mind reminding the night staff to wake Mum up to take her medication?' Nothing happened, and I didn't hear anything back from the staff. Then I went in to visit Mum and she told me that at the dinner table the woman next door said to her, 'Did you hear what happened with the tablets?', and Mum said, 'No', and her neighbour said, 'They've been coming in and waking me up and giving me half a tablet, and it should have been for you!' So I think because I complained, they'd spoken to the staff and they said they were doing it and then they must have done some investigating and it turned out that they were giving the medication to the lady in the next room. As it turns out, the lady next door has a very similar name to my mother and also suffers from Parkinson's.

I think my Mum and her neighbour both thought it was quite funny, but it could have been quite serious – I don't really know how serious, but it did concern me that they had made such a mistake and had not told me or my mother about it. I never received any communication from the facility about the mistake, but they did remedy the error by commencing the medication again for my mother.

Reflective questions

1. In this example, no disclosure has occurred. Describe what should have happened, referring to the five elements of open disclosure as set out in the *Australian Open Disclosure Framework*. Note that open disclosure is not mandatory in the aged care setting but is still considered best practice, as endorsed by the Australian College of Nursing and all state and federal health ministers.
2. If you were Richard in this example, what would you have done upon hearing about the mistake from your mother?
3. How do you think the aged care facility should have responded to Richard's concerns, had he expressed them?
4. Reflect on the importance of healthcare services engaging in open disclosure. Do you think it should be the responsibility of patients or their families to identify errors or request information about errors? Why or why not?

Reflective questions

1. Ask friends and family if they have ever experienced a healthcare incident. If they have, ask if the incident was explained to them. If it was, ask them how the explanation was given, whether they got an apology, and whether they found discussion satisfactory. If not, ask them how they feel about being denied an explanation. Record all your answers.
2. Imagine you are a clinician who has made a medication error and you have to tell the patient. What kind of apology might you use? Answer this question after reading the following excerpt from the Australian Open Disclosure Framework on 'saying sorry'.

Saying sorry (*Australian Open Disclosure Framework*)
Apology and/or expressions of regret are a key component of open disclosure, but it is also the most sensitive. 'Saying sorry' must occur with great care. The exact wording and phrasing of an apology (or expression of regret) will vary in each case. The following points should be considered:
- The words 'I am sorry' or 'we are sorry' should be included.
- It is preferred that, wherever possible, people directly involved in the adverse event also provide the apology or expression of regret.
- Sincerity is the key element for success. The effectiveness of an apology or expression of regret hinges on the way it is delivered, including the tone of voice, as well as non-verbal communication such as body language, gestures and facial expressions. These skills are often not innate, and may need to be practised. Training and education in open disclosure should address this (see Section 6.4).
- The apology or expression of regret should make clear what is regretted or being apologised for, and what is being done to address the situation.

- An apology or expression of regret is essential in helping patients, their family and carers cope with the effects of a traumatic event. It also assists clinicians in their recovery from adverse events in which they are involved.

It is important to note that apology or expression of regret alone is insufficient, and must be backed up by further information and action to ensure effective open disclosure.

Further reading

Berlinger, N. (2005). *After harm: Medical error and the ethics of forgiveness*. Baltimore: Johns Hopkins Press.

This book offers an overview of the ethical and practical demands that clinicians confront when they are involved in avoidable patient harm. Berlinger's book is unique because it brings together patients' narratives about harm they experienced and clinicians' narratives about being involved in or even having occasioned incidents.

Truog, R., Browning, D., Johnson, J., & Gallagher, T. H. (2011). *Talking with patients and families about medical error: A guide for education and practice*. Baltimore: Johns Hopkins University Press.

Truog and colleagues' book focuses on incident disclosure communication, outlining the various challenges that clinicians and health service managers need to overcome, setting out a range of models for preparing the healthcare workforce for disclosure discussions, and specifying the communicative behaviours that satisfy the requirement to be open and honest. This book is the most detailed and informative guide for health services and heath professionals charged with conducting incident disclosure.

Wu, A. W., McCay, L., Levinson, W., Iedema , R.Wallace, G., Boyle, D. et al. (2014). Disclosing adverse events to patients: International norms and trends. *Journal of Patient Safety 04*. doi:10.1097/PTS.0000000000000107

The authors reviewed trends in policy and practice in five countries with extensive experience with adverse event disclosure and they identified five themes that reflect key challenges to disclosure: (1) the challenge of putting policy into large-scale practice, (2) the conflict between patient safety theory and patient expectations, (3) the conflict between legal privilege for quality improvement and open disclosure, (4) the challenge of aligning open disclosure with liability compensation, and (5) the challenge of measurement related to disclosure.

Web resources

Agency for Health Research and Quality: http://psnet.ahrq.gov/primer.aspx?primerID=2
Australian Commission on Safety and Quality in Health Care: http://www.safetyandquality. gov.au/our-work/open-disclosure/implementing-the-open-disclosure-framework/open-disclosure-resources-for-clinicians-and-health-care-providers

Hear me, a segment from a play about a death in hospital: http://www.youtube.com/watch?v=2ymWvnUjb2E

....

References

Australian Commission on Quality and Safety in Health Care. (2012). *National safety and quality health service standards*. Sydney: Australian Commission on Quality and Safety in Health Care.

Australian Commission on Safety and Quality in Health Care. (2012). *Australian Open Disclosure Framework – consultation draft*. Sydney: Australian Commission on Safety and Quality in Health Care.

—— (2013). *The Australian Open Disclosure Framework*. Sydney: Australian Commission on Safety and Quality in Health Care.

Australian Council for Safety and Quality in Health Care. (2003). *Open disclosure standard: A national standard for open communication in public and private hospitals following an adverse event in health care*. Canberra: Commonwealth of Australia.

Berlinger, N. (2005). *After harm: Medical error and the ethics of forgiveness*. Baltimore: Johns Hopkins Press.

Braithwaite, J. (2002). *Restorative justice theory*. New York, NY: Oxford University Press.

Classen, D., Resar, R. K., Griffin, F., Federico, F., Frankel, T., Kimmel, N. et al. (2011). 'Global Trigger Tool' shows that adverse events may be ten times greater than previously measured. *Health Affairs, 34*(4), 581–589.

Iedema, R., Allen, S., Britton, K., & Gallagher, T. (2011). What do patients and relatives know about problems and failures in care? *BMJ Qual Saf, 12*(21), 198–205.

Iedema, R., Allen, S., Britton, K., Grbich, C., Piper, D., Baker, A. et al. (2011). Patients' and family members' views on how clinicians enact and how they should enact open disclosure – the '100 Patient Stories' qualitative study. *British Medical Journal, 343*: 1–9.

Iedema, R., Mallock, N., Sorensen, R., Manias, E., Tuckett, A., Williams, A. et al. (2008). The national open disclosure pilot: Evaluation of a policy implementation initiative. *Medical Journal of Australia, 188*(7): 397–400.

Lazare, A. (2004). *On apology*. New York: Oxford University Press.

McDonald, T., Helmchen, L. A., Smith, K. M., Centomani, N., Gunderson, A., Mayer, D., & Chamberlin, W. H. (2010). Responding to patient safety incidents: The 7 pillars. *Quality and Safety in Health Care*. doi:10.1136/qshc.2008.031633

Tavuchis, N. (1991). *Mea culpa: A sociology of apology and reconciliation*. Stanford: Stanford University Press.

—— (2004). Analysis of clinical incidents: A window on the system not a search for root causes. *Quality and Safety in Health Care, 13*(4), 242–243.

—— (2010). *Patient safety* (2nd ed.). Oxford: Wiley-Blackwell.

Vincent, C., Aylin, P., Dean Franklin, B., Holmes, A., Iskander, S., Jacklin, A., & Moorthy, K. (2008). Is health care getting safer? *British Medical Journal, 337*(November), 1205–1207.

Vincent, C., Young, M., & Phillips, A. (1994). Why do people sue doctors? A study of patients and relatives taking legal action. *The Lancet, 343*, 1609–1613.

Wilson, R., Runciman, W. B., Gibberd, R. W., Harrison, B., Newby, L., & Hamilton, J. (1995). The Quality in Australian Health Care study. *Medical Journal of Australia, 163*(9), 458–471.

23

The role of the law in communicating patient safety

Donella Piper, Tina Cockburn, Bill Madden, Prue Vines and Janine McIlwraith

Learning objectives

This chapter will enable you to:

- define 'patient safety law' and understand the role of the law in communicating patient safety;
- describe some of the ways the law facilitates patient safety via the imposition of preventative measures such as registration and accreditation;
- describe some of the ways the law communicates patient safety via the disclosure of patient safety issues;
- describe some of the ways the law improves patient safety by responding to patient safety issues;
- analyse the arguments for reform of the legal system to better facilitate and communicate patient safety.

Key terms

Accountability
Adverse event
Apology
Civil liability
Criminal prosecution
Harm
Law
Open disclosure
Patient safety incident
Patient safety law

Overview

This chapter considers the role of the **law** in communicating patient safety. Downie and colleagues' (2006) 'preventing, knowing and responding' theoretical framework is adopted to classify the different elements of patient safety law. Rather than setting out all relevant patient safety laws in detail, this chapter highlights key legal strategies which are employed to prevent the occurrence of a **patient safety incident** ('preventing'); support the discovery and open discussion of patient safety incidents when they do occur ('knowing'); and guide responses after they occur ('responding') (Downie et al., 2006).

> **law**
> legislation (enacted by Australian parliaments) and case law (law made by judges hearing a case).
>
> **patient safety incident**
> 'an event or circumstance that could have resulted, or did result, in unnecessary harm to a patient' (WHO, 2009, p. 22). Incidents include adverse events, near misses, and no-harm incidents.

After highlighting some legal strategies used to communicate patient safety, two practice examples are presented. The practice examples highlight different aspects of **patient safety law** and are indicative of communication issues commonly faced in practice. The first practice example focuses on the role of the coroner in communicating patient safety. It highlights the investigative role of the law in relation to patient safety (knowing). It also showcases the preventing element in respect of the significant number of communica-

> **patient safety law**
> a body of law that functions to protect the patient by reducing patient safety incidents within the healthcare system (Downie et al., 2006).

tion errors that can occur in a multidisciplinary, networked health system. The main focus of the second practice example is responding to health service providers' and professionals' miscommunication (and subsequent incidents) during treatment; however, it also touches upon knowing and preventing.

Introduction

Law is increasingly being used as an instrument for improving system-wide performance in the interest of patient safety (Healy, 2011). This involves, on the one hand, greater legal focus on prevention and avoidance of incidents and provider-caused **harm**. On the other hand, it involves the more traditional legal approach of identifying negligence and compensating injured patients after an incident occurs.

> **harm**
> impairment of structure or function of the body and/or any deleterious effect arising therefrom, including disease, injury, suffering, disability and death; and may be physical, social or psychological (WHO, 2009, p. 23).

The law communicates patient safety in three main ways: *preventing* patient safety incidents, *knowing* when they do occur, and *responding* to them (Downie et al., 2006).

Patient safety law that aims to prevent patient safety incidents can generally be said to do so by controlling or influencing one of three variables: *where* care is delivered, *who* delivers care, and *what* is delivered.

'Knowing' relates to how the law can be seen to work to support the discovery and open discussion of patient safety incidents (Downie et al., 2006). To achieve this, the law engages in two related yet somewhat contradictory practices: protecting certain information from being publicly promulgated and, at the same time, ensuring information is disclosed.

When a patient has received unsafe care resulting in harm, legal attention shifts to ensuring both **accountability** and compensation to redress the wrong (Downie et al., 2006; Vines, 2005, 2007). This is the responding dimension of the law. That is, the law responds by holding those who are responsible for the act and the harm accountable, whether through coronial investigation, disciplinary action or, on rare occasions, criminal prosecution (Yeung & Horder, 2014). In appropriate cases, the law provides compensation to the person who has been harmed. The preventing, knowing and responding elements of the how law communicates patient

> **accountability**
> holding of responsibility by individuals, organisations, and government for their actions and omissions.

safety are discussed in more detail in the 'Theoretical links' section later in this chapter.

With this as brief background, let us turn to the first practice example, focusing on a child death in hospital and the coroner's findings about the case.

Practice example 23.1

Role of the Coroner's Court in communicating patient safety: inquest into the death of Jacob Belim (Mitchell, 2011)

Jacob Belim, aged 8 years, died of septic shock from a ruptured appendix on 28 March 2009. The events leading up to his death are set out by New South Wales Deputy State Coroner Mitchell in his findings of 15 August 2011 (*Jacob Belim*, 0839/09).

On 23 March 2009, Jacob complained of abdominal pain and vomiting. His mother took him to First Care Medical Centre (FCMC) where Dr Khan, a general practitioner (GP), examined him and prescribed an elixir to settle the pain. Dr Khan did not diagnose Jacob's appendicitis.

As Jacob's symptoms persisted, a couple of days later he was taken back to FCMC to see Dr Gounder, his regular doctor. Dr Gounder diagnosed appendicitis, and thought Jacob's appendix may have ruptured, requiring urgent surgery. She phoned an ambulance to take Jacob to hospital; it arrived promptly. At the ambulance handover Dr Gounder gave the officers a referral letter describing Jacob's 'distended, tender, rigid' abdomen and diagnosed 'appendicitis'. Dr Gounder did not identify a specific service, and Jacob was therefore taken to Liverpool Hospital (hereafter called 'Liverpool'). The treating ambulance officer chose Liverpool because it was one of the closest hospitals capable of taking paediatric patients, and had not exceeded its admissions quota. The officer had not been told that sick children requiring surgery should not be taken to Liverpool. As he seemed 'reasonably stable', Jacob was categorised as 'non-urgent'.

continued ›

Practice example 23.1 continued ›

About three hours after Jacob left, Dr Gounder phoned Liverpool and told the nurse in the Paediatric Emergency Department, 'This boy looks like having a ruptured appendix. Please investigate.' This message failed to draw anybody's attention to Dr Gounder's correct diagnosis.

Jacob arrived at Liverpool at about 10:22 a.m. The ambulance officers handed over the referral. He was marked 'category 2' ('to be seen within 10 minutes') at triage, but waited about 80 minutes to be seen by the Emergency Department Registrar, Dr Ferreira, and was only seen then because a nurse asked that he be seen out of turn. Dr Ferreira ordered some tests, but not an abdominal ultrasound, despite Jacob's mother urgings given the GP's statements about appendicitis. Soon after the tests, Dr Ferreira knew (by 11:30 a.m.) that an operation was highly likely, and that it would need to be undertaken elsewhere. Test results showed possible shock and dehydration. Dr Ferreira also knew Jacob's C reactive protein level was at 380.0 mg/L, which was grossly elevated and consistent with appendicitis and/or peritonitis. At about 3:30 p.m. Dr Ferreira telephoned the visiting medical officer, who directed her to transfer Jacob to Royal Alexandra Hospital for Children at Westmead (hereafter called 'Westmead').

Dr Ferreira telephoned Westmead and spoke to Dr Patel, stating that Jacob required paediatric surgical review for a possible bowel obstruction, but did not mention appendicitis, peritonitis or possible septic shock. Despite knowing that surgery was inevitable and urgent, and a decision having already been made to transfer Jacob, Dr Ferreira asked paediatric registrar, Dr Nassar, to review him and assess treatment urgency. Dr Nassar appeared on the ward at about 2:10 p.m., but did not review Jacob until about 40 minutes later. He agreed Jacob had an acute abdomen and should be transferred to Westmead. During Dr Nassar's half-hour review, he examined Jacob, took a history from Mrs. Belim, but did not speak to Jacob. He did not see Dr Gounder's referral (although it was with the hospital notes), or read the ambulance notes. Dr Nassar's notes recorded that Jacob had 'acute abdomen – bowel obstruction' secondary to faecalith, malrotation and/or infection, but did not mention appendicitis or peritonitis despite Jacob's mother's urgings. Dr Nassar told Mrs Belim that Jacob needed surgery at Westmead because they did not operate on children at Liverpool. By then Jacob had been at Liverpool for about four and a half hours.

Jacob left Liverpool by ambulance at about 5:23 p.m., almost seven and a half hours after arriving. He arrived at Westmead just after 6:00 p.m. The Liverpool misdiagnosis of 'bowel obstruction' was recorded on the admission documents at Westmead, and the triage nurse repeated that 'X-ray shows bowel obstruction'. No mention was made of appendicitis. Jacob underwent further tests, some of which had already been undertaken at Liverpool. Despite ample evidence Jacob was suffering from a burst appendix, the decision to operate was not taken until around 9:00 p.m., after an ultrasound. Surgery commenced at 11:00 p.m., some twelve and a half hours after Jacob's arrival at Liverpool and about five hours after his arrival at Westmead.

While at Westmead, Jacob was treated by several doctors. Dr Hale determined that postoperatively Jacob was to remain in the ward with hourly observations. This was found

continued ›

> **Practice example 23.1** continued ›
>
> to be inadequate given the severity of his condition, including a very high heart rate post-surgery and the high volume of fluid required during surgery (indicating possible septic shock). Dr Thacker, Paediatric Registrar on duty, saw Jacob at 4:30 a.m. the next morning and then again, due to a concern, at 6:30 a.m. On both occasions, the heart rate was 162 – 'worryingly high'. Dr Thacker did not refer Jacob to the Intensive Care Unit (ICU) immediately, but telephoned the ICU, and was told to wait for the ICU registrar's review. When the ICU registrar arrived, he recommended more fluid but before Dr Thacker could respond, Dr Patel came on to the ward and responsibility passed to him. Dr Patel was surprised to see that the ICU review had not taken place but, shortly after, handed over Jacob and went off duty. Jacob remained on the ward until late on 27 March 2009 with his condition steadily deteriorating.
>
> The nursing shift handover occurred at around 2:00 p.m. Nurse Idquival reviewed Jacob at 4:00 p.m. and again at 4:20 p.m. She was worried about his condition, so asked about Jacob's treatment plan. The duty doctor said the plan was to bring down Jacob's temperature. Because Nurse Idquival thought more should be done, she called paediatric ICU (PICU) and said Jacob was very sick, and asked for help. Then, after consulting with a nurse practitioner, she 'called an arrest' (to escalate the request for immediate care). The medical arrest team arrived quickly, but Jacob's eyes rolled back, he passed out and could not be wakened. He was then transferred to PICU.
>
> Jacob was admitted to PICU after about 6:30 p.m. on 27 March 2009. He 'was in a critical and perilous condition. He was in profound shock, only minimally responsive with groaning to deep pain, had very poor peripheral perfusion, tachycardia and wide pulse pressure. He had marked abdominal distension … [and] life threatening septic shock and/or ischaemic gut.'
>
> As Jacob was not responding to the maximum ICU treatment, once stabilised with a heartbeat of 134 and a temperature of 36 degrees C, he was taken back to theatre for an emergency laparotomy where he died at about 2:28 a.m. on 28 March 2009.

Analysis and reflection

Jacob's death was investigated by the coroner. The *Coroners Act* in each jurisdiction requires coroners to inquire into certain kinds of deaths (such as where a person's death was not the reasonably expected outcome of a health-related procedure carried out in relation to the person). Coronial investigations aim to determine a number of factors, including how they died and the medical cause of death. It is not the coroner's role of find people guilty of criminal or civil offences. (See the coroners' links in 'Web resources' at the end of the chapter).

The coroner found Jacob died when his heart failed as a result of septic and/or hypervolaemic shock consequent on a burst appendix leading to peritonitis. The coroner stated that the treatment Jacob received for his perforated appendix was inadequate in several respects, including communication and clinical issues leading to failure to suspect appendicitis, and unnecessary delays.

Communication and clinical issues leading to failure to suspect appendicitis

The coroner found that it should have been obvious to any medical practitioner dealing with Jacob at Liverpool that his situation was very serious, and that he needed urgent surgery without delay. The coroner found Dr Ferreira's care to be wanting in several respects. Some concerns related to communication issues – for example, Dr Ferreira's failure to adequately consult the notes and read the GP's referral letter during her examination.

Other concerns related to clinical failings, which affected communication with subsequent treating health professionals, including Dr Ferreira's failure to consider appendicitis, at least as a differential diagnosis, and her failure to arrange an ultrasound. This contributed uncertainty, confusion and delays in Jacob's subsequent treatment. The coroner also mentioned Dr Nassar's communication and clinical failures, including his failure to speak to Jacob on examination; his failure to read Dr Gounder's letter or the ambulance notes; his description of the boy as being only 'mildly unwell'; the paucity of his notes on examination; and his failure to draw any conclusion from the rigidity of Jacob's abdomen (a diagnostic marker for a ruptured appendix). All this suggested Dr Nassar's 'fixed view', producing a less than adequate care intervention.

Unnecessary delays

The coroner found that communication issues also underpinned the unnecessary delays during the almost seven hours Jacob spent at Liverpool en route to surgery at Westmead. More specifically, while at Liverpool, Jacob's history was taken, ignoring or missing his mother's concerns and his treating GP's findings. X-rays were taken, but not an ultrasound (a better diagnostic tool). Jacob was misdiagnosed and was left significantly dehydrated; antibiotic medication was delayed; surgical review was missed; and his transfer to Westmead occurred hours later than required. The coroner concluded that '[i]n short, his visit to Liverpool was a tragic waste of time'. In addition, communication problems underpinned the unnecessary delays during the almost four and a half hours that Jacob was at Westmead before going to theatre. In particular, it was found that performing a laparotomy for peritonitis earlier would have significantly increased Jacob's likelihood of survival.

Implications for practice

Based upon their investigation, coroners are empowered to make recommendations to improve public health and safety (see Studdert & Cordner, 2010, and the coroners' links in the 'Web resources' section at the end of the chapter). It appears, however, that coronial recommendations are not always implemented by health services or other policy-makers such as government (Sutherland et al., 2014). The coroner made a number of specific recommendations, namely that:

- steps be taken to ensure the ready availability to medical and nursing staff at the hospital emergency departments;
- a guideline be developed regarding the circumstances in which appendicitis may call for urgent surgical treatment and the steps to be taken in such instances;
- a protocol be developed to ensure the prompt and efficient transfer of paediatric patients requiring surgery not to be performed at the hospital;
- steps be taken to keep paediatricians, general practitioners and the New South Wales Ambulance Service advised of the availability of paediatric surgical services.

Both Liverpool and Westmead have sought to implement the coroner's recommendations. Liverpool has made a number of systemic changes based upon the recommendations. For example, the hospital has reinforced and improved access to surgical review, regardless of the age of the patient. The Ministry of Health (New South Wales) has also released a policy directive entitled *Recognition and management of patients who are clinically deteriorating* (NSW Health, 2013), which sets out principles for improving the recognition, response to and management of all patients who are clinically deteriorating. The directive includes a clinical emergency response system and escalation matrix (Appendix 8.2) that describes the role delineations of staff and the appropriate response and escalation process for all patients in Ministry of Health facilities, including paediatric patients.

Theoretical links

As noted in the introduction to this chapter, the law plays a role in preventing incidents and harm ('preventing'), ensuring we have information about what goes wrong in health care ('knowing'), and responding to **adverse events** ('responding'). These three dimensions form a theoretical link between law and communication in patient safety. This section elaborates on these three dimensions.

> **adverse events**
> incidents in which harm resulted to a person receiving health care (WHO, 2009, p. 23).

Preventing

Patient safety law that aims to prevent patient safety incidents can generally be said to do so by controlling or influencing one of three variables: *where* care is delivered, *who* delivers care, and *what* is delivered.

In Australia, *where* care is delivered is regulated by the Australian Commission on Safety and Quality in Health Care (ACSQHC): an organisation does not automatically qualifiy as a healthcare provider. ACSQHC's National Safety and Quality Health Service Standards ensure that heath care services are accredited against its standards (ACSQHC, 2011).

Who delivers care is set out under the *Health Practitioner Regulation National Law Act 2009* (hereafter the 'National Law'), as adopted in each state and territory (see the 'Web resources' section at the end of the chapter). *It is important to note that the National Law has been modified in some jurisdictions. You should refer to the legislation relevant to the jurisdiction where you work*. The National Law provides for accreditation, registration, and performance and conduct standards to be applied to health service providers (for example, see Parts, 6, 7 and 8 of the *Health Practitioner Regulation National Law (NSW) No 86a*). The Australian Health Practitioner Regulation Agency (AHPRA) is responsible for the implementation of people's registration, which currently applies to 14 health professions. The registration requirements regulate health professionals' training and registration to prevent unsafe care. Disciplinary processes, which focus on the health, performance and conduct of individuals, determine who should and should not be entitled to deliver care. This regulatory framework is therefore preventive in that it seeks to protect the public by imposing minimum standards that all registered health practitioners must meet.

The law also prescribes *what* can be delivered in the *Therapeutic Goods Act 1989* (Cth). In aiming to prevent patient safety incidents, the Therapeutic Goods Administration is responsible for ensuring that medicines and medical devices (therapeutic goods) available for supply in Australia are safe and fit for their intended purpose prior to their consumption and usage.

Knowing

'Knowing' relates to how the law can support the discovery and open discussion of patient safety incidents (Downie et al., 2006). What constrains knowing are healthcare providers' fears about the consequences of acknowledging patient safety incidents. One such fear is damage to one's reputation, and another is exposure to civil liability (Studdert, Piper & Iedema, 2010).

Qualified privilege protects the confidentiality of certain documents and communications against demands for disclosure in legal proceedings (Studdert & Richardson, 2010). The policy rationale for this protection is to encourage candour and the free flow of information for investigation of adverse events, where this is in the public interest. There are subtle variations however between state jurisdictions as to the nature and extent of qualified privilege protection (Studdert & Richardson, 2010).

Similarly, '**apology** laws' contained in civil liability legislation provide protection for health professionals who offer apologies (as defined in each jurisdiction's legislation) to patients involved in incidents. Like qualified privilege legislation, apology laws vary between state jurisdictions (Vines, 2005, 2007, 2013; McLennan & Truog, 2013). Apology laws are focused on reassuring healthcare providers that apologies are not determinative of liability.

> **apology**
> a statement of regret that includes the word 'sorry'. There is a difference between 'We are sorry that this happened' and 'We are sorry that we did the wrong thing'. The latter expression is admissible in some states' courts of law as constituting an acknowledgement of liability (all states except New South Wales and the Australian Capital Territory).

It should be clear to you by now that there is a tension between qualified privilege and apology laws (serving to protect healthcare providers and their communications) on the one hand and disclosure, transparency and public accountability (encouraging open discussion of care problems) on the other hand. To address this tension, legal instruments are *also* used to encourage the public availability of incident and complaint information, and the disclosure of adverse events to patients.

The first element of knowing is therefore disclosure. Adverse events are acknowledged and discussed through **open disclosure** (see Chapter 22) by providers to patients, peers or the public through data gathering and publication processes (Downie et al., 2006). Open disclosure policy presents providers with legal and ethical obligations to inform patients of adverse events.

> **open disclosure**
> 'The open discussion of adverse events that result in harm to a patient while receiving health care with the patient, their family and carers' (Australian Commission on Safety and Quality in Health Care, 2013, p. 11). Open disclosure includes an apology, explanation, patient views, consequences, and steps taken to prevent similar incidents.

The legal obligations may stem from civil law obligations as expressed by the courts (Madden & Cockburn, 2007). There are also a number of data-gathering and reporting requirements, such as clinical audits and adverse event reporting systems imposed under accreditation requirements (ACSQHC, 2010; 2012), where accreditation refers to the process of assessing services' fitness to provide patient care.

The ethical obligations derive from the code of conduct for each health profession (available from the 'National boards' websites set out in the 'Web resources' section at the end of the chapter).

Another means of discovering patient safety incidents is through patient complaint mechanisms. Complaints can be a valuable patient safety communication and learning tool when handled appropriately (Downie et al., 2006). In Australia, all states and territories have a complaints commissioner and an ombudsman (see the 'Web resources' section at the end of the chapter), enabling patients and their families to complain about the care they have received. Although the legislation differs across jurisdictions, the complaints commissioner or ombudsman share a common objective: the independent, impartial resolution of health complaints as one means of improving the safety and quality of health care (ACSQHC, 2009). A high proportion of complaints received relate to inappropriate or substandard communication from the provider to the patient (ACSQHC, 2009, Chapter 5; Health Care Complaints Commission (HCCC), 2013, p. 16).

Complaints commissioners or ombudsman offices can respond to complaints in a variety of ways, including investigation of complaints that raise serious issues or public health or safety or assisting in the resolution of other complaints. **Civil liability** claims or criminal prosecutions usually lead to the involvement of lawyers, police and courts (Healy, 2011). For serious health, performance or conduct matters requiring orders protective of the public, the national boards work with AHPRA to investigate and prosecute complaints (National Law, Part 8), although in some states the complaints commissioners take this role. In this way the law attempts to act as a catalyst for improvement by communicating the standards expected and the outcomes if they are not met.

> **civil liability**
> legal responsibility to provide financial compensation for a patient safety incident.

Inquiry is a further mechanism by which the law sets about knowing. For example, the coroners' courts throughout Australia communicate safety and quality by investigating unexpected deaths in health services (Middleton & Buist, 2014; Studdert & Cordner, 2010). The coroner may make recommendations for system improvement (adding a 'responding' and preventing 'role' to 'knowing'). In some but not all jurisdictions, health service providers must report to the coroner on the action taken on coronial recommendations (Freckleton & Ranson, 2006). However, research suggests that only about one-third of coronial recommendations are acted upon by authorities (Sutherland et al., 2014).

Coronial inquest findings are shared by the National Coroners Information System (NCIS). NCIS is a database that includes information from all Australian coroners' cases since 2000, including the medical cause of deaths and the circumstances surrounding deaths. According to Downie and colleagues (2006) '[i]nformation from the system has been used in the context of patient safety in areas such as deaths associated with pregnancy, the insertion of naso-gastric tubes, and the administration of medication in nursing homes'.

Parliaments in Australia also have the power to order inquiries under special commissions of inquiry legislation, and have done so on a number of occasions in relation to safety and quality in healthcare matters, for example Walker (2004), Hughes & Walters (2007), and Garling (2008). Each of these inquiries has produced important reports, communicating with the public and government about significant problems in the health system, and culminating in recommendations for systems improvement (Stewart & Dwyer, 2009). The Garling inquiry is discussed by Skinner and colleagues (2009).

Responding

The law responds to incidents by holding those who are responsible for the act and the harm accountable. It may do so through civil liability, disciplinary action or, on rare occasions, **criminal prosecution** (Yeung & Horder, 2014).

Civil liability for medical injury in Australia is contingent on a finding of fault on the part of the health professional and/or provider. This happens through patients commencing litigation, usually alleging negligence. To prove negligence it must be established that healthcare providers or professionals

> **criminal prosecution**
> a legal process initiated by the state (or Crown) seeking imposition of a penalty for a behaviour.

acted in ways that fell below the standard of reasonable care, causing harm to the patient. The harm may be such as to justify monetary compensation ('damages') (Madden & McIlwraith, 2013).

Litigation may be expensive and time consuming, however. This raises a question about equity: a considerable number of injured patients do not make a claim. They are perhaps unaware of their rights, or the incident was not disclosed to them (Gilmour, 2011).

By the same token, this focus on **liability** and negligence of healthcare professionals (and sometimes of institutional healthcare providers such as hospitals) creates a tendency towards blaming and penalising individuals (Downie et al., 2006). Some commentators argue that suing individual professionals does not have a positive effect on their behaviour. They suggest that court judgments may not communicate

> **liability**
> someone's legal responsibility for an action.

better practices, such as the need to be more careful and to avoid adverse incidents. Rather, court judgments encourage health professionals to keep errors from patients and providers, thereby preventing openness and learning (Gilmour, 2011; Healy, 2011). Further, the focus on individual liability and negligence fails to acknowledge the complexity of contemporary care, where individual professionals' work depends heavily on the work of many of their colleagues. Thus, claims which focus on individuals may fail to analyse these more complex 'systems' factors, and how they played a role in bringing about the patient's injuries.

There are some options for avoiding these challenges. For example, to enable harmed patients to get on with their lives, we could offer compensation immediately after registering the incident (Boothman & Hoyler, 2013), make increased use of mediation (Ong, 2013), or put in place 'specialist health courts' aimed at streamlining the compensation process (Howard & Maine, 2013). We could also improve access for harmed patients to currently privileged or protected information, and introduce a 'no-fault compensation system'. Under a no-fault compensation system, a person suffering a health-service-caused injury may be awarded a government payment. This approach has been in place in New Zealand since 1976, in the form of the Accidents Compensation Commission. An approach to no-fault compensation focused on serious disability and necessary supports is developing in Australia under the National Disability Insurance Scheme, and this scheme may be expanded with a National Injury Insurance Scheme (Madden, McIllwraith & Brell, 2013).

Conclusion

Jacob Belim's case study demonstrates the significant role that coroners' courts play in communicating safety and quality. These courts investigate deaths (the responding element) where a death was not the reasonably expected outcome of a health-related procedure (the knowing element), and then make recommendations based upon this investigation for system improvement (a preventing role).

Jacob's case provides a good example of the problems in health care created by poor communication. Coronial findings highlight the numerous communication errors that can occur in a multidisciplinary networked health system. These communication issues related to the failure to communicate about where specific kinds of paediatric surgery are to occur; ineffective communication on clinical handover, including not creating accurate medical records and documentation such as referrals, and not ensuring access and consultation of those records by subsequent treating practitioners.

The coroner's findings also identified clinical errors: errors in diagnosing appendicitis and recognising the need for urgent surgical treatment; a lack of protocols to ensure prompt and efficient transfers of patients; a failure to recognise patient deterioration, and inadequate postoperative care.

Practice example 23.2 — The case of Mr Clive Impu

When you read practice example 23.2, think about how the 'preventing, knowing and responding' framework applies. You will see that, like practice example 23.1, it demonstrates the significant role that coroners' courts play in knowing and preventing. However, the main focus of this second practice example is the role of civil courts in providing accountability, an aspect of responding.

Specifically, the case highlights systemic communication problems in the healthcare services provided to a patient. The problems in question pertain to health services having inadequate administrative procedures in place to communicate with patients who fail to attend appointments relating to potentially serious conditions.

In this case, the system in place was described by the judge hearing the case as 'inherently unreliable', which meant that the Central Australian Aboriginal Congress Inc. (CAACI) was held in breach of its duty of care to its patient (*Young v Central Australian Aboriginal Congress Inc & Ors* [2008] NTSC 47). The decision demonstrates that healthcare providers must not only provide reasonable medical advice and treatment, but also their administrative practices must ensure that appropriate communication between provider and patient occurs, so that patients are in a position to make fully informed decisions about their ongoing health care. The case also demonstrates that while patients have rights, they also have responsibilities to take reasonable care for their own safety.

The facts of the case are as follows. In March 2000, Mr Impu (the deceased), aged 25 years, attended a clinic operated by CAACI and was initially diagnosed with a potentially serious heart problem. The recommended action was to undergo a fasting cholesterol test to determine whether he had ischaemic heart disease. The patient failed to attend scheduled appointments, but did attend the clinic a number of times over the next few months for other unrelated complaints. Administrative errors prevented CAACI from following up the initial diagnosis and recommended treatment. The following January the patient attended the clinic complaining about heart pain, was given tablets, and then turned away, but no reference was made to the original diagnosis. Later that day he died from coronary thrombosis, aged 26. He was survived by his wife (then aged 30) and three young children (then aged seven, five and two years).

An inquest into his death was held in the Coroner's Court in Alice Springs in 2001 (Cavanagh, 2001). The coroner determined that the deceased died from coronary thrombosis due to coronary atherosclerosis (Cavanagh, 2001). The coroner stated that 'although there is a high rate of death from ischaemic heart disease the level of diagnosis remains low [amongst Aboriginal people]' (Cavanagh, 2001, p. 33). Accordingly, the coroner made a recommendation that 'all medical practitioners in Central Australia undergo a specific orientation in respect of the greater prevalence of chronic disease amongst Aboriginal people

continued ›

Practice example 23.2 continued ›

than in the wider population, including the prevalence of ischaemic heart disease as soon as possible after commencement of medical practice' (Cavanagh, 2001, p. 34).

Mr Impu's widow initiated a negligence claim, which is explained in the judgment of *Young v Central Australian Aboriginal Congress Inc & Ors* [2008] NTSC 47. The deceased's widow claimed compensation for herself and their children under legislation that enables claims to be brought by the dependants of people whose death is a result of the negligence of another. She claimed that the CAACI was negligent by failing to follow up the initial diagnosis and treatment. She also claimed two of the doctors who ordered the test were negligent by failing to properly diagnose the deceased and/or treat him. The defendant (CAACI) claimed 'contributory negligence', meaning that the deceased patient failed to take reasonable care for his own safety, and that he should bear some responsibility.

Evidence was also presented about administrative procedures in the clinic at the time the deceased attended. Patients who attended the clinic often saw different doctors each time they visited. A physicians' clinic was held once a fortnight for tests or follow-up treatment. When a doctor ordered a test or follow-up treatment, they would complete a pink form that was placed in the file for an appointment to be made at the clinic. The patient was notified of the appointment and once the test or treatment was completed, the referring doctor would receive written notification. If a patient failed to attend an appointment, the clinic would follow up with the patient and attempt to arrange another time. Alternatively, the file would be marked and the test would be carried out the next time the patient visited the clinic.

In this case, a number of administrative errors occurred. This meant that the patient was not followed up about his missed appointment, and no record was made on his file for the test to be carried out on his next visit. In particular, there was another patient with the same name as him and, as no steps had been taken to note this, the wrong file was retrieved. The deceased attended the clinic on a number of occasions after the referring doctor had arranged the test, but did not see that doctor again and did not mention the test to the other doctors.

The court found that the referring doctor was not negligent in his treatment of the deceased. It was the responsibility of the clinic coordinator, not the referring doctor, to follow-up patients who missed appointments. In fact, the referring doctor was the only treating doctor who had correctly diagnosed the deceased's condition.

As to CAACI's liability, the court found that it 'had a responsibility to put administrative procedures in place for the situation that arose in this case where a patient fails to attend for a fasting cholesterol test which is part of the treatment plan for a potentially serious condition' (*Young v Central Australian Aboriginal Congress Inc & Ors* [2008] NTSC 47, p. 58 per Thomas J). This was especially so given the evidence that approximately 30–50% of Indigenous patients failed to attend due to social problems. The clinic had

continued ›

Practice example 23.2 continued ›

'a direct responsibility and duty to the deceased to exercise reasonable care and skill in the administration and management of the deceased's treatment and care by its employed general practitioners, nursing and administrative support staff' (*Young v Central Australian Aboriginal Congress Inc & Ors* [2008] NTSC 47, p. 84 per Thomas J). It was found that there was no system in place to follow up whether a person had attended for appointments other than picking it up next time the patient came in. This 'opportunistic follow-up system' was held to be inherently unreliable (*Young v Central Australian Aboriginal Congress Inc & Ors* [2008] NTSC 47, p. 85 per Thomas J).

The administrative errors leading to a failure in communication included:
- The deceased's congress file number was not written in the appointment book.
- The receptionist retrieved the 'incorrect' Mr Impu file.
- The receptionist did not check the file for the pink 'referral within Congress form' (referring practitioners were required to put a pink slip referral form on file). There was no pink referral form in the 'incorrect' Mr Impu file and its absence should have given rise to a query.
- The files were not marked to indicate there were two files in the name of 'Clive Impu' (as about 10% of the patients had the same names, it was the practice to mark the files of patients with the same names with coloured texta, stating that another file existed that bore the same name, but this did not happen in this case).
- There was a note made on the 'incorrect' Mr Impu file to sort out his referral at his next visit, but this did not occur.
- The practitioners who saw Mr Impu when he attended CAACI following 21 March 2000 did not properly refer to the notes to alert them to the fact that the deceased had not attended important tests.
- When Mr Impu attended the clinic on 26 January 2001, shortly before his death, the attending doctor did not have his file.

The judge held that the administrative errors were a breach of duty owed by the clinic to the deceased (that is, the clinic was negligent). The failures by the clinic to exercise reasonable care towards the deceased were found to be a direct cause of his death, for which CAACI should be held responsible by a damages award to his dependants.

On the question of contributory negligence, the court held that the deceased failed to exercise reasonable care for his own safety and that, taking into account all the circumstances, the damages award should be reduced by 50%. Relevant circumstances in this case were that the referring doctor fully explained the seriousness of the suspected heart condition and the importance of the follow-up appointments to the deceased, and the deceased had a good understanding of English, was employed and not unsophisticated or uneducated such that he could not have failed to understand the significance of the advice given. Accordingly, the failures by the deceased to attend for the test and tell other clinic doctors about it were failures to exercise reasonable care for his own safety, health and well-being, which contributed to the harm suffered.

Reflective questions

The preamble to the Australian Medical Association (AMA) *Code of ethics 2004* (editorially revised 2006) (https://ama.com.au/sites/default/files/documents /AMA_Code_of_Ethics_2004._Editorially_Revised_2006.pdf) includes the following statement:

> The doctor–patient relationship is itself a partnership based on mutual respect and collaboration. Within the partnership, both the doctor and the patient have rights as well as responsibilities.

The AMA recently published a position statement called *Patient follow-up, recall and reminder systems – 2013* (https://ama.com.au/position-statement/patient-follow-recall-and-reminder-systems-2013). After reading this document, consider the following questions:

1. Sometimes patients do not take care of themselves. How should health care be managed if there is a clear danger of a patient not taking care of themselves?
2. In the case example the clinic had taken a number of steps to try and create follow-up but they failed. What should they have done?
3. How does the law strike a balance between promoting patient safety by holding healthcare providers accountable for failure to implement follow-up and recall systems and respecting patient autonomy and holding patients responsible for the consequences of a decision not to return?

Further reading

Brooks, L. (2013). *Cultural diversity and the failure of doctors to follow up.* http://www. mauriceblackburn.com.au/about/media-centre/newsletters/medical-law/spring-2013/ culturaldiversity-and-the-failure-of-doctors-to-follow-up-with-patients

Madden, B., & McIlwraith, J. (2013) *Australian medical liability* (2nd ed.). Sydney: LexisNexis.

McIlwraith, J., & Madden, B. (2014). *Health care & the law* (6th ed.). Pyrmont: Thomson Reuters.

These texts provide a more comprehensive coverage of medical liability and health law issues presented in this chapter and beyond.

Luntz, H., Hambly, D., Burns, K., Dietrich, J., & Foster, N. (2013) *Torts: Cases and commentary* (7th ed.). Sydney: LexisNexis Butterworths.

Sappideen, C., Vines, P., & Watson, P. (2012). *Torts: Commentary and cases* (11th ed.). Pyrmont: Thomson Reuters.

Both these texts provide detailed explanation and analysis of the law of negligence including but not limited to medical negligence.

Web resources

ABC News, *Coroner urges paediatric reform after Jacob's death*: http://www.youtube.com/watch?v=ZZe72hspmrg

Inter-professional Education for Quality Use of Medicines – Vanessa Anderson module: http://www.ipeforqum.com.au/modules/vanessa-anderson

Complaints commissions and ombudsmen

Australian Capital Territory – ACT Human Rights Commission: http://www.hrc.act.gov.au

New South Wales – Health Care Complaints Commission: http://www.hccc.nsw.gov.au

Northern Territory – Health and Community Services Complaints Commission (HCSCC): http://www.hcscc.nt.gov.au

Queensland – Office of the Health Ombudsman: http://www.hqcc.qld.gov.au

South Australia – Health and Community Services Complaints Commissioner (HCSCC): http://www.hcscc.sa.gov.au

Tasmania – Health Complaints Commissioner: http://www.healthcomplaints.tas.gov.au

Victoria – Office of the Health Services Commissioner: http://www.health.vic.gov.au/hsc

Western Australia – Health and Disability Services Complaints Office (HaDSCO): http://www.hadsco.wa.gov.au/home

Privacy commissioners

Information and Privacy Commission New South Wales: http://www.ipc.nsw.gov.au

Office of the ACT Human Rights Commission: http://www.hrc.act.gov.au

Office of the Australian Information Commissioner: http://www.privacy.gov.au

Office of the Information Commissioner Northern Territory: http://www.privacy.nt.gov.au

Office of the Information Commissioner Queensland: http://www.oic.qld.gov.au

Office of the Victorian Privacy Commissioner: http://www.privacy.vic.gov.au/domino/privacyvic/web2.nsf/pages/home

Ombudsman Tasmania: http://www.ombudsman.tas.gov.au

Coroners' courts

Australian Capital Territory: http://www.courts.act.gov.au/magistrates/courts/coroners_court

National Coronial Information System: http://www.ncis.org.au

New South Wales: http://www.coroners.lawlink.nsw.gov.au/coroners/index.html

Northern Territory: http://www.nt.gov.au/justice/courtsupp/coroner/index.shtml

Queensland: http://www.courts.qld.gov.au/courts/coroners-court

South Australia: http://www.courts.sa.gov.au/OurCourts/CoronersCourt/Pages/default.aspx

Tasmania: http://www.magistratescourt.tas.gov.au/divisions/coronial

Victoria: http://www.coronerscourt.vic.gov.au

Western Australia: http://www.coronerscourt.wa.gov.au

Coroners' cases

Inquest into the death of Vanessa Anderson: http://www.ipeforqum.com.au/modules/
vanessa-anderson

The national law as enacted in each state and territory

Australian Capital Territory – *Health Practitioner Regulation National Law (ACT) Act 2010*:
http://www.legislation.act.gov.au/a/db_39269

New South Wales – *Health Practitioner Regulation (Adoption of National Law) Act 2009 No
86*: http://www.legislation.act.gov.au/a/db_39269

Northern Territory – *Health Practitioner Regulation (National Uniform Legislation) Act 2010*:
http://www.austlii.edu.au/au/legis/nt/num_act/hprula20102o2010642

Queensland – *Health Ombudsman Act 2013*: http://www.austlii.edu.au/au/legis/qld/consol_
act/hoa2013162

South Australia – *Health Practitioner Regulation National Law (SA) Act 2010*: http://www.
legislation.sa.gov.au/LZ/C/A/Health%20Practitioner%20Regulation%20National%20
Law20%28South%20Australia%29%20Act%202010.aspx

Tasmania – *Health Practitioner Regulation National Law (Tas) Act 2010*: http://www.thelaw.
tas.gov.au/tocview/index.w3p;cond=ALL;doc_id=2%2B%2B2010%2BAT%40EN%2B201
11019100000;histon=;prompt=;rec=;term=Health%20Practitioners

Victoria – *Health Practitioner Regulation National Law (Victoria) Act 2009*: http://www.
parliament.vic.gov.au/static/www.legislation.vic.gov.au-lawtoday.html

Western Australia – *Health Practitioner Regulation National Law (WA) Act 2010*: http://
www.slp.wa.gov.au/legislation/statutes.nsf/main_mrtitle_12107_homepage.html

National boards

Aboriginal and Torres Strait Islander Health Practice Board of Australia: http://www.
atsihealthpracticeboard.gov.au

Chinese Medicine Board of Australia: http://www.chinesemedicineboard.gov.au

Chiropractic Board of Australia: http://www.chiropracticboard.gov.au

Dental Board of Australia: http://www.dentalboard.gov.au

Medical Board of Australia: http://www.medicalboard.gov.au

Medical Radiation Practice Board of Australia: http://www.medicalradiationpracticeboard.gov.au

Nursing and Midwifery Board of Australia: http://www.nursingmidwiferyboard.gov.au

Occupational Therapy Board of Australia: http://www.occupationaltherapyboard.gov.au

Optometry Board of Australia: http://www.optometryboard.gov.au

Osteopathy Board of Australia: http://www.osteopathyboard.gov.au

Pharmacy Board of Australia: http://www.pharmacyboard.gov.au

Physiotherapy Board of Australia: http://www.physiotherapyboard.gov.au

Podiatry Board of Australia: http://www.podiatryboard.gov.au

Psychology Board of Australia: http://www.psychologyboard.gov.au

National agencies and schemes

Australian Commission on Safety and Quality in Health Care (ACSQHC): http://www.
safetyandquality.gov.au

Australian Government Department of Health Therapeutic Goods Administration: http://www.
   tga.gov.au/index.htm
Australian Health Practitioner Regulation Agency (AHPRA): http://www.ahpra.gov.au
National Disability Insurance Scheme: http://www.ndis.gov.au
National Safety and Quality Health Service Standards: http://www.safetyandquality.gov.
   au/publications/national-safety-and-quality-health-service-standardshttp://www.
   safetyandquality.gov.au/wp-content/uploads/2011/09/NSQHS-Standards-Sept-2012.
   pdf

....

References

Australian Commission on Safety and Quality in Health Care (ACSQHC). (2009). *Learning from complaints: Windows into safety and quality.* Sydney: Author.

——. (2010). *Reporting for safety: Use of hospital data to monitor and improve patient safety: Windows into safety and quality.* Sydney: Author.

——. (2011). *National safety and quality health service standards.* Sydney: Author.

——. (2012). *Safety and Quality Improvement Guide Standard 1: Governance for safety and quality in health service organisations.* Sydney: Author.

——. (2013). *Australian Open Disclosure Framework.* Sydney: Author.

Boothman, R., & Hoyler, M. (2013). The University of Michigan's early disclosure and offer program. *Bulletin of the American College of Surgeons, 98*(3), 21–25.

Cavanagh, G., Senior Magistrate (Northern Territory Coroner). (2001). *Inquest into the death of Clive Henry Impu* [2001] NTMC 72, A0005/2001, Alice Springs, NT Coroners Court. Retrieved February 4, 2015 from http://www.nt.gov.au/justice/courtsupp/coroner/findings/2001/impu.pdf

Downie, J., Lahey, W., Ford, D., Gibson, E., Thomson, M., Ward, T. et al. (2006). Patient safety law: From silos to systems. Retrieved from http://eprints.qut.edu.au/62121/1/HLI_Patient_Safety-Main_Report_(final).pdf

Freckelton, I., & Ranson, D. (2006). *Death investigation and the coroner's inquest.* Melbourne: Oxford University Press.

Garling, P. (2008). *Final report of the Special Commission of Inquiry: Acute care services in NSW public hospitals.* Sydney: NSW Government. Retrieved from http://www.lawlink.nsw.gov.au/lawlink/Special_Projects/ll_splprojects.nsf/pages/acsi_finalreport

Gilmour, J. M. (2011). Patient safety and the law in Canada. In J. Tingle & B. Bark (Eds.), *Patient safety, law policy and practice* (pp. 177–195). London: Routledge.

Health Care Complaints Commission. (2013). *Health Care Complaints Commission annual report 2012–13.* Sydney: Author.

Healy, J. (2011). *Improving health care safety and quality: Reluctant regulators.* Law, Ethics and Governance series. Farnham: Ashgate.

Howard, P., & Maine, R. (2013). Health courts may be best cure for what ails the liability system. *Bulletin of the American College of Surgeons, 98*(3), 29–31. Retrieved from http://bulletin.facs.org/2013/03/health-courts-best-cure/

Hughes, C., & Walters, W. (2007). *Report of inquiry into the care of a patient with threatened miscarriage at Royal North Shore Hospital on 25 September 2007.* Sydney: NSW Health. Retrieved from http://www.health.nsw.gov.au/pubs/2007/pdf/inquiry_rnsh.pdf

Madden, B, & Cockburn, T. (2007). Bundaberg and beyond: Duty to disclose adverse events to patients. *Journal of Law and Medicine, 14*(4) 501–527.

Madden, B., & McIlwraith , J. (2013). *Australian medical liability* (2nd ed.). Sydney: LexisNexis.

Madden, B., McIlwraith, J., & Brell, R. (2013). *The national disability insurance scheme handbook.* Sydney: LexisNexis.

McLennan, S., & Truog , R. (2013). Apology laws and open disclosure. *Medical Journal of Australia, 198*(8), 411–412.

Middleton, S., & Buist, M. (2014). The coronial reporting of medical setting deaths: A legal analysis of the variation in Australian jurisdictions. *Melbourne University Law Review, 37*(3), 699–735.

Mitchell, S. Magistrate (New South Wales Deputy State Coroner) (2011). *Inquest into the death of Jacob Belim 0839/09,* Sydney: NSW State Coroners' Court.

NSW Health (2013). *Recognition and management of patients who are clinically deteriorating.* Sydney: NSW Health. Retrieved March 13, 2015 from: http://www0.health.nsw.gov.au/policies/pd/2013/PD2013_049.html

Ong, C. (2013). Medical mediation: Bringing everyone to the table. *Bulletin of the American College of Surgeons, 98*(3), 17–20. http://bulletin.facs.org/2013/03/medical-mediation

Skinner, C., Braithwaite, J., Frankum, B., Kerridge, R., & Goulston, K. (2009). Reforming New South Wales public hospitals: An assessment of the Garling inquiry. *Med J Aust, 190* (2), 78–79.

Stewart, G., & Dwyer, J. (2009). Implementation of the Garling recommendations can offer real hope for rescuing the New South Wales public hospital system. *Med J Aust, 190* (2), 80–82.

Studdert, D., & Cordner, S. (2010). Impact of coronial investigations on manner and cause of death determinations in Australia, 2000–2007. *Med J Aust, 192,* 444–447.

Studdert, D., Piper, D., & Iedema, R. (2010). Legal aspects of open disclosure II – Findings from a national survey. *Med J Aust, 193*(5), 351–355.

Studdert, D., & Richardson, M. (2010). Legal aspects of open disclosure: A review of Australian law. *Med J Aust, 193*(5), 273–276.

Sutherland, G., Kemp, C., Bugeja, L.Sewell, G., Pirkis, J., & Studdert, D. (2014). What happens to coroners' recommendations for improving public health and safety? Organisational responses under a mandatory response regime in Victoria, Australia. *BMC Public Health 14*(732), 1–8. doi:10.1186/1471–2458–14–732

Vines, P. (2005). Apologising to avoid liability: Cynical civility or practical morality? *Sydney Law Review, 27*(5), 483–505.

—— (2007). The power of apology: Mercy, forgiveness or corrective justice in the civil liability area, 1. *Public Space: The Journal of Law and Social Justice, 1,* Art 5, 1–51.

—— (2013). The apology in civil liability: Underused and undervalued? *Precedent, 115,* 29–31.

Walker, B. (2004). *Final report of the Special Commission of Inquiry into Campbelltown and Camden Hospitals*. Sydney: New South Wales Attorney General's Department.

World Health Organization (WHO), World Alliance for Patient Safety. (2009). *More than words: Conceptual framework for the international classification of patient safety, version 1.1, final technical report*. Geneva: Author. Retrieved February 4, 2015 from http://www.who.int/patientsafety/taxonomy/icps_full_report.pdf

Yeung, K., & Horder, J. (2014). How can the criminal law support the provision of quality in healthcare? *BMJ Qual Saf 23*(6), 519–524.

Young v Central Australian Aboriginal Congress Inc & Ors [2008] NTSC 47. Retrieved February 4, 2015 from http://www.supremecourt.nt.gov.au/doc/judgements/2008/ntsc/pdf/NTSC47%20Young%20v%20CAACI%20%26%20Ors%20%5B2008%5D%2019Nov.pdf

Index